Mosby's

Pocket Guide for

Basic Skills and Procedures

Mosby's
Pocket Guide for
Basic Skills and Procedures
Sixth Edition

Anne Griffin Perry, RN, MSN, EdD, FAAN
Professor and Chairperson
Department of Primary Care and Health Systems Nursing
Southern Illinois University
Edwardsville, Illinois

Patricia A. Potter, RN, PhD, FAAN, CMAC
Research Scientist
Siteman Cancer Center
Barnes-Jewish Hospital
St. Louis, Missouri

With 224 illustrations

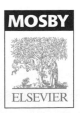

MOSBY

ELSEVIER

MOSBY
ELSEVIER

11830 Westline Industrial Drive
St. Louis, Missouri 63146

Mosby's Pocket Guide for Basic Skills and Procedures   ISBN-13: 978–0–323–04610–7
ISBN-10: 0–323–04610–X
Copyright © 2007 by Mosby, Inc., an affiliate of Elsevier Inc.

NOTICE

Nursing is an ever-changing field. Standard safety precautions must be followed, but as new research and clinical experience broaden our knowledge, changes in treatment and drug therapy may become necessary or appropriate. Readers are advised to check the most current product information provided by the manufacturer of each drug to be administered to verify the recommended dose, the method and duration of administration, and contraindications. It is the responsibility of the licensed prescriber, relying on experience and knowledge of the patient, to determine dosages and the best treatment for each individual patient. Neither the publisher nor the author assumes any liability for any injury and/or damage to persons or property arising from this publication.

Previous editions copyrighted 2003, 1998, 1994, 1990, 1986

ISBN-13: 978–0–323–04610–7
ISBN-10: 0–323–04610–X

Executive Editor: Susan R. Epstein
Senior Developmental Editor: Robyn L. Brinks
Publishing Services Manager: John Rogers
Project Manager: Douglas Turner
Designer: Amy Buxton

Printed in China

Working together to grow
libraries in developing countries
www.elsevier.com | www.bookaid.org | www.sabre.org
ELSEVIER   BOOK AID International   Sabre Foundation

Last digit is the print number: 9   8   7   6   5   4   3   2

Preface

Mosby's Pocket Guide to Basic Skills and Procedures, sixth edition, is a practical, portable reference for students and practitioners in the clinical setting. Grouped alphabetically, more than 80 commonly performed skills are presented in a clear, step-by-step format that includes:

- Purpose for performing each skill
- Delegation guidelines to help students in delegating tasks to assistive personnel
- List of equipment required
- Rationales to explain why specific techniques are used
- Photographs and drawings to provide visual reinforcement

In addition, Nurse Alerts are included in the skills to highlight important information about patient safety and effective performance. Current Standard Precautions guidelines from the Centers for Disease Control and Prevention are incorporated throughout. Preprocedure and postprocedure protocols are conveniently located on the inside back cover.

Features of This Edition

- New Skills are offered on Aspiration Precautions, Automated External Defibrillator, Fall Prevention in a Health Care Facility, Restraint Application, Restraint-Free Environment, and Seizure Precautions.
- A-to-Z organization of skills makes this an easy-to-use reference.
- Recording and Reporting guidelines are provided for each skill.
- A gloving logo identifies when gloves should be worn.

For a more complete discussion of information presented in this book, refer to Perry and Potter: *Clinical Nursing Skills and Techniques,* sixth edition.

Anne Griffin Perry
Patricia A. Potter

Contents

E

F

H

I

M

S

T

U

V

W

Acapella Device

An acapella or flutter device is a ready-to-use, small, hand-held device that mobilizes airway secretions. The device acts by applying alternately a positive and then a negative pressure to a client's airway to assist in clearing retained bronchopulmonary secretions. The vibratory features of a flutter valve and the resistive features of positive expiratory pressure shake free mucous plugs that a client can then cough up. The device is shown to be a better alternative to chest percussion and postural drainage.

Delegation Considerations

This skill may be delegated to assistive personnel (AP) in special circumstances. The nurse is responsible for (1) determining that the procedure is appropriate and that the client is able to tolerate the procedure and (2) evaluating the client's response to the procedure.

- Instruct AP to be alert for the client's tolerance of procedure, such as comfort level and changes in breathing pattern, and to immediately report changes to the nurse.
- Instruct AP about specific client precautions.

Equipment

- Stethoscope
- Pulse oximeter
- Trendelenburg hospital bed or tilt table
- Water in pitcher and glass
- Chair (for draining upper lobes)
- One to four pillows
- Tissues and paper bag
- Clear, graduated, screw-top container
- Suction equipment (if client unable to cough and clear own secretions)
- Acapella device
- Client education materials
- Clean gloves

Step	Rationale
1. Complete preprocedure protocol.	
2. Prepare acapella device: Turn acapella frequency adjustment dial	This initial setting helps client adjust to device and benefit from treatment.

Step	Rationale
counterclockwise to lowest resistance setting. As client improves or becomes more proficient, adjust proper resistance level upward by turning dial clockwise.	

3. Instruct client to (Fink and Mahlmeister, 2002):
   a. Sit comfortably.
   b. Take in breath that is larger than normal but not to fill lungs completely.
   c. Position mouthpiece, maintaining tight seal.
   d. Hold breath for 2 to 3 seconds.
   e. Try not to cough and to exhale slowly for 3 to 4 seconds through device, while it is vibrating.

   Vibrations seem to reduce the viscosity of mucus, which improves client's ability to cough up and expectorate secretions (Langenderfer, 1998; Volsko, DiFiore, Chatburn, 2003).

   f. Repeat cycle for 10 to 20 breaths as tolerated.
   g. Remove mouthpiece and have client perform 2 to 3 "huff" coughs.
   h. Repeat steps *a* through *g* as ordered.
4. Auscultate lung fields, obtain vital signs and pulse oximetry.
5. Complete postprocedure protocol.

Recording and Reporting

■ Record level of resistance and client's tolerance.

Unexpected Outcomes	Related Interventions
1. Client unable to maintain mouth seal.	• Reinstruct or demonstrate.

Apical-Radial Pulse

An inefficient contraction of the heart that fails to transmit a pulse wave to the peripheral pulse site creates a pulse deficit. Pulse deficits are frequently associated with dysrhythmias and warn of potential alteration of cardiac output. Assessment for a pulse deficit requires two persons. One nurse assesses a radial pulse rate while a second nurse assesses the apical pulse rate simultaneously. Compare the measurements. The difference between the rates is the pulse deficit.

Delegation Considerations

The skill of radial pulse palpation may be delegated to assistive personnel (AP) while the nurse assesses the apical pulse. However, the nurse is responsible for determining the presence of a pulse deficit and follow-up assessments.

Equipment

- Stethoscope
- Watch with second hand or digital display
- Pen or pencil
- Vital sign flowsheet or record form
- Alcohol swab

Step	Rationale
1. Complete preprocedure protocol.	
2. Assist client to supine or sitting position. Move aside bed linen and gown to expose sternum and left side of chest.	
3. Locate apical and radial pulse sites. If two nurses are available, one nurse auscultates apical pulse and one nurse palpates radial pulse.	Simultaneous measurement allows for comparison of the two pulse rates.

Step	Rationale
4. Nurse measuring radial pulse and holding watch states "start."	Ensures that pulse rates are measured simultaneously.
5. Both nurses count pulse rate for 60 seconds simultaneously. Count ends when nurse taking radial pulse states "stop." Sixty seconds is required when discrepancy between pulse sites is expected or rhythm is irregular.	
6. Subtract radial rate from apical rate to obtain pulse deficit. Pulse deficit reflects number of ineffective cardiac contractions in 1 minute.	Reveals problem with cardiac contractions.
7. If pulse deficit is noted, assess for other signs and symptoms of decreased cardiac output.	
8. Discuss findings with client as needed.	
9. Complete postprocedure protocol	

Recording and Reporting

- Record apical pulse, radial pulse and site, and pulse deficit in nurses' notes.
- Inform nurse in charge or physician of presence of pulse deficit.

Unexpected Outcomes	Related Interventions
1. Pulse deficit exists.	• Report findings to physician. • Anticipate physician's order for an electrocardiogram. • Reassess for deficit at next scheduled assessment.

Aquathermia and Heating Pads

Aquathermia and heating pads are forms of dry heat therapy. Both devices are covered and applied directly to the skin's surface. For this reason you must take extra precautions to prevent burns. Adjust the temperature setting of an aquathermia pad by inserting a plastic key into the control unit. Set the temperature regulators to the recommended temperature—approximately 40.5° to 43° C (105° to 109.4° F). Because of the constant temperature, aquathermia pads are safer than heating pads. If distilled water in the unit runs low, simply add more distilled water to the reservoir at the top of the control unit. Rubber and plastic conduct heat, so enclose the pad in a towel or pillowcase to avoid direct exposure to the skin.

The conventional heating pad is not used in health care settings but may be seen in the client's home. This type of heating pad consists of an electric coil enclosed in a waterproof cover. A cotton or flannel cloth covers the outer pad. The pad connects to an electrical cord that has a temperature-regulating unit for high, medium, or low settings. Because it is so easy to readjust temperature settings on heating pads, instruct clients not to turn the setting higher once they have adapted to the temperature. Avoid using the highest setting.

Delegation Considerations

The skill of applying an aquathermia or heating pad may be delegated to assistive personnel (AP). As the nurse, assess the condition of the area to be treated and explain the purpose of the treatment.

- Caution AP to maintain proper temperature of the application throughout the treatment and to keep the application in place for only the length of time specified based on physician order or hospital policy.
- Caution AP to check the client's skin for excessive redness and pain during application and to report any changes to the nurse.
- Instruct AP to report when the treatment is complete so that you can evaluate the client's response.

Equipment

- Aquathermia (acute care) or heating pad (home care)
- Electrical control unit
- Distilled water (for aquathermia pad)
- Bath towel or pillowcase
- Tape, ties, or gauze roll

Step	Rationale
1. Complete preprocedure protocol.	
2. Check electrical plugs and cords for obvious fraying or cracking.	Prevents injury from accidental electrical shock.
3. Determine client's or family members' knowledge of procedure, including steps for application and safety precautions.	Heating pads are frequently used in home. Assessment determines extent of health teaching required.
4. Position client comfortably so area to be treated may be exposed.	Client must be able to assume position for several minutes during application.
5. For aquathermia or uncovered heating pad, cover or wrap affected area with bath towel or enclose pad with pillowcase.	Prevents heated surface from touching client's skin directly and increasing risk for injury to client's skin.

NURSE ALERT Do not pin the wrap to the pad because this may cause a leak in the device.

Step	Rationale
6. Place pad over affected area (Fig. 3-1), and secure with tape, tie, or gauze as needed.	Pad delivers dry warm heat to injured tissues. Pad should not slip onto different body part.

NURSE ALERT Never position the client so that the client is lying directly on the pad. This position prevents dissipation of heat and increases risk of burns.

Step	Rationale
7. Turn heating pad on to low or medium setting. Check	Prevents exposure of client to temperature extremes.

Step	Rationale

Fig. 3-1 Aquathermia pad applied.

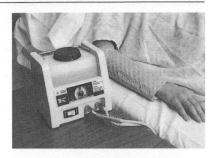

temperature of aquathermia pad.

8. Monitor condition of skin every 5 minutes during application, and question client regarding sensation of burning.

Determines if heat exposure is resulting in burn.

9. After 20 to 30 minutes (or time ordered by physician), remove pad and store.

Continued exposure will result in burns. Some clients should not have access to pad without supervision.

10. Complete postprocedure protocol.

11. Observe client apply pad during next application.

Measures level of learning.

Recording and Reporting

- Record site of application, duration of therapy, and client's response; describe any instruction given and client's success in demonstrating procedure.
- Report changes in skin integrity such as burns.

Unexpected Outcomes	Related Interventions
1. Skin is reddened and sensitive to touch. Symptoms indicate first-degree burn.	• Remove pad, and reassess in 5 to 10 minutes. • If symptoms continue, notify nurse in charge or contact physician.
2. Edema and inflammation are increased. Applying heat too soon after injury can increase edema through vasodilation.	• Notify nurse in charge, or contact physician.
3. Body part is painful to move. Movement stretches burn-sensitive nerve fibers in skin.	• Discontinue aquathermia or heating pad use. Wait for swelling to resolve before attempting to reapply. • Notify nurse in charge, or contact physician.
4. Client applies pad incorrectly.	• Reinstruct client as necessary.

Aspiration Precautions

Aspiration in the adult client usually occurs as a result of difficulties in swallowing (dysphagia). Swallowing dysfunction, or dysphagia, is associated with multiple neurogenic, myogenic, and obstructive causes. Characteristics of dysphagia include cough and/or voice change after swallow; abnormal lip closure and tongue movement; lingual discoordination; hoarse voice; slow, weak, imprecise, or uncoordinated speech; abnormal gag; abnormal volitional cough; delayed oral and pharyngeal transit; incomplete oral clearance; regurgitation; pharyngeal pooling; delayed or absent trigger of swallow; and inability to speak consistently (Groher, 1997). Any one of these characteristics may warrant referral to a specialist for evaluation of dysphagia (Box 4-1).

Complications of dysphagia include increased length of stay, chest infections, disability/decreased functional status, decreased nutritional status, increased likelihood of discharge to long-term care, and increased mortality (Elmstahl and others, 1999). The "silent aspiration," or aspiration that occurs without a cough, is a serious concern with dysphagic individuals and is often the cause of complications (Hammond and others, 2001). Silent aspiration accounts for 40% to 70% of aspiration in clients with dysphagia (Daniels and others, 2000).

Dysphagia screening is a procedure designed to detect any clinical indication of potential neurological deglutition dysfunction (Perry and Love, 2001). Registered dietitians, speech therapists, and registered nurses can screen for dysphagia. Dysphagia can be noted by observing a client at a meal for change in voice quality, posture and head control, percentage of meal consumed, eating time, drooling of liquids and solids, cough during/after a swallow, facial or tongue weakness, difficulty with secretions, pocketing, and presence of voluntary and dry cough (Brody and others, 2000b).

Delegation Considerations

The assessment of the client's risk for aspiration and determination of positioning should not be delegated to assistive personnel (AP).

- Instruct AP to report to the nurse in charge, as soon as possible, any onset of coughing, gagging, or pocketing of food.

Equipment

- Chair or electric bed (to allow client to sit upright)
- Thickening agents as needed (rice, cereal, yogurt, gelatin, commercial thickening agent)

BOX 4-1   Criteria for Dysphagia Referral

Before referral:
If the answer is "yes" to either of the following two questions, the referral at this time is not appropriate.
- Is the client unconscious or drowsy?
- Is the client unable to sit in an upright position for a reasonable length of time?

Consider the next two questions before making the referral:
- Is the client near end of life?
- Does the client have an esophageal problem that will require surgical intervention?

When observing the client or giving mouth care, look for:
- Open mouth (weak lip closure)
- Drooling liquids or solids
- Poor oral hygiene/thrush
- Facial weakness
- Tongue weakness
- Difficulty with secretions
- Slurred, indistinct speech
- Change in voice quality
- Poor posture or head control
- Weak, involuntary cough
- Delayed cough (up to 2 minutes after swallow)
- General frailty
- Confusion/dementia
- No spontaneous swallowing movements

- Tongue blade
- Penlight

Step	Rationale
1. Complete preprocedure protocol.	
2. Assess clients who are at increased risk of aspiration for signs and symptoms of dysphagia (see Box 4-1).	Clients at risk include those who have neurological or neuromuscular diseases and those who have had trauma to or surgical procedures of the oral cavity or throat (Dangerfield and Sullivan, 1999).

Step	**Rationale**
3. Observe chest during mealtime for signs of dysphagia, and allow client to attempt to feed self. Note at end of meal if client fatigues.	Detects abnormal eating patterns such as frequent clearing of throat or prolonged eating time. Fatigue increases risk of aspiration.
4. Ask client about any difficulties with chewing or swallowing various textures of food.	Be alert for symptoms such as coughing, dyspnea, or drooling that suggest difficulty handling food, especially thin liquids.
5. Report signs and symptoms of dysphagia to physician.	Client may need to have evaluation performed by radiologist or speech language pathologist (Perry, 2001a).
6. Place identification on client's chart or Kardex indicating dysphagia.	Identifying client as dysphagic reduces risk of his or her receiving oral nutrients without supervision.
7. Using penlight and tongue blade, gently inspect mouth for pockets of food.	Pockets of food in mouth can indicate difficulty swallowing.
8. Position client so that hips are flexed at 90-degree angle and head is flexed slightly forward.	Reduces risk of aspiration.
9. Observe client consume: foods and liquids of various consistencies.	Difficulty managing foods may indicate dysphagia. Referral to dietitian is appropriate.
10. Ask client to remain sitting upright for at least 30 minutes after meal.	Reduces risk of gastroesophageal reflux, which can cause aspiration.
11. Help client perform hand hygiene and perform mouth care.	Mouth care after meals helps prevent dental caries.
12. Return client's tray to appropriate place, and perform hand hygiene.	Reduces spread of microorganisms.
13. Monitor client's food and fluid intake.	Client may avoid certain types and textures of food that are difficult to swallow.

Step	Rationale
14. Weigh client weekly.	Determines if weight is stable and reflects adequate caloric level.
15. Observe client's oral cavity after meal to detect pockets of food.	Determines presence of pockets of food when meal has included foods of various textures.
16. Complete postprocedure protocol.	

Recording and Reporting

- Document in client's chart: client's tolerance of various food textures, amount of assistance required, position during meal, absence or presence of symptoms of dysphagia, and amount eaten.
- Report any coughing, gagging, choking, or swallowing difficulties to nurse in charge or physician.

Unexpected Outcomes	Related Interventions
1. Client coughs, gags, complains of food "stuck in throat," or has pockets of food in mouth.	• Client may require a swallowing evaluation (see Box 4-1). • Consider consultation with speech therapist for swallowing exercises and techniques to improve swallowing and reduce risk of aspiration. • Notify physician of any symptoms that occurred during meal and which foods caused symptoms.
2. Client avoids certain textures of food.	• Change consistency and texture of food (Table 4-1).

TABLE 4-1   Stages of National Dysphagia Diet

Stage	Description	Examples
Dysphagia Puree	Uniform Pureed	Smooth hot cereals cooked to "pudding" consistency
	Cohesive "Puddinglike" texture	Mashed potatoes Pureed meat Pureed pasta or rice Pureed vegetable Yogurt
Dysphagia Mechanically altered	Moist Soft textured Easily forms bolus	Cooked cereals Dry cereals moistened with milk Canned fruit (excluding pineapple) Moist ground meat Well-cooked noodles in sauce/gravy Well-cooked, diced vegetables
Dysphagia Advanced	Regular foods (with exception of very hard, sticky, or crunchy foods)	Moist breads (with butter, jelly, etc.) Well-moistened cereals Peeled soft fruits (peach, plum, kiwi) Tender, thin-sliced meats Baked potato (without skin) Tender, cooked vegetables
Regular	All foods	No restrictions

Data from National Dysphagia Diet Task Force: *National dysphagia diet: standardization for optimal care*, Chicago, 2002, American Dietetic Association.

Assistive Device Ambulation (Use of Crutches, Cane, and Walker)

Clients who have been immobile for even a short time may require assistance with ambulation. Assistance may mean walking alongside the client while providing support or the client may require the use of an assistive device such as a crutch or walker. Safety precautions are important before and during ambulation of clients to ensure they do not fall as a result of orthostatic hypotension. Selection of an appropriate assistive device depends on the client's age, diagnosis, muscular coordination, and ease of maneuverability (Hoeman, 2002). Use of assistive devices may be temporary, such as during recuperation from a fractured extremity or orthopedic surgery, or permanent, as in the case of a client with paralysis or permanent weakness of the lower extremities.

Delegation Considerations

The skill of assisting clients with crutch walking or use of a walker may be delegated to assistive personnel (AP).

- Remind AP to safely ease a dizzy or fainting client into a sitting position in a chair or on the floor.
- Instruct AP to immediately return the client to the bed or chair if the client is nauseated, dizzy, pale, or diaphoretic. Report these signs and symptoms immediately.
- Discuss the importance of applying safe, nonskid-soled shoes and ensuring that the environment is free of clutter and there is no moisture on the floor before ambulating the client.

Equipment

- Ambulation device (crutch, walker, cane)
- Safety device (gait belt)
- Well-fitting, flat, nonskid shoes for client
- Robe

Step	Rationale
1. Complete preprocedure protocol.	
2. Assess degree of assistance client needs.	For safety, another person may be needed initially to assist with client ambulation.
3. Prepare client for procedure:	
a. Explain reasons for exercise, and demonstrate specific gait technique.	Teaching and demonstration enhance learning, reduce anxiety, and encourage cooperation.
b. Decide with client how far to ambulate.	Consider client's personal preferences and tolerance to exercise.
c. Schedule ambulation around client's other activities.	Scheduled rest periods between activities reduce client fatigue.
d. Apply gait belt. Place bed in low position, and slowly assist client to Fowler's upright position. If in chair, have client sit upright with feet flat on floor.	Allows few minutes for circulation to equilibrate. Prevents orthostatic hypotension and potential injuries (Kenny, 2000).
e. Assist client in bed to dangling position on side of bed. Let client sit for few minutes, taking a few deep breaths, until balance is gained. Have client move legs and feet while dangling. Assist sitting client to standing position and allow to stand.	Movement of legs in dangling position promotes venous return.
f. Ask if client feels dizzy or light-headed. If client appears light-headed, recheck blood pressure.	Allows nurse to detect orthostatic hypotension before ambulation begins.
g. Use caution if client has intravenous (IV)	Allows client to ambulate unencumbered.

Step	**Rationale**
tubing or a Foley catheter. Obtain IV pole with wheels that can be pushed as client walks. Urinary catheter drainage bags must stay at or below level of bladder.	Urine in tubing must not reenter bladder, which increases infection risk.
4. If ambulation device is used, make sure it is appropriate height:	
a. *Crutch measurement:* Includes three areas—client's height, distance between crutch pad and axilla, and angle of elbow flexion. Use one of two methods:	Promotes optimal support and stability.
(1) *Standing:* Position crutches with crutch tips at 15 cm (6 inches) to side and 6 inches in front of client's feet and crutch pads 5 cm (2 inches) below axilla (Hoeman, 2002).	Radial nerve passes under axillary area superficially. If crutch is too long, it can cause pressure on axilla and radial nerve. Injury to radial nerve causes paralysis of elbow and wrist extensors, commonly called *crutch palsy*. Also, if crutch is too long, shoulders are forced upward and client cannot push body off ground. If ambulation device is too short, client will be bent over and uncomfortable.
(2) *Supine:* Crutch pad should be approximately 2 inches or 2 to 3 finger-widths under axilla with crutch tips positioned 15 cm (6 inches)	

Step	Rationale
lateral to client's heel (Hoeman, 2002) (Fig. 5-1).	
(3) Instruct client to report any tingling or numbness in upper torso.	May mean that crutches are being used incorrectly or that they are wrong size.
(4) Following correct crutch adjustment, 2 to 3 fingers should fit between top of crutch and axilla (Fig. 5-2).	Adequate space prevents crutch palsy.
(5) With either measurement method, elbows should be flexed 15 to 30 degrees. Elbow flexion is verified with goniometer (Fig. 5-3).	Angle ensures that arms can push body off ground.

Fig. 5-1   Supine method.

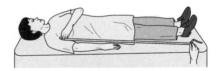

Fig. 5-2   Top of crutch.

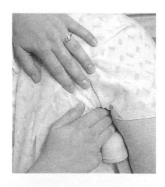

Step	Rationale

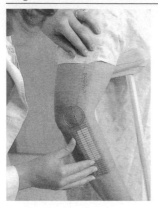

Fig. 5-3 Elbows flexed. Verification of elbow flexion.

(6) In addition to overall *length* of axillary crutch, *height* of handgrip is important. Adjust handgrip so that client's elbow is slightly flexed.

If handgrip is too low, radial nerve damage can occur even if overall crutch length is correct because extra length between handgrip and axillary bar can force bar up into axilla as client stretches down to reach handgrip. If handgrip is too high, client's elbow is sharply flexed and strength and stability of arms are decreased.

b. *Cane measurement:* Client should hold cane on uninvolved side 10 to 15 cm (4 to 6 inches) to side of foot. Cane should extend from greater trochanter to floor while cane is held 15 cm (6 inches) from foot (Hoeman, 2002). Allow approximately 15 to 30 degrees of elbow flexion.

Offers most support when cane is placed on stronger side of body. Cane and weaker leg work together with each step. If cane is too short, client will have difficulty supporting weight and be bent over and uncomfortable. As weight is taken on by hand and affected leg is lifted off floor, complete extension of elbow is necessary.

c. *Walker measurement:* Upper bar of walker

Ensures stable support as client stands and moves walker.

Step	**Rationale**
should be slightly below client's waist. Elbows should be flexed at approximately 15 to 30 degrees when client is standing inside walker with hands on handgrips.	
5. Make sure ambulation device has rubber tips.	Prevents device from slipping.
6. Make sure surface that client walks on is clean and dry. Remove any obstacles or objects that might obstruct pathway. Avoid crowds.	Prevents injuries. Crowds increase risk of crutch, cane, or walker being kicked or jarred and client losing balance.
7. Ambulation with crutches:	
a. Assist client in crutch-walking by choosing appropriate crutch gait (note: in most facilities physical therapist selects gait):	To use crutches, client supports self with hands and arms; therefore strength in arm and shoulder muscles, ability to balance body in upright position, and stamina are necessary. Type of gait client uses depends on amount of weight client is able to support with one or both legs.
(1) Four-point gait:	This is most stable of crutch gaits because it provides at least three points of support at all times. Requires bearing weight on both legs. Each leg moves alternately with each opposing crutch so that three points of support are on floor all the time.
(a) Begin in tripod position. Place crutches 15 cm (6 inches) in front and 15 cm to side	Improves client's balance by providing wide base of support. Client should have posture of erect head and neck, straight vertebrae, and extended hips and knees.

Step	Rationale
of each foot. Place client's weight on handgrips, not under arms (Fig. 5-4).	
(b) Move right crutch forward 10 to 15 cm (4 to 6 inches) (Fig. 5-5, *A*).	Crutch and foot position is similar to arm and foot position during normal walking.
(c) Move left foot forward to level of left crutch (see Fig. 5-5, *B*).	
(d) Move left crutch forward 10 to 15 cm (4 to 6 inches) (see Fig. 5-5, *C*).	
(e) Move right foot forward to level of right crutch (see Fig. 5-5, *D*).	
(f) Repeat above sequence.	
(2) Three-point gait: May be useful for	Requires client to bear all weight on one foot. Weight is borne on

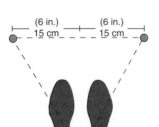

Fig. 5-4 Tripod position.

Step	Rationale

Fig. 5-5 Four-point gait. Solid feet and crutch tips show foot and crutch tip movement in each of the four phases. **A,** Right tip moves forward. **B,** Left foot moves toward left crutch. **C,** Left crutch tip moves forward. **D,** Right foot moves toward right crutch.

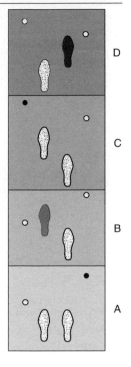

client with broken leg or sprained ankle.

(a) Begin in tripod position (Fig. 5-6, *A*).
(b) Advance both crutches and affected leg (see Fig. 5-6, *B*).
(c) Move stronger leg forward, stepping on floor (see Fig. 5-6, *C*).

uninvolved leg and then on both crutches. Affected leg does not touch ground during early phase of three-point gait.

Improves client's balance by providing wide base of support.

Step	Rationale

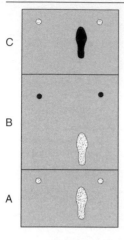

Fig. 5-6 Three-point gait with weight borne on unaffected right leg. Solid foot and crutch tips show weight bearing in each phase.

(d) Repeat sequence.	
(3) Two-point gait:	Requires at least partial weight bearing on each foot. Requires more balance because only two points support body at one time (Hoeman, 2002).
(a) Begin in tripod position (Fig. 5-7, *A*).	Improves client's balance by providing wide base of support.
(b) Move left crutch and right foot forward (see Fig. 5-7, *B*).	Crutch movements are similar to arm movement during normal walking as client moves crutch at same time as opposing leg.
(c) Move right crutch and left foot forward (see Fig. 5-7, *C*).	
(d) Repeat sequence.	
(4) Swing-to gait: Frequently used by clients whose lower extremities are paralyzed or who wear weight-	This is easier of two swinging gaits. It requires ability to partially bear body weight on both legs.

Step	Rationale

Fig. 5-7 Two-point gait. Solid areas indicate weight-bearing leg and crutch tips.

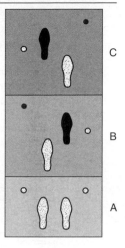

       supporting braces
on their legs.
- (a) Begin in tripod position.
- (b) Move both crutches forward.
- (c) Lift and swing legs to crutches, letting crutches support body weight.
- (d) Repeat two previous steps.

(5) Swing-through gait:

Requires that client have ability to bear partial weight on both feet.

- (a) Begin in tripod position.

Improves client's balance by providing wide base of support.

- (b) Move both crutches forward.

Initial placement of crutches is to increase client's base of support so that when body swings forward, client is moving center of gravity toward additional support provided by crutches.

Step	Rationale
(c) Lift and swing legs through and beyond crutches.	
b. Assist client in climbing stairs with crutches:	
(1) Begin in tripod position.	Improves client's balance by providing wide base of support.
(2) Client transfers body weight to crutches (Fig. 5-8).	Prepares client to transfer weight to unaffected leg when ascending first stair.
(3) Client advances unaffected leg to stair (Fig. 5-9).	Crutch adds support to affected leg. Client then shifts weight from crutches to unaffected leg.
(4) Both crutches are aligned with unaffected leg on stairs (Fig. 5-10).	Maintains balance and provides wide base of support.
(5) Repeat sequence until client reaches top of stairs.	

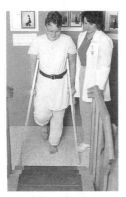

Fig. 5-8 Transfer body weight to crutches.

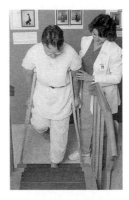

Fig. 5-9 Advance unaffected leg to stair.

Step	Rationale

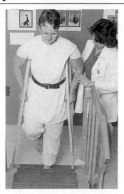

Fig. 5-10 Align crutches with unaffected leg.

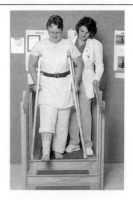

Fig. 5-11 Body weight is transferred to unaffected leg.

   c. Assist client in descending stairs with crutches:

(1) Begin in tripod position.	Improves client's balance by providing wide base of support.
(2) Client transfers body weight to unaffected leg (Fig. 5-11).	Prepares client to release support of body weight maintained by crutches.
(3) Move crutches to stair, and instruct client to begin to transfer body weight to crutches (Fig. 5-12) and move affected leg forward.	Maintains client's balance and base of support.
(4) Client moves unaffected leg to stair and aligns with crutches (Fig. 5-13).	Maintains balance and provides base of support.
(5) Repeat sequence until stairs are descended.	

Step   **Rationale**

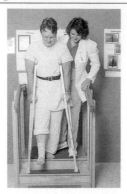

Fig. 5-12   Transfer weight to crutches.

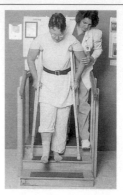

Fig. 5-13   Move unaffected leg, and align with crutches.

8. Ambulation with walker: Walker is used by clients who are able to bear partial weight.

Client needs sufficient strength to be able to pick up walker. Four-wheeled model does not need to be picked up; however, it is not as stable (Hoeman, 2002).

a. Have client stand in center of walker and grasp handgrips on upper bars.

Client balances self before attempting to walk.

b. Lift walker, move it 15 to 20 cm (6 to 8 inches) forward, and then set it down, making sure all four feet of walker stay on floor. Take step forward with either foot. Then follow through with other leg.

Provides broad base of support between walker and client. Client then moves center of gravity toward walker. Keeping all four feet of walker on floor is necessary to prevent tipping of walker.

c. If there is unilateral weakness, after walker

Step	**Rationale**
is advanced, instruct client to step forward with weaker leg, support self with arms, and follow through with uninvolved leg. If client is unable to bear weight on one leg, after advancing walker have client swing into it, supporting weight on hands.	
9. Ambulation with cane (same steps are taught for standard or quad cane) (Fig. 5-14):	
a. Begin by placing cane on uninvolved side.	Provides added support for weak or impaired side.
b. Place cane forward 15 to 25 cm (6 to 10 inches), keeping body weight on both legs.	Distributes body weight equally.
c. Move involved leg forward, even with cane.	Body weight is supported by cane and uninvolved leg.

Fig. 5-14   Client walking properly with cane.

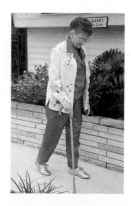

Step	Rationale
d. Advance uninvolved leg past cane.	Body weight is supported by cane and involved leg.
e. Move involved leg forward, even with uninvolved leg.	Aligns client's center of gravity. Returns client's body weight to equal distribution.
f. Repeat these steps.	
10. Complete postprocedure protocol.	

Recording and Reporting

- Record in nurses' notes type of gait client used, amount of assistance required, distance walked, and activity tolerance.
- Immediately report to nurse in charge or physician any injury sustained during attempts to ambulate, alteration in vital signs, or inability to ambulate.

Unexpected Outcomes	Related Interventions
1. Client is unable to ambulate.	• Possible reasons include fear of falling, physical discomfort, upper body muscles that are too weak to use ambulation device, and lower extremities that are too weak to support body.
	• Initiate isometric exercise program to strengthen upper body muscles.
	• Provide analgesic if needed.
2. Client sustains injury.	• Obstacles in client's path, incorrect technique used, or proper safety precautions not taken.
	• Notify physician. Return client to bed if injury stable.

Automated External Defibrillator

An automated external defibrillator (AED) administers an electrical shock through the chest wall to the heart in clients who have a cardiac arrest. It contains built-in computers programmed to assess the victim's heart rhythm and to determine if defibrillation is needed. The advantage of the AED is that laypersons or health care providers trained in basic life support, who have less training than advanced cardiac life support (ACLS) personnel, can defibrillate. The device attaches to a client by two adhesive pads and connecting cables. Most AEDs are stand-alone boxes with a very simple three-step function (Fig. 6-1) and verbal prompts to guide the responder. All AEDs offer the automated rhythm analysis comparing the client's rhythm with thousands of other rhythms stored in the AED's computer software. Upon rhythm identification, some AEDs will automatically provide the electrical shock after a verbal warning (fully automated). Other AEDs recommend a shock, if needed, and then prompt the responder to press the shock button.

Delegation Considerations

Basic life support certification provides hands-on training with an AED for laypersons, assistive personnel (AP), and licensed health care professionals. Most hospitals using AEDs have given the authority to use an AED to all CPR-trained personnel, including AP (see hospital policy).

Equipment

- AED
- Pair of AED adhesive pads

Step	Rationale
1. Establish loss of consciousness, and call for help.	This information assists nurse in determining if client is unconscious rather than asleep, intoxicated, or hearing impaired.

Step	Rationale

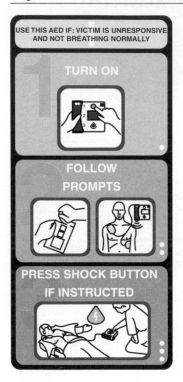

Fig. 6-1 Power panel with prompts. (Courtesy Philips Medical Systems.)

2. Establish absence of respirations and lack of circulation: no pulse, no respirations, no movement.

NURSE ALERT Apply an AED only to a client who is unconscious, breathless, and pulseless. An AED should NOT be used on children younger than 8 years, unless the AED and AED pads have been specially designed for children younger than 8 years (AHA, 2000).

3. Activate code team in accordance with	First available person to bring resuscitation cart and AED.

Step	Rationale

hospital policy and
procedure.

4. Place AED next to client
   near chest or head.
5. Start chest compressions
   until AED arrives and
   is ready to be attached.

NURSE ALERT It is essential that the AED be applied as soon as possible even if chest compressions are interrupted. If the AED is immediately available, attach the AED to the client before chest compressions.

Step	Rationale
6. Turn on power (Fig. 6-1).	Turning on power begins verbal prompts to guide you through next steps.
7. Attach device. Stop CPR before attaching pads. Place first AED pad on upper right sternal border directly below clavicle. Place second electrode pad lateral to left nipple with top of pad a few inches below axilla. Ensure that cables are connected to AED. Do not attach pads to wet surface, over medication patch, or over pacemaker or implanted defibrillator.	Survival rates after ventricular fibrillation arrest decrease approximately 7% to 10% with every minute that defibrillation is delayed (AHA, 2000). Wet surface, implanted defibrillator, and medication patch may reduce effectiveness of defibrillation attempt and result in complications.
8. Allow AED to analyze rhythm. Some devices will require that an analysis button be pressed. Clear rescuers and bystanders from victim, and ensure that no one is touching victim. AED will take approximately 5 to 15 seconds to analyze rhythm.	Each brand of AED is different, so familiarity with model is important. Clearing victim prevents artifact errors, avoids all movement during analysis (Cummins, 2001), and prevents shock from being delivered to bystanders.
9. Deliver shock in series of three as indicated by AED.	Series of three repeated shocks decreases intrathoracic

Step	Rationale
Before pressing shock button, announce loudly to clear victim, and perform visual check to ensure that no one is in contact with victim. Do not resume CPR until AED verbal prompts instruct you to do so.	pressure to electrical current (AHA, 2000). Clearing client ensures safety for those involved in rescue efforts.
10. After three shocks, check pulse, respirations, movement. If no pulse, resume CPR for 1 minute and then begin shock sequence again as prompted by AED.	Most AEDs will analyze heart rhythm between each shock. If rhythm conversion occurs, AED will prompt you to check for signs of circulation before end of three-shock series.
11. Inspect pad adhesion to chest wall between series of shocks.	If pads are not in good contact with chest wall, remove AED pads and apply new set. Attach new set of pads to AED.
12. Continue resuscitative efforts until client regains pulse or until physician determines cessation of efforts.	
13. Complete postprocedure protocol.	

Recording and Reporting

- Immediately report arrest, indicating exact location of victim.
- Cardiopulmonary arrest requires precise documentation. Most hospitals use form designed specifically for in-hospital arrests.
- Record in nurses' notes or on designated CPR worksheet: onset of arrest, time and number of AED shocks (you will not know exact energy level used by AED), time and energy level of manual defibrillations, medications given, procedures performed, cardiac rhythm, use of CPR, and client's response.

Unexpected Outcomes	Related Interventions
1. Client's heart rhythm does not convert into stable rhythm with pulse after defibrillation.	• Assess pad contact on client's chest wall. • Do not touch client during AED's rhythm analysis. • Avoid placing AED pads over medication patches, pacemaker, or implantable defibrillator generators.
2. Client's skin has burns under AED pads.	• Assess AED pad contact on chest. • Ensure that chest is dry before applying pads to chest.

Bladder Volume Measurement

BladderScan®, or bladder volume measurements with ultrasound, are noninvasive methods to determine urinary bladder volume in the client who requires monitoring of bladder volume or post-voiding residual volume. Bladder volume measurement reduces the need for urinary catheterizations to determine residual volume. As a result, the risk of urinary tract infections is also reduced (Schott-Baer and Reaume, 2001). Clinical studies comparing the measurement of urine volume in the bladder through the use of a BladderScan® and intermittent catheterizations for residual volumes showed no significant difference between the two forms of measurement (Borrie and others, 2001; Schott-Baer and Reaume, 2001). In addition, bladder volume measurement is effective in managing bacteriuria and urinary incontinence in some clients (Barabas and Molstad, 2005).

Delegation Considerations

The skill of bladder volume measurement may be delegated to assistive personnel (AP) in some situations. However, the nurse is responsible for determining that the procedure is appropriate and for evaluating the information obtained. The nurse provides AP with the following directions:

- Instruct AP to inform the nurse about the client's complaints of discomfort, inability to void completely, or fever.
- Instruct AP to inform the nurse immediately about any increase in residual urine volume.

Equipment

- BladderScan® or bladder ultrasound device (Fig. 7-1)
- Ultrasound transmission gel
- Alcohol wipes
- Tissues or washcloth

Step	Rationale
1. Complete preprocedure protocol.	

Step	Rationale
2. Determine need for bladder volume measurement:	
a. Used in clients suspected of having increased residual bladder volume.	BladderScan® is a noninvasive measure to determine bladder volume.
b. Assesses need for intermittent catheterization.	Clients with spinal cord injuries or other neurological conditions may not perceive full bladder and may not be able to voluntarily empty their bladder. BladderScan® can assist in identifying specific bladder volume to indicate need for catheterization (Borrie and others, 2001).
c. Identify contraindications to BladderScan® (e.g., not recommended for pregnant women, clients with open abdominal wounds, clients with indwelling catheters).	Affects accuracy of ultrasound transmission and subsequent results.

NURSE ALERT BladderScan® should not be used on clients with abdominal scar tissue, sutures, or staples.

Step	Rationale
3. Palpate client's bladder.	Detects bladder distention.
4. Ask client to empty bladder.	Clients who are receiving a BladderScan® measurement for post-voiding residuals must empty bladder 10 to 20 minutes before scanning.
5. Assess client for presence of bladder spasms and discomfort.	Provides information about any bladder irritation.
6. Assess client's knowledge regarding purpose of bladder volume measurement.	Reveals need for client instruction.
7. Turn BladderScan® on and press scan button.	

| Step | Rationale |

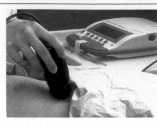

Fig. 7-1   Correct placement of BladderScan®. (Courtesy Verathon Inc., Bothell, Washington, USA.)

8. Press "Male" or "Female" button.

Indication of gender allows BladderScan® to exclude uterus.

NURSE ALERT If a woman has had a hysterectomy, select "Male" as per the manufacturer's directions.

9. Apply gel to clean scan head.

10. Palpate abdomen, and place scan head 3 cm ($1^1/_2$ inches) above symphysis pubis (Fig. 7-1).

11. Locate "ultrasound waveform" icon/button on probe. Make sure top of icon or head of icon is pointed toward head of client.

Orients ultrasound device correctly.

12. Firmly apply scan head to client's abdomen and press "ultrasound waveform" icon/button until audible beep or other sound is heard.

Firm pressure is necessary to ensure contact of ultrasound head to client's abdomen.

13. While observing screen, tilt head of scanner until bladder image is aligned in cross hair of screen or according to manufacturer's instructions.

Alignment of bladder with screen is necessary to ensure accurate measure of bladder volume.

Step	Rationale
14. Once bladder is aligned in screen, obtain measurement and press "Done" when finished.	BladderScan® will automatically save largest scan.

NURSE ALERT If a hard copy of the scan result is needed, press "Print" and attach the result to the client's chart.

Step	Rationale
15. Turn scan off, wipe off gel from client's abdomen, and perform hygiene as needed.	Reduces transmission of microorganisms.

NURSE ALERT Some clients may have an order to obtain post-scan voiding or catheterization. This should be performed immediately after obtaining the scan.

Step	Rationale
16. Clean scan head with alcohol wipes.	Alcohol wipes adequately clean scan head. DO NOT immerse scan head or use other solvents to clean.
17. Return BladderScan® to charger.	Maintains charge on BladderScan® battery.
18. Complete postprocedure protocol.	

Recording and Reporting

- Record and report amount voided before BladderScan®, BladderScan® volume, and any subsequent amount voided or obtained from catheterization.
- Note characteristics of urine output, and record information on intake and output (I&O) sheet.

Unexpected Outcomes	Related Interventions
1. Unable to obtain bladder volume.	• Examine connections on equipment.
2. Client complains of bladder fullness, increase in bladder spasms.	• Verify presence of ultrasound gel. • Obtain scan as ordered. • Notify physician.

Blood Administration

Blood administration or transfusion therapy is the intravenous (IV) administration of whole blood or blood products. The physician determines which blood component is needed to treat a client's medical condition. Blood products are ordered to restore circulating blood volume, to improve hemoglobin levels, or to correct serum protein deficiencies. Clinical indications differ among blood products, and the nurse is responsible for understanding which components are appropriate in various situations.

Delegation Considerations

This skill may not be delegated to assistive personnel (AP). The nurse is responsible for assessing and monitoring the client's status during the initial phase of the transfusion. After the transfusion has been started and the client is stable, AP can monitor the client's vital signs. AP should be taught the signs and symptoms of a transfusion reaction and the importance of immediately reporting if any signs or symptoms occur. Depending upon the agency's policy, AP may:

- Obtain blood components from the blood bank.
- Assist in the verification procedure before the initiation of blood therapy; many inpatient facilities require two licensed professionals to verify blood units.

Equipment

- Blood administration set
- 0.9% NaCl (normal saline) IV solution
- Alcohol wipes
- Disposable clean gloves
- Tape
- Blood pressure cuff and stethoscope
- Thermometer
- Signed transfusion consent form

If Needed

- Rapid infusion pump
- Leukocyte-depleting filter
- Blood warmer

- Pressure bag
- Pulse oximeter

For Perioperative Blood Salvage
- Cell saver or continuous collection container and appropriate tubing

For Postoperative Salvage via Drainage Tubes
- Drainage collection and reinfusion device
- 0.9% NaCl IV solution
- Anticoagulant, if needed
- Transfer bag and tubing
- Label
- Disposable gloves

Step	Rationale
1. Complete preprocedure protocol.	
2. Verify that IV cannula is patent and without complications such as infiltration or phlebitis. In emergency situations that require rapid transfusions, 16- or 18-gauge cannula is preferred; however, transfusions for therapeutic indications may be infused with cannulas ranging from 20 to 24 gauge.	Patent IV ensures that transfusion will be initiated and infused within established time guidelines. Gauge of IV cannula should be appropriate for accommodating infusion of blood and/or blood components (Intravenous Nurses Society, 2000). Large cannulas, such as 18 gauge, promote optimal flow of blood components. Use of smaller cannula such as 22 to 24 gauge may require blood bank to divide unit so that each half can be infused within allotted time or may require pressure-assisted devices. Infiltration or signs of infection at IV site contraindicate use of that line.
3. Obtain client's transfusion history.	Identifies client's prior response(s) to transfusion of blood components. If client has experienced reaction in past,

Step	Rationale
	anticipate similar reaction and be prepared to rapidly intervene.
4. Review physician's order for blood component transfusion. Check that transfusion consent has been properly completed and signed by client.	Physician's order must be present before transfusing blood product. Verifying order helps ensure that appropriate blood component will be administered. Because of inherent risks, most agencies require clients to sign consent forms before receiving blood component therapy.
5. Obtain and record vital signs, including temperature, immediately before initiation of transfusion.	Change from baseline vital signs during infusion will alert nurse to potential transfusion reaction or adverse effect of therapy.
6. ▰ Preadministration:	
a. Obtain blood component from blood bank following agency protocol.	Timely acquisition ensures that product is safe to administer. Agency protocol usually encompasses safeguards to ensure quality control throughout transfusion process.
b. Correctly verify product and identify client with person considered qualified by your agency (e.g., RN, licensed practical nurse [LPN], client care technician):	Strict adherence to verification procedures before administration of blood or blood components reduces risk of administering wrong blood to client. Most hemolytic transfusion reactions are caused by clerical errors (AABB, 2002).
(1) Check client's first and last names by having client state name, if able. Also, check client's identification number and date of birth on armband and client record.	When discrepancy is noted during verification procedure, do not administer product. Notify blood bank and appropriate personnel as indicated by agency policy.

Step	**Rationale**
(2) Verify that component received from blood bank is component ordered by physician.	Ensures that client receives correct therapy.
(3) Check that client's blood type and Rh type are compatible with donor blood type and Rh type. Be sure that transfusion product is not discolored, clotted, or leaking and does not have bubbles present.	Verifies accurate donor blood type. Air bubbles, clots, or discoloration may indicate bacterial contamination or inadequate anticoagulation of stored component and would be contraindications to transfusion of that product.
(4) Check that unit number on unit of blood and on form from blood bank match.	Prevents accidental administration of wrong component.
(5) Check expiration date and time on unit of blood.	Expired blood should never be used, because cell components deteriorate and may contain excess citrate ions.
(6) Record verification process as directed by agency policy.	Documentation on legal medical record.
c. Empty urine drainage collection container, or have client void.	If transfusion reaction occurs, urine specimen containing urine produced after initiation of transfusion will be sent to laboratory.
7. 🖼 Administration:	
a. Autologous transfusion only:	Allows collection of client's blood for reinfusion, storage (no longer than 6 hours), or washing and spinning.
(1) Connect drainage tubes to collection container or cell-processing system.	

Step	Rationale
(2) Minimize air bubbles by establishing secure connections. Follow agency's and manufacturer's procedure for setup and maintenance of system.	
b. Open Y tubing blood administration set.	Y tubing is used to facilitate maintenance of IV access in case client will need more than 1 unit of blood. Both a unit of blood and a container of 0.9% NaCl are connected to system. With Y tubing, normal saline can be easily infused at keep-vein-open (KVO) rate (10 to 12 gtt/min) to maintain venous patency while obtaining next transfusion unit following each transfusion (follow manufacturer's guidelines regarding number of units that can be given before tubing must be changed). If client is to receive only 1 unit of blood, piggyback infusion of 0.9% NaCl IV solution should be connected with blood administration set, using stopcock or needleless valve. Saline should be readily available in case of transfusion reaction.
c. Set roller clamp(s) to "off" position.	Moving roller clamps to "off" position prevents accidental spilling and wasting of product.
d. Spike 0.9% NaCl IV bag with one of Y tubing spikes (Fig. 8-1). Invert filter, open roller	Primes tubing with fluid to eliminate air on both sides of Y tubing. Inverting filter to fill from top to bottom reduces

Step	Rationale

Fig. 8-1 Blood administration set is primed with normal saline.

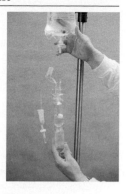

clamps of IV bag and component side of Y, keeping common tubing clamp below filter closed. Set IV bag on table, and gently press down to squeeze IV bag to fill both sides of Y tubing. Close tubing clamp of component side of Y, and open common tubing clamp below filter. Continue to press down on IV saline bag to completely fill filter and half of drip chamber. Close both tubing clamps. All three tubing clamps should be closed.

formation of air pockets. Closing roller clamp prevents spillage and waste of fluid.

e. Hang on IV pole. Open common tubing clamp to finish priming tubing to distal end of tubing connector. Close tubing clamp when tubing is

This will completely prime tubing with saline, and IV line is ready to be connected to client's vascular access device (VAD).

Step	Rationale

filled with saline.
Maintain protective
sterile cap on tubing
connector.

f. Prepare blood
component for
administration.
Remove protective
covering from access
port. Spike blood
component unit with
other Y connection
(Fig. 8-2). Hang on IV
pole. Open clamp of Y
connected to blood
unit, and open common
tubing clamp to prime
tubing with blood.
Allow saline in tubing
to flow into receptacle,
being careful to ensure
that any blood spillage
is contained in Blood
Precaution container.

Protective barrier drape may be
used to catch any potential blood
spillage. Tubing is primed with
blood unit and ready for
transfusion into client.

NURSE ALERT Normal saline is compatible with blood products, unlike
solutions that contain dextrose, which cause coagulation of donor blood.

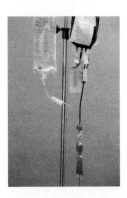

Fig. 8-2   Unit of blood connected to Y
tubing.

Step	Rationale
g. Maintaining asepsis, attach primed tubing to client's VAD. Open common tubing clamp.	This initiates infusion of blood product into client's vein.
h. Remain with client during first 5 to 15 minutes of transfusion. Initial flow rate during this time should be 2 ml/min, or 20 gtt/min.	Most transfusion reactions occur within first 5 to 15 minutes of transfusion. Infusing small amount of blood component initially minimizes volume of blood to which client is exposed, thereby minimizing severity of reaction.

NURSE ALERT If signs of a transfusion reaction occur, stop the infusion, start normal saline with new primed tubing directly into VAD at KVO (5–10 ml/hr), and notify the physician immediately.

i. Monitor client's vital signs 5 minutes after blood product has begun infusing and per agency policy after that.	Frequent monitoring of vital signs will help to quickly alert nurse to transfusion reaction.
j. Regulate rate of transfusion according to physician's orders. (Drop factor for blood tubing is 10 gtt/ml.)	Maintaining prescribed rate of flow decreases risk of fluid volume excess while restoring vascular volume.

NURSE ALERT A unit of whole blood should not hang for more than 4 hours because of the danger of bacterial growth.

k. After blood has infused, clear IV line with normal saline and discard blood bag according to agency policy.	Infusing IV saline solution infuses remainder of blood in IV tubing and keeps IV line patent for supportive measures in case of transfusion reaction.
l. Appropriately dispose of all supplies. Remove gloves, and perform hand hygiene.	Standard Precautions during transfusion reduce transmission of microorganisms.

Step	Rationale
8. Monitor IV site and status of infusion each time vital signs are taken.	Detects presence of infiltration or phlebitis and verifies continuous and safe infusion of blood product.
9. Observe for any changes in vital signs and for chills, flushing, itching, dyspnea, rash, or other signs of transfusion reaction.	These may be early signs of transfusion reaction.
10. Complete postprocedure protocol.	

Recording and Reporting

- Record type of blood component and amount administered, along with client's response to therapy. This may be documented on transfusion record itself, in nurses' notes, medication administration record, and/or intake and output sheet, depending on agency policy.
- Report signs and symptoms of transfusion reaction immediately.

Unexpected Outcomes	Related Interventions
1. Client displays signs and symptoms of transfusion reaction, which include fever with or without chills, tachycardia, tachypnea, wheezing, dyspnea, headache, flushing of skin, hives or itching, hypotension, or gastrointestinal symptoms. These occur when donor blood is incompatible with recipient's blood	• Stop transfusion. • Normal saline should be connected at VAD hub to prevent any subsequent blood from infusing from tubing. Disconnect blood tubing at VAD hub, and cap distal end with sterile connector to maintain sterile system. Keep vein open with slow infusion of normal saline at 10 to 12 gtt/min to ensure venous patency and maintain venous access for medication or to resume transfusion. It is important to regulate flow rate to minimize administration of excess IV fluid, especially in clients who are prone to fluid overload such as clients

Unexpected Outcomes	Related Interventions
or when recipient has sensitivity to a plasma protein in transfused (donor's) blood.	with cardiac and renal disorders, pediatric clients, and older adults. Notify physician.
2. Client develops infiltration or phlebitis at venipuncture site.	• Remove IV, and insert new VAD in different site. Product may be restarted if remainder can be infused within 4 hours of initiation of transfusion. • Institute nursing measures to reduce discomfort at infiltrated or infected site.
3. Fluid overload occurs, and/or client exhibits difficulty breathing or has crackles upon auscultation.	• Slow or stop transfusion, elevate head of bed, and inform physician of physical findings. • Administer diuretics, morphine, and/or oxygen as ordered by physician. • Continue frequent assessments, and closely monitor vital signs, intake and output.

Blood Pressure by Auscultation: Upper Extremities, Lower Extremities, Palpation

The standard unit for measuring blood pressure (BP) is millimeters of mercury (mm Hg). The measurement indicates the height to which the BP can sustain the column of mercury. The most common technique of measuring BP is auscultation using a sphygmomanometer and stethoscope. As the sphygmomanometer cuff is deflated, the five different sounds heard over an artery are called *Korotkoff phases*. The sound in each phase has unique characteristics (Fig. 9-1). BP is recorded with the systolic reading (first Korotkoff sound) before the diastolic (beginning of the fifth Korotkoff sound) (Beevers and others, 2001b). The difference between systolic pressure and diastolic pressure is the pulse pressure. For a BP of 120/80, the pulse pressure is 40.

Delegation Considerations

The skill of BP measurement may be delegated to assistive personnel (AP) unless the client is considered unstable. However, it is the nurse's responsibility to analyze and act on client assessment data. Before delegating this skill, the nurse must:

- Inform AP of the usual BP values for the client and the frequency of BP measurement for select client.
- Inform AP if the client has alterations affecting the appropriate limb for BP measurement.
- Provide AP the appropriate-size BP cuff for the designated extremity.
- Notify AP if the client is at risk for orthostatic hypotension.
- Instruct AP of the need to report any abnormalities that should be reconfirmed by the nurse.

Equipment

- Aneroid sphygmomanometer
- Cloth or disposable vinyl pressure cuff of appropriate size for client's extremity
- Stethoscope

Fig. 9-1 The sounds auscultated during blood pressure (BP) measurement can be differentiated into five Korotkoff phases. In this example, the BP is 140/90 mm Hg.

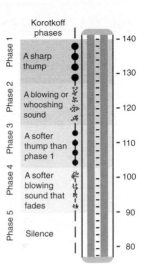

- Alcohol swab
- Pen, pencil, vital sign flowsheet or record form

Step	Rationale
1. Complete preprocedure protocol.	
2. Assess for factors that influence BP (e.g., age, gender, history of smoking, medication, weight).	Normal average BP varies throughout life. Smoking results in vasoconstriction— narrowing of blood vessels. BP rises acutely and returns to baseline in about 15 minutes after stopping smoking (Joint National Committee, 2003).
3. Determine proper cuff size and best site for BP assessment (Fig. 9-2). Avoid applying cuff to (1) extremity in which intravenous (IV) fluids or arteriovenous shunt or fistula is present, (2) extremity on same side on which breast	Inappropriate site selection may result in poor amplification of sounds, causing inaccurate readings. Application of pressure from inflated bladder temporarily

Step	Rationale

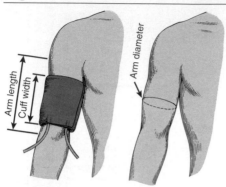

Arm length
Cuff width
Arm diameter

Fig. 9-2
Guidelines for proper blood pressure cuff size. Cuff width = 20% more than upper arm diameter, or 40% of circumference and two thirds of upper arm length.

or axillary surgery has been performed.	impairs blood flow and can further compromise circulation in extremity that already has impaired blood flow.

4. Obtain BP:
   a. Assessing BP by auscultation: upper extremities:

(1) With client sitting or lying, position client's forearm, supported if needed, at heart level, with palm turned up. If sitting, client should be instructed to keep feet flat on floor without legs crossed.	Placement of arm above level of heart causes false low reading. Even in supported position, diastolic pressure effort up to 3 to 4 mm Hg can occur for each 5-cm change in heart level (Netea and others, 2003).
(2) Expose upper arm fully by removing constricting clothing.	Ensures proper cuff application. Do not place BP cuff over clothing.
(3) Palpate brachial artery (Fig. 9-3, *A*). Position cuff 2.5 cm (1 inch) above site of brachial pulsation (antecubital space). Apply bladder of cuff above artery by	Inflating bladder directly over brachial artery ensures that proper pressure is applied during inflation. Loose-fitting cuff causes false high readings.

Step	**Rationale**

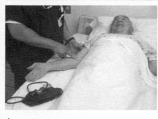

A

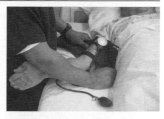

B

C

Fig. 9-3 **A,** Nurse palpating client's brachial artery. **B,** Center bladder of cuff above artery. **C,** Blood pressure cuff wrapped around upper arm.

centering arrows marked on cuff over artery (see Fig. 9-3, *B*). If no center arrows are on cuff, estimate center of bladder and place this center over artery. With cuff fully deflated, wrap cuff evenly and snugly around upper arm (see Fig. 9-3, *C*).	
(4) Position manometer vertically at eye level. Observer should be no farther than 1 meter (approximately 1 yard).	Looking up or down at scale can result in distorted readings.
(5) Measure BP:	
(a) Two-step method:	
1) Relocate brachial pulse. Palpate artery distal to cuff with fingertips	Estimating systolic pressure prevents false low readings, which may result in presence of an

Step	Rationale
of nondominant hand while inflating cuff. Note point at which pulse disappears, and continue to inflate cuff to pressure 30 mm Hg above that point. Note pressure reading. Slowly deflate cuff, and note point when pulse reappears. Deflate cuff fully, and wait 30 seconds.	auscultatory gap. Maximal inflation point for accurate reading can be determined by palpation. If unable to palpate artery because of weakened pulse, ultrasonic stethoscope can be used. Deflating cuff prevents venous congestion and false high readings.
2) Place stethoscope earpieces in ears, and be sure sounds are clear.	Each earpiece should follow angle of ear canal to facilitate hearing.
3) Relocate brachial artery, and place the bell or diaphragm of stethoscope over it. Do not allow chest piece to touch cuff or clothing.	Proper stethoscope placement ensures optimal sound reception. Stethoscope improperly positioned causes muffled sounds that often result in false low systolic and false high diastolic readings. Bell will give better sound reproduction, whereas diaphragm is easier to secure with fingers and covers larger area (Beevers and others, 2001b).
4) Close valve of pressure bulb clockwise until tight.	Tightening valve prevents air leak during inflation.

Step	Rationale
5) Quickly inflate cuff to 30 mm Hg above client's estimated systolic pressure.	Rapid inflation ensures accurate measurement of systolic pressure.
6) Slowly release pressure bulb valve, and allow manometer needle to fall at rate of 2 to 3 mm Hg/sec. Make sure there are no extraneous sounds.	Too rapid or slow a decline can cause inaccurate readings. Noise interferes with precise hearing of Korotkoff phases.
7) Note point on manometer when first clear sound is heard. The sound will slowly increase in intensity.	First Korotkoff sound reflects systolic blood pressure.
8) Continue to deflate cuff gradually, noting point at which sound disappears in adults. Note pressure to nearest 2 mm Hg. Listen for 20 to 30 mm Hg after the last sound, and then allow remaining air to escape quickly.	Beginning of fifth Korotkoff sound is recommended as indication of diastolic pressure in adults (Joint National Committee, 2003). Fourth Korotkoff sound involves distinct muffling of sounds and is recommended as indication of diastolic pressure in children.
(b) One-step method:	
1) Place stethoscope earpieces in ears, and be sure	Earpieces should follow angle of ear canal to facilitate hearing.

Step	Rationale
	sounds are clear, not muffled.	
2)	Relocate brachial artery, and place bell or diaphragm of stethoscope over it. Do not allow chest piece to touch cuff or clothing.	Proper stethoscope placement ensures optimal sound reception.
3)	Close valve of pressure bulb clockwise until tight. Quickly inflate cuff to 30 mm Hg above client's usual systolic pressure.	Tightening of valve prevents air leak during inflation. Inflation above systolic level ensures accurate measurement of systolic pressure.
4)	Slowly release pressure bulb valve, and allow manometer needle to fall at rate of 2 to 3 mm Hg/sec. Note point on manometer when first clear sound is heard. Sound will slowly increase in intensity.	Too rapid or slow decline in mercury level can cause inaccurate readings. First Korotkoff sound reflects systolic pressure.
5)	Continue to deflate cuff gradually, noting point at which sound disappears in adults. Note pressure to nearest 2 mm Hg. Listen for 10 to 20 mm Hg	Beginning of fifth Korotkoff sound is recommended as indication of diastolic pressure in adults (Joint National Committee, 2003). Fourth Korotkoff sound involves distinct muffling of sounds and is

Step	**Rationale**
after last sound, and then allow remaining air to escape quickly and remove cuff.	recommended as indication of diastolic pressure in children.
(6) The Joint National Committee (2003) recommends the average of two sets of BP measurements, 2 minutes apart. Use second set of BP measurements as your baseline.	Two sets of BP measurements help prevent false positives based on client's sympathetic response (alert reaction). Averaging minimizes effect of anxiety, which often causes first reading to be higher than subsequent measures (Joint National Committee, 2003).

b. Assessing BP by auscultation: lower extremities:

Step	**Rationale**
(1) Assist client to prone position. If unable to assume position, assist client to supine position with knee slightly flexed.	Prone position provides best access to popliteal artery.
(2) Move aside bed linen and any constrictive clothing from leg.	Ensures proper cuff positioning.
(3) Locate popliteal artery behind knee.	Artery palpation site lies just below client's thigh, behind knee in popliteal space.
(4) Apply large leg cuff 2.5 cm (1 inch) above popliteal artery around posterior aspect of middle thigh. Center arrows marked on cuff over artery (Fig. 9-4).	Proper cuff size is necessary for accurate reading. Cuff must be wide and long enough to allow for larger girth of thigh. Narrow cuff causes false high readings.

Step	Rationale

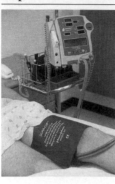

Fig. 9-4   Blood pressure cuff applied around thigh.

(5) Position manometer vertically at eye level. Observer should be no farther than 1 meter (approximately 1 yard).	Looking up or down at scale can result in distorted readings.
(6) Using popliteal artery, follow Step (5) (b) (p. 53) of one-step method for auscultation of upper extremity.	
(7) If this is first assessment of client, repeat procedure on other leg.	Comparison of BP in both legs detects circulatory problems.

c. Assessing blood pressure by palpation:

(1) Follow Steps 4a (p. 50) (1) through (4) of auscultation method for upper extremity.	
(2) Locate and then continually palpate either brachial or radial artery with fingertips of one hand. Inflate cuff to pressure 30 mm Hg above point at which pulse can no longer be palpated. *Optional:* Palpation of	Ensures accurate detection of true systolic pressure once pressure valve is released.

Step	Rationale

popliteal artery can also be done with leg cuff.

NURSE ALERT If the artery cannot be palpated because of a weakened pulse, a Doppler ultrasonic stethoscope can also be used.

(3) Slowly release valve and deflate cuff, allowing manometer needle to fall at rate of 2 mm Hg/sec. Note point on manometer when pulse is again palpable. — Too rapid or slow a decline can result in inaccurate readings. Palpation can identify systolic pressure only.

(4) Deflate cuff rapidly and completely. Remove cuff from client's extremity unless measurement must be repeated. — Continuous cuff inflation causes arterial occlusion, resulting in numbness and tingling of client's arm.

(5) Assist client in returning to comfortable position, and cover upper arm if previously clothed. — Restores comfort and promotes sense of well-being.

5. If BP is assessed for the first time, establish BP as baseline if it is within acceptable range. — Used to compare future BP measurements.

6. Compare BP reading with client's previous baseline and usual BP for client's age. — Allows nurse to assess for change in condition. Provides comparison with future BP measurements.

7. Complete postprocedure protocol.

Recording and Reporting

- Record BP and site assessed on vital sign flowsheet or nurses' notes.
- Record any signs or symptoms of BP alterations in narrative form in nurses' notes.
- Report abnormal findings to nurse in charge or physician.

Unexpected Outcomes	Related Interventions
1. BP is above acceptable range.	• Repeat measurement: • Verify correct BP cuff size. • Assess BP in other arm or extremity, and compare findings.

2. BP is hypotensive, and BP is not sufficient for adequate perfusion and oxygenation of tissues.	• Place client in supine position to enhance circulation, and restrict activity that may decrease BP further.
	• Observe for symptoms associated with hypotension related to decreased cardiac output:
	  • Tachycardia.
	  • Weak, thready pulse.
	  • Weakness, dizziness, confusion.
	  • Cool, pale, dusky, or cyanotic skin.

Blood Pressure: Automatic

Many different styles of electronic blood pressure (BP) machines are available to determine BP automatically. Electronic BP machines rely on an electronic sensor to detect the vibrations caused by the rush of blood through an artery.

Although electronic BP machines are fast and free up the care provider for other activities, the nurse must consider the advantages and limitations of electronic BP machines. The devices are used when frequent assessment is required, such as in critically ill or potentially unstable clients, during or after invasive procedures, or when therapies require frequent monitoring.

Delegation Considerations

The skill of automatic BP measurement may be delegated to assistive personnel (AP) unless the client is considered unstable. Before delegating this skill, the nurse must:

- Provide AP with the client's current and/or normal values, the appropriate limb, and the frequency of BP measurement.
- Instruct AP of the need to report any abnormalities that should be reconfirmed by the nurse.

Equipment

- Electronic BP machine
- BP cuff of appropriate size as recommended by manufacturer

Assessment

1. Complete preprocedure protocol.
2. Determine appropriateness of using electronic BP measurement. Clients with irregular heart rate, peripheral vascular disease, seizures, tremors, or shivering are not candidates for this device.
3. Locate *on/off* switch, and turn on machine to enable device to self-test computer systems.
4. Select appropriate site and cuff size for client extremity (see Skill 9, Step 3, p. 49) and appropriate cuff for machine. Electronic BP cuff and machine must be matched by manufacturer and cannot be interchanged.
5. Expose upper arm fully by removing constricting clothing, which ensures proper cuff application.

6. Prepare BP cuff by manually squeezing all air out of cuff and connecting cuff to connector hose.
7. Wrap flattened cuff snugly around extremity, verifying that only one finger can fit between cuff and client's skin. Make sure "artery" arrow marked on outside of cuff is correctly placed.
8. Verify that connector hose between cuff and machine is not kinked. Kinking prevents proper inflation and deflation of cuff.
9. Following manufacturer's directions, set frequency control for *automatic* or *manual* and then press *start* button. The first BP measurement will pump cuff to peak pressure of about 180 mm Hg. After this pressure is reached, machine begins deflation sequence that determines BP. First reading determines peak pressure inflation for additional measurements.
10. When deflation is complete, digital display will provide most recent values and flash time in minutes that has elapsed since measurement occurred.

NURSE ALERT   If unable to obtain the BP with the electronic device, verify the machine connections (e.g., plugged into working electrical outlet, hose-cuff connections tight, machine on, correct cuff). Repeat the electronic BP measurement; if unable to obtain, use the auscultatory technique (see Skill 9, Step 4a, p. 50).

11. Set frequency of BP measurements and upper and lower alarm limits for systolic, diastolic, and mean BP readings. Intervals between BP measurements can be set from 1 to 90 minutes. Nurse determines frequency and alarm limits based on client's acceptable range of BP, nursing judgment, and physician order.
12. Additional readings, which may be needed for unstable clients, can be obtained at any time by pressing *start* button. Pressing *cancel* button immediately deflates cuff.
13. If frequent BP measurements are required, cuff may be left in place. Remove cuff every 2 hours to assess underlying skin integrity and, if possible, alternate BP sites. Clients with abnormal bleeding tendencies are at risk for microvascular rupture from repeated inflations. When electronic BP machine no longer is used, clean BP cuff according to facility policy to reduce transmission of microorganisms.
14. Complete postprocedure protocol.

Central Venous Access Device Care: CVC, Ports

To manage long-term intravenous (IV) therapy effectively, the nurse must be familiar with the various types of central venous access devices (CVADs). Knowing the type of CVADs can be confusing because catheters are often referred to by brand name instead of type and placement (e.g., Hickman, Groshong, Raaf, Port-a-Cath). For this skill these CVADs will be divided into three types: tunneled and percutaneous central venous catheters (CVCs) and implanted infusion ports. Both types of CVCs, tunneled and percutaneous, are threaded into a large vein, typically the internal or external jugular or the superior vena cava that leads to the right atrium of the heart (Figs. 11-1 and 11-2).

The implanted infusion port consists of a portal body, a central septum, a reservoir, and a catheter (Fig. 11-3). The port is also available with a double-lumen catheter. The physician implants the infusion port under sterile conditions in an operating room with the client under local anesthesia. The port can be easily palpated to determine placement. Specially designed non-coring Huber needles (straight or with 90-degree angles) are inserted through the skin to enter the port (see Fig. 11-3, *B*). The infusion port usually rests in a subcutaneous pocket in the infraclavicular fossa, and the catheter is inserted into a large vein and threaded into the superior vena cava (see Fig. 11-3, *C*).

Delegation Considerations

The skill of caring for a CVAD *in an acute care setting* should not be delegated to assistive personnel (AP). However, the nurse provides information and direction, including:

- Instructing AP in the signs and symptoms of CVC complications to report.

Equipment
Blood Drawing

- Antimicrobial swabs (e.g., chlorhexidine, povidone-iodine, alcohol preparation swabs)
- Four to five syringes (10 ml)
- Sterile drape
- Saline flush

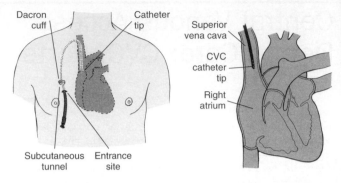

Fig. 11-1 Catheter tip from CVAD lies in superior vena cava.

Fig. 11-2 Tunneled CVC placed in jugular vein.

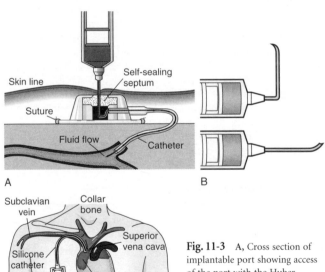

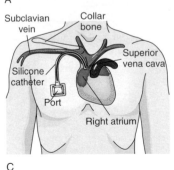

Fig. 11-3 A, Cross section of implantable port showing access of the port with the Huber needle. B, Two Huber needles used to enter implanted port. The 90-degree needle is used for top-entry ports for continuous infusion. C, Implant port and catheter.

- Heparin flush (100 units/ml)
- Plastic clamp
- Sterile Huber needle, injectable (20 to 22 gauge)
- Sterile needle, injectable (20 to 22 gauge)
- Blood tubes, labels, requisitions
- Gloves, gowns, masks

Administration of Drugs, Fluids, Blood Products

- Antimicrobial swabs (e.g., chlorhexidine, povidone-iodine, alcohol preparation swabs)
- Drug, fluid, blood product to be infused
- Sterile IV tubing
- IV pole, infusion pump, or blood pump
- Sterile drape
- Saline flush
- Sterile Huber safety needle (infusion port only)
- Sterile needleless access
- Dressing supplies as indicated
- Gloves, gowns, masks

Dressing Change

- Antimicrobial swabs (e.g., chlorhexidine, povidone-iodine, alcohol preparation swabs)
- Gloves (clean and sterile), mask
- Tape
- Transparent occlusive dressing (transparent dressing)
- Sterile gauze 4×4 or 2×2 sponges (gauze dressing)

Heparinization

- Antimicrobial swabs (e.g., chlorhexidine, povidone-iodine, alcohol preparation swabs)
- Access syringe (5 ml or 10 ml—see agency policy)
- Saline flush
- Heparin flush (100 units/ml)
- Plastic clamp
- Sterile needleless access

Discontinuance of Percutaneous CVC

- Antimicrobial swabs (e.g., chlorhexidine, povidone-iodine, alcohol preparation swabs)
- Petroleum-based or antimicrobial ointment
- Gloves and gown, mask, goggles (based on risk)

- Sterile gauze 4 × 4 or 2 × 2 sponges
- Sterile hypoallergenic tape
- Suture removal kit (if sutures are in place)

Step	Rationale
1. Complete preprocedure protocol.	
2. Assess type of CVAD in place and need to use CVAD for blood sampling.	Care and management depend on type of catheter. Scheduling sampling needs allows nurse to minimize number of times CVAD system is entered and allows for timely collection of specimens to evaluate therapy.

NURSE ALERT In most situations, several tests can be run from one blood tube sample. For example, potassium, calcium, and magnesium test results can all be obtained from one full tube of blood versus three separate tubes. Always anticipate the need for a blood test (e.g., blood cultures if a client has developed an elevated temperature). If your next task is to draw blood for electrolyte results, you could eliminate reaccessing the peripherally initiated central catheter (PICC) later by asking the physician if blood cultures are to be drawn. Consultation with the laboratory services can provide and confirm specific instructions.

Step	Rationale
3. Assess CVAD placement site for skin integrity and signs of infection (i.e., redness, swelling, tenderness, exudates, bleeding).	Clients requiring long-term IV therapy often have conditions placing them at risk for alterations in skin integrity and immune function. CVAD site is insult to skin integrity and provides access for pathogens through skin as well as pathogens to migrate from catheter.
4. Assess need for irrigation and dressing change by referring to medical record, nurses' notes, agency policies, and manufacturer's	Provides guidelines for maintaining catheter patency and preventing infection.

Step	Rationale
recommended guidelines for use.	
5. Administration of infusions or sampling of blood from implanted infusion port:	
a. Mask self and client. Not all institutions require masking client. Client may, instead, be asked to turn head away from port site. Refer to agency policy.	Reduces transfer of microorganisms; prevents spread of airborne microorganisms while access to system is exposed.
b. Prepare sterile field, and open sterile supplies. Prepare 10-ml syringe filled with saline.	Provides workspace for use of sterile items.
c. Using antimicrobial swab, prepare client's skin overlying port septum, moving first in horizontal pattern, next with vertical plane, and final swab in circular pattern moving outward in concentric circles from insertion site out. Allow to dry.	Rigorous skin preparation is necessary to prevent introducing microbes into system. This pattern allows penetration of antiseptic solutions into cracks and fissures of epidermal layer of skin (Crosby and Mares, 2001).
d. Apply sterile gloves.	Prevents transmission of microorganisms by nurse's hands.
e. Apply sterile drape to port site (may be optional in some agencies).	Provides sterile work area.
f. Attach one end of sterile extension tubing to syringe, and attach appropriate-size Huber needle to other end. Fill	Removes all air from tubing, reducing risk of air embolus.

Step	Rationale
	tubing with saline solution.
g. Palpate port septum with nondominant hand, observing aseptic technique (Fig. 11-4, *A*).	Septum port must be located to ensure proper Huber safety needle entry.
h. While holding wings or needle hub, insert *Huber safety needle* through skin at 90-degree angle and push firmly down until needle penetrates silicone septum and is in portal chamber (Fig. 11-4, *B*).	Do not push too hard. If tip of needle bends, septum can be damaged upon removal of needle. Safety needle device should be used.
i. Check for proper placement by aspirating blood return with attached syringe (Fig. 11-5).	
j. If blood return is good, flush tubing with remaining saline in syringe. If no blood return, fill another syringe and attempt to flush port with 10 ml normal saline.	If cannot aspirate blood, it may signal presence of clots in catheter lumen and/or at catheter tip. Forceful irrigation against resistance may propel clotted blood into client's vascular system.

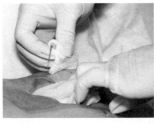
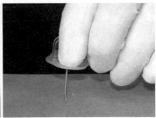

A   B

Fig. 11-4 **A,** Palpate port septum before inserting Huber needle. **B,** Close-up of insertion of Huber needle. (B Courtesy B. Braun Medical, Inc.)

Step	Rationale

Fig. 11-5   Aspirate blood return
from port.

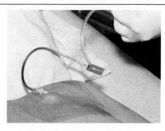

k. Observe for swelling. If
swelling occurs around
needle insertion site,
stop procedure and
notify physician.

This may indicate that needle is
not in port but, rather, in
surrounding subcutaneous tissue
or that there is tear in catheter.

l. To draw blood samples,
first aspirate and
discard 5 ml of serous
fluid.

Avoids dilution of sample.

m. Withdraw necessary
blood for each sample,
using two 10-ml
syringes equal to total
volume withdrawn.

Eliminates repeated need to
puncture infusion port for
sampling.

n. Flush port with 10 ml
normal saline. (Refer to
agency policy.)

Any fluid other than normal
saline has potential for clotting
blood or precipitating in
catheter.

o. If continuous infusion
is not indicated,
heparinize port by
flushing with 3 ml
heparin (100 units/ml)
flush solution or amount
and solution per agency
policy, using positive
pressure or injection
cap valve.

Prevents clot formation.

p. If IV fluid will be
continuously

Prevents accidental dislodging of
needle at insertion site.

Step	Rationale
administered, secure Huber needle with Steri-Strips or commercial securing device. Cover Huber needle and insertion site with transparent dressing. If Huber needle does not sit flush on skin, place folded 2 × 2 gauze under hub and then cover with dressing.	Gauze underneath transparent dressing is considered gauze dressing and should be changed every 48 hours.
q. Connect IV infusion tubing with sterile tubing connected to Huber needle.	IV infusion system should be closed to maintain sterility.
r. Regulate IV infusion as ordered.	Maintains desired fluid intake and patency of catheter.
s. If infusion is intermittent, turn off infusion and de-access port by withdrawing needle (Fig. 11-6). Discard needle in appropriate safety container. Remove sterile gloves.	Avoids needle-stick injury. Reduces transmission of microorganisms.
6. Administration of infusion or sampling of blood from central venous catheter:	

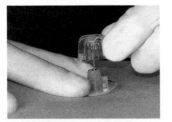

Fig. 11-6   Demonstration of how to de-access port; first stabilize base, and then withdraw needle. The safety clip will automatically activate. (Courtesy B. Braun Medical, Inc.)

Step	Rationale
a. ![icon] Don gown and goggles (check agency policy) if blood sampling.	Prevents transfer of body fluids.
b. Use antimicrobial preparation swabs to cleanse injection cap or catheter hub according to agency policy.	Prevents introduction of microorganisms into catheter.
c. Prepare two syringes with 10 ml normal saline each.	Used to flush catheter.
d. If injection cap will be removed, clamp catheter.	Catheter must be clamped if injection cap is removed, to prevent entrance of air.
e. If injection cap is in place, insert needleless access of syringe containing 10 ml normal saline, aspirate for blood return, and, if present, flush. If injection cap is removed, connect syringe tip to catheter hub, release clamp, aspirate for blood return, and, if present, flush with positive pressure, and reclamp.	Aspiration of blood return indicates catheter placement in venous system. Flushing ensures patency of catheter. Catheter must always be clamped during change of syringe or tubing to prevent exposure to air.

NURSE ALERT If the catheter is occluded and resistance is felt, do not force flushing. Vigorous flushing may cause catheter rupture or catheter emboli.

| f. Connect syringe for blood sampling, and release clamp. Aspirate 5 ml fluid, reclamp, and discard aspirate. | Avoids diluting sample. |

Step	Rationale
g. Attach or insert syringe of size equal to volume of blood sample needed to catheter. Release clamp. Withdraw necessary blood for samples, and reclamp.	Samples should be collected at one time to minimize time with open catheter system.
h. Attach or insert syringe filled with 10 ml normal saline to catheter. If clamp is present, release, flush vigorously, and reclamp.	Catheter should be cleared of all blood or medications that may clog catheter lumen or precipitate with additives in IV fluids.
i. Follow Step 5 o through s.	
j. Secure all tubing connections.	Prevents accidental tubing disconnection and catheter displacement. Luer-Lok connections should be used.
7. Dressing change:	
a. Mask self and client, if indicated (check agency policy).	Prevents exposure of catheter exit or placement site to airborne microorganisms (CDC, 2002).
b. Carefully remove old dressing in direction catheter was inserted.	Remove tape carefully because clients frequently have alterations in skin integrity.
c. Inspect placement or exit site for signs of redness, swelling, inflammation, tenderness, or exudates.	This is potential site of infection. Drainage or inflammation indicates catheter site infection (CDC, 2002).
d. If catheter is tunneled, palpate Dacron cuff in subcutaneous tunnel.	Documenting position of cuff verifies proper placement.
e. Inspect catheter and hub for intactness, and remove clean gloves.	Catheter may become torn, cut, displaced, cracked, or split.
f. Perform hand hygiene, and open dressing kit in sterile manner. Most agencies have dressing	

Step	Rationale
kits that contain all needed dressing change supplies.	
g. Apply sterile gloves.	Prevents direct transmission of microorganisms to skin exit site.
h. Clean placement or exit site with antimicrobial swab, moving first in horizontal pattern, then with vertical plane, and final swab in circular pattern moving outward in concentric circles from insertion site out. Allow to dry (Fig. 11-7).	It is impossible to sterilize skin. Organisms that accumulate must be eliminated by mechanical and chemical means. Mechanical friction in this pattern allows penetration of antiseptic solution into cracks and fissures of epidermal layer of skin (Crosby and Mares, 2001). Antiseptic solutions should be allowed to air-dry completely to effectively reduce microbial counts (INS, 2000). If antiseptic agents are used in combination, allow each to air-dry separately.
i. Redress site using sterile gauze and tape or transparent dressing as indicated (see Skill 19, p. 124).	Prevents entrance of bacteria into exit or placement site.
j. Secure connections. Remove sterile gloves.	Prevents accidental pulling and displacement. Luer-Lok connections should be used.
k. Label date, time of dressing change, and size of cannula in place.	Documents dressing change. Provides guideline for time of next change.

Fig. 11-7   Cleanse central venous access device site.

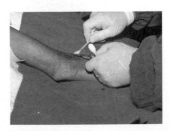

Step	Rationale
8. Discontinuance of percutaneous CVC:	
a. Place client in supine position. If client has difficulty tolerating supine position, may delay positioning until actual withdrawal.	Reduces gravitational release of venous fluid at exit site.
b. ⚡ Remove dressing, being careful not to remove CVC.	Dressing removal exposes CVC site and provides unobstructed access.
c. Apply antimicrobial swabs starting at CVC site and working outward.	Cleanses CVC site to avoid introduction of microorganisms.
d. If sutures are present, use sterile scissors to remove. Dispose of scissors in sharps container.	Sutures must be removed before removal of CVC. Immediate sharps disposal reduces risk of injury.
e. Place 2 × 2 gauze sponge with petroleum-based or antimicrobial ointment on CVC site.	Provides protected covering when CVC is removed to absorb blood and serous fluid (INS, 2000).
f. Have client perform Valsalva maneuver as you slowly and steadily remove CVC.	Promotes negative intrathoracic pressure, thus reducing risk of introduction of air into venous system.
g. When CVC completely removed, apply firm pressure on IV site.	Pressure on IV site assists in clot formation. Clients who have been on anticoagulant therapy may require 5 minutes of pressure.
h. Position sterile gauze (4 × 4 or 2 × 2) over site, and secure with sterile hypoallergenic tape.	Protects insertion site from microorganisms.

Step	Rationale
i. Inspect integrity of catheter tip.	CVCs may fracture or shear.
9. When continuous infusions are administered, observe and calculate drip rate hourly. Note ease with which fluid rate can be increased.	To maintain proper fluid infusion, desired drip rate should be regulated continuously. Gradual slowing in rate or inability to increase rate may indicate catheter occlusion.
10. Routinely assess vital signs of client, noting changes symptomatic of infection.	Catheter-related sepsis can cause fever, chills, flushed skin, tachycardia.
11. Observe catheter or port exit or placement site when sites are exposed.	Continual monitoring for signs of inflammation or infection is essential.
12. Inspect condition of catheter and connection tubing daily for leaks, holes, tears, splits, or cracked hubs.	Break in integrity of system predisposes client to hemorrhage or air embolus.
13. Consult x-ray examination reports for catheter placement.	Routine chest x-ray examination can locate position of catheter tip.
14. Complete postprocedure protocol.	

Recording and Reporting

- On medical record, record date and time of medications, blood products, parenteral fluids given, and blood samples obtained. Record condition of exit site or port insertion site, including skin integrity, signs of infection, placement, patency, integrity, and functionality of catheter. Record dressing change procedure; label date, time, type, and size of Huber needle in port.
- Record date, time, and condition of CVC when discontinued, description of site, and how site was dressed.

Unexpected Outcomes	Related Interventions
1. Occlusion: thrombus, precipitation, malposition.	• Reposition client. • Have client cough and deep breathe. • Administer thrombolytics if ordered. • Remove catheter (CVC requires order). • Obtain x-ray examination as ordered. • Do not use 1-ml syringe to instill saline because pressure exceeds 200 psi.
2. Infection: exit site, tunnel, thrombus, port pocket.	• Administer antibiotic therapy as ordered. (Draw blood cultures first when ordered.) • Remove catheter (CVC requires order). • Administer thrombolytic agent if ordered. • Replace catheter. • Obtain blood cultures peripherally and from CVC if ordered.
3. Infiltration, extravasation	• Apply cold/warm compresses according to specific vesicant protocol. • Obtain x-ray examination if ordered. • Use antidotes per protocol. • Discontinue IV fluids.

Chest Tube Care

A chest tube is a catheter inserted through the thorax to remove fluid and/or air and promote lung reexpansion. A pleural chest tube is inserted when air or fluid enters the pleural space, compromising oxygenation or ventilation (e.g., chest trauma, open chest surgery, large pleural leak). A closed chest drainage system with or without suction is attached to the chest tube to promote drainage of air and fluid. Lung reexpansion occurs as the fluid or air is removed from the pleural space.

Delegation Considerations

This skill may not be delegated to assistive personnel (AP). However, AP may assist with other aspects of the client's care, such as monitoring vital signs. Before delegating aspects of care, the nurse should inform AP about:

- Proper positioning of the client with chest tubes to facilitate chest tube drainage and optimal functioning of the system.
- How to ambulate and transfer the client with chest drainage.
- Informing the nurse of any changes in vital signs, chest pain, or sudden shortness of breath, excessive bubbling in the water-seal chamber or disconnection of system, change in type and amount of drainage, sudden bleeding, or sudden cessation of bubbling.

Equipment

- Disposable chest drainage system as ordered
- Suction source and setup (wall canister or portable):
  - *Water suction system:* add sterile water or normal saline (NS) solution to cover the lower 2.5 cm (1 inch) of water-seal U tube, sterile water or NS to pour into the suction control chamber if suction is to be used (see manufacturer's directions)
  - *Waterless system:* add vial of 30 ml injectable sodium chloride or water, 20-ml syringe, 21-gauge needle, and antiseptic swab
- Nonsterile gloves
- Sterile gauze sponges
- Local anesthetic, if this is not an emergent procedure
- Chest tube tray (all items are sterile): knife handle (1), chest tube clamp, small sponge forceps, needle holder, knife blade No. 10, 3-0 silk sutures, tray liner (sterile field), curved 8-inch Kelly clamps (2), 4 × 4 sponges (10), suture scissors, hand towels (3)

- Dressings: petrolatum gauze, split chest-tube dressings, several 4 × 4 gauze dressings, large gauze dressings (2), and 4-inch tape or elastic bandage (Elastoplast)
- Head cover
- Face mask/face shield
- Sterile gloves
- Rubber-tipped hemostats for each chest tube (2)
- 1-inch adhesive tape for taping connections

Step	Rationale
1. Complete preprocedure protocol.	
2. Obtain baseline and serial vital signs, oxygen saturation (SpO_2), and level of orientation.	Baseline vital signs are essential for any invasive procedure. Clients requiring chest tube insertion frequently have respiratory distress, and vital signs are taken serially. Changes in level of orientation may indicate decreased levels of oxygen and/or hypoxia.
3. Assess pulmonary status.	Clients in need of chest tubes have impaired oxygenation and ventilation.
4. Assess client for known allergies. Ask clients if they have had problem with medications, latex, or anything applied to skin.	Povidone-iodine is antiseptic used to cleanse skin. Lidocaine is local anesthetic administered to reduce pain. Chest tube will be held in place with tape. Iodine, lidocaine, and tape are common allergens.
5. Review client's medication record for anticoagulant therapy.	Anticoagulation therapy such as aspirin, warfarin, heparin, or platelet aggregation inhibitors such as ticlopidine can increase procedure-related blood loss.
6. For clients who have chest tubes, observe:	
a. Chest tube dressing and site surrounding tube insertion.	Ensures that dressing is intact and occlusive seal remains without air or fluid leaks and that area surrounding insertion site is free

Step	Rationale
	of drainage or skin irritation (Carroll, 2002).
b. Tubing for kinks, dependent loops, or clots.	Maintains patent, freely draining system, preventing fluid accumulation in chest cavity. Presence of kinks, dependent loops, or clotted drainage increases client's risk for infection, atelectasis, and tension pneumothorax (Allibone, 2003).
c. Chest drainage system, which should be upright and below level of tube insertion.	Facilitates drainage; system must be in this position to function properly.
7. Set up prescribed drainage system. *Open system when physician is ready to insert chest tube.*	Premature opening of sterile chest drainage system increases risk of contamination of sterile equipment.
a. Water-seal system (check manufacturer's guidelines):	Permits displaced air to pass into atmosphere.
(1) Obtain chest drainage system. Remove wrappers, and prepare to set up system.	Maintains sterility of system. System is packaged in this manner so it can be used under sterile operating room conditions (Carroll, 1991).
(2) While maintaining sterility of drainage tubing, stand system upright and add sterile water or NS to appropriate compartments:	Reduces possibility of contamination.
(a) For two-chamber system (without suction), add sterile solution to water-seal chamber (second	Maintains water seal.

TABLE 12-1 Physician's Role and Responsibility in Chest Tube Placement

Role and Responsibility	Rationale
Explain purpose, procedure, and possible complications to client, and have client sign consent form.	Provides informed consent.
Perform hand hygiene. Cleanse chest wall with antiseptic.	Reduces transmission of microorganisms.
Don mask and gloves.	Maintains surgical asepsis.
Drape area of chest tube insertion with sterile towels.	Maintains surgical asepsis.
Inject local anesthetic, and allow time to take effect.	Decreases pain during procedure.
Use blunt or sharp dissection to create incision in skin and chest wall.	Opens chest for insertion of chest tube. Trocar is no longer used and increases risk of tissue damage.
Thread clamped chest tube through incision. Physician clamps chest tube until system is connected to water seal.	Inserts chest tube into intrapleural space. Clamping prevents entry of atmospheric air into chest and worsening of pneumothorax.
Suture chest tube in place, if suturing is policy or physician preference.	Secures chest tube in place.
Cover chest insertion site with sterile petrolatum gauze, 4 × 4 gauze, and large dressing to form occlusive dressing supported with elastic bandage (Elastoplast).	Holds chest tube in place and occludes site around chest tube. Helps stabilize chest tube and holds dressing tightly in place. Helps prevent bacteria entry and air leak.
Water-seal system:	
Remove connector cover from client's end of chest drainage tubing with sterile technique. Secure drainage tubing to chest tube and drainage system.	Physician is responsible for making certain that system is set up properly, proper amount of water is in water seal, dressing is secure, and chest tube is securely connected to drainage system.
Water-seal suction:	
Connect system to suction, or supervise nurse connecting it to suction, if suction is to be used.	Physician is responsible for determining and checking amount of fluid that is to be added to suction control chamber and prescribing suction setting.

TABLE 12-1 Physician's Role and Responsibility in Chest Tube Placement—cont'd

Role and Responsibility	Rationale
Waterless system:	
Remove connector cover from client's end of chest drainage tubing with sterile technique. Secure drainage tubing to chest tube and drainage system.	Physician is responsible for making certain that system is set up properly and chest tube is securely connected to drainage system.
Waterless suction:	
Turn on suction source. Set float ball level to prescribed setting.	Physician is responsible for prescribing level of float ball and prescribing suction setting.
Physician or nurse adds sterile water or NS to diagnostic indicator.	Allows quick assurance that system is functioning properly.
Unclamp chest tube.	Connects chest tube to drainage.
In both systems, physician orders and reviews chest x-ray studies.	Verifies correct chest tube placement.

Step	Rationale
chamber), bringing fluid to required level as indicated.	
(b) For three-chamber system (with suction), add sterile solution to water-seal chamber (second chamber). Add amount of sterile solution prescribed by physician to suction control (third chamber), usually 20 cm	Depth of fluid level dictates highest amount of negative pressure that can be present within system (Shuster, 1998). For example, 20 cm of water is approximately −20 cm of water pressure.

Step	**Rationale**
(8 inches). Connect tubing from suction control chamber to suction source.	
(3) Suction control chamber vent must be without occlusion when suction is used.	Provides safety factor of releasing excess negative pressure into atmosphere through suction control vent. Too little suction prevents lung reexpansion and increases client's risk for infection, atelectasis, and tension pneumothorax. Too much suction damages lung tissue and perpetuates existing air leaks (Allibone, 2003).
b. Waterless system (check manufacturer's guidelines):	
(1) Remove sterile wrappers, and prepare to set up equipment.	Maintains sterility of system. System is packaged in this manner so it can be used under sterile operating room conditions.
(2) For two-chamber system (without suction), nothing is added or needs to be done to system.	The waterless two-chamber system is ready for connecting to client's chest tube after opening wrappers.
(3) For three-chamber waterless system with suction, connect tubing from suction control chamber to suction source.	Suction source provides additional negative pressure to system.
(4) Instill 15 ml of sterile water or NS into diagnostic indicator injection	Instillation of water into injection port enables nurse to observe for rise and fall in diagnostic air-leak window. Constant left-to-right

Step	**Rationale**
port located on top of system. NOTE: This step is not necessary for mediastinal drainage because there will be no tidaling. Also, in emergency, it is not necessary because system does not require water for setup.	bubbling or rocking is abnormal and may indicate air leak.
8. Provide two shod hemostats or approved clamps for each chest tube, attached to top of client's bed with adhesive tape. Chest tubes are clamped only under the following specific circumstances per physician order or nursing policy and procedure: a. To assess air leak (Table 12-2).	Shod hemostats have covering to prevent hemostat from penetrating chest tube once clamped. Use of these shod hemostats or other clamps prevents air from reentering pleural space (Allibone, 2003).

TABLE 12-2 Problem Solving With Chest Tubes

Assessment	Intervention
Air leak can occur at insertion site, connection between tube and drainage, or within drainage device itself. Continuous bubbling is noted in water-seal chamber and water seal.	Locate leak by clamping tube at different intervals along tube. Leaks are corrected when constant bubbling stops.
Assess for location of leak by clamping chest tube with two rubber-shod or toothless clamps close to chest wall. If bubbling stops, air leak is	Unclamp tube, reinforce chest dressing, and notify physician immediately. Leaving chest tube clamped can cause collapse of lung, mediastinal shift, and

Continued

TABLE 12-2 Problem Solving With Chest Tubes—cont'd

Assessment	Intervention
inside client's thorax or at chest insertion site.	eventual collapse of other lung from buildup of air pressure within pleural cavity.
If bubbling continues with clamps near chest wall, gradually move one clamp at a time down drainage tubing away from client and toward suction control chamber. When bubbling stops, leak is in section of tubing or connection between clamps.	Replace tubing, or secure connection and release clamps.
If bubbling still continues, this indicates leak is in drainage system.	Change drainage system. Make sure chest tubes are patent: remove clamps, eliminate kinks, or eliminate occlusion.
	Notify physician immediately, and prepare for another chest tube insertion.
Assess for tension pneumothorax, indicated by: ■ Severe respiratory distress ■ Low oxygen saturation ■ Chest pain ■ Absence of breath sounds on affected side ■ Tracheal shift to unaffected side ■ Hypotension and signs of shock ■ Tachycardia	Obstructed chest tubes trap air in intrapleural space when air leak originates within thorax. Flutter (Heimlich) valve or large-gauge needle may be used for short-term emergency release of pressure in intrapleural space. Have emergency equipment, oxygen, and code cart available because condition is life-threatening.
Water-seal tube is no longer submerged in sterile fluid because of evaporation.	Add sterile water to water-seal chamber until distal tip is 2 cm under surface level.

Step	Rationale
b. To quickly empty or change disposable systems; performed by nurse who has received education in procedure.	

Step	Rationale
c. To assess if client is ready to have chest tube removed (which is done by physician's order); monitor client for recurrent pneumothorax	
9. Position client: during chest tube insertion, client will need to be positioned so client's back or side in which tube will be placed is accessible to physician.	Permits optimal drainage of fluid and/or air.
10. ✈ Administer parenteral premedications, such as sedatives or analgesics, as ordered.	Reduces client anxiety and pain during procedure.

NURSE ALERT Sedatives and analgesics may alter vital signs, depending on the dose and client's tolerance. Monitor closely for changes in blood pressure and respirations.

11. Assist physician in providing psychological support to client. (See physician's responsibilities in Table 12-1.)	
a. Reinforce preprocedure explanation.	Reduces client anxiety and assists in efficient completion of procedure.
b. Coach and support client throughout procedure.	
12. Show local anesthetic to physician. Hold anesthetic solution bottle upside down with label facing physician. Physician will withdraw solution and inject into client's skin. Physician places chest tube.	Allows physician to read label of drug before administering it to client. Allows physician to withdraw solution properly while maintaining surgical asepsis.

Step	Rationale
13. Help physician attach drainage tube to chest tube.	Connects drainage system and suction (if ordered) to chest tube.
14. After chest tube is inserted, tape all connections in double-spiral fashion with 1-inch adhesive tape (taping of chest tube is usually done by physician at time of tube placement).	Secures chest tube to drainage system and reduces risk of air leak causing breaks in airtight system.
Then check systems for proper functioning by:	Provides chance to ensure airtight system before connecting it to client. Allows correction or replacement of system if it is defective before connecting it to client.
a. Clamping drainage tubing that will connect client to system.	
b. Connecting tubing from float ball chamber to suction source.	NOTE: Bubbling will be seen at first because air is in tubing and system initially. This should stop after few minutes unless there are other sources of air entering system.
c. Turning on suction to prescribed level.	

NURSE ALERT If bubbling continues, check connections and locate source of the air leak, as described in Table 12-2.

Step	Rationale
15. Turn off suction source, and unclamp drainage tubing before connecting client to system.	Having client connected to suction when it is being inserted could damage pleural tissues from sudden increase in negative pressure. Suction source is turned on again after client is connected to three-chamber system.
16. Check patency of air vents in system:	
a. Water-seal vent must not be occluded.	Permits displaced air to pass into atmosphere.

Step	**Rationale**
b. Suction control chamber vent must not be occluded when suction is used.	Provides safety factor of releasing excess negative pressure into atmosphere.
c. Waterless systems have relief valves without caps.	Provides safety factor of releasing excess negative pressure.
17. Coil excess tubing on mattress next to client. Secure with rubber band and safety pin or system's clamp.	Prevents excess tubing from hanging over edge of mattress in dependent loop. Drainage could collect in loop and occlude drainage system.
18. Adjust tubing to hang in straight line from chest tube to drainage chamber.	Promotes drainage and prevents fluid or blood from accumulating in pleural cavity.
19. If chest tube is draining fluid, indicate on the drainage chamber's write-on surface date and time (e.g., 0900) that drainage was begun.	Provides baseline for continuous assessment of type and quantity of drainage.

NURSE ALERT Check institutional policy before stripping or milking chest tubes. This practice is being discontinued at most institutions because it is believed that stripping the tube greatly increases intrapleural pressure, which could damage the pleural tissue and cause or worsen an existing pneumothorax. However, even though the literature is contradictory, stripping or milking may be done in selected clients (e.g., fresh postoperative thoracic surgery, chest trauma). The rationale for this selective use of stripping or milking is that the presence of clotted tube drainage causes decreased rate of reexpansion and increases risk of tension pneumothorax (Allibone, 2003). In these selected cases, the benefits outweigh the risks.

20. After tube is placed, assist client to comfortable position:	Reduces client anxiety and promotes cooperation.
a. Semi-Fowler's to high-Fowler's position to evacuate air (pneumothorax).	Air rises to highest point in chest. Pneumothorax tubes are usually placed on anterior aspect at midclavicular line, second or

Step	Rationale
	third intercostal space (Woodruff, 1999).
b. High-Fowler's position to drain fluid (hemothorax).	Permits optimal drainage of fluid. Posterior tubes are placed on midaxillary line, fifth or sixth intercostal space.
21. Complete postprocedure protocol.	
22. Monitor vital signs, oxygen saturation, and insertion site every 15 minutes for first 2 hours.	Provides immediate information about procedure-related complications such as respiratory distress.
23. Monitor chest tube drainage:	
a. Assessment after chest tube insertion is done every 15 minutes for first 2 hours. This assessment interval then changes *on basis of client's status.* Mark time and level of drainage on calibrated write-on strip periodically.	Permits timely and efficient account of amount of drainage from chest tube. Drainage is marked at specified periods of time and documented on nurses' notes and on intake and output (I&O) sheet. Ensures early detection of complications.
b. *Expected drainage in adult:* less than 50 to 200 ml/hr immediately after surgery in mediastinal chest tube. Approximately 500 ml in first 24 hours.	Dark-red drainage is expected only during immediate postoperative period. This drainage turns serous over time.
c. *Expected drainage in adult:* between 100 and 300 ml of fluid may drain from pleural tube during first 3 hours after insertion. 24-hour rate is 500 to 1000 ml.	Reexpansion of lungs forces drainage into tube. Coughing can also cause large gushes of drainage or air. Acute bleeding indicates hemorrhage.

NURSE ALERT If drainage suddenly increases or is bright red or if there is more than 100 ml/hr of bloody drainage (except for the first 3 hours

Step	**Rationale**

postoperatively), the nurse should notify the physician and remain with the client and assess vital signs and cardiopulmonary status.

24. Observe:

a. Chest tube dressing and drainage.	Ensures that dressing is occlusive.
b. Tubing should be free of kinks and dependent loops.	Straight and coiled drainage tube positions are optimal for pleural drainage. However, when dependent loop is unavoidable, periodic lifting and draining of tube also will promote pleural drainage (Schmelz and others, 1999).
c. Chest drainage system should be upright and below level of tube insertion. Note presence of clots or debris in tubing.	System must be in this position to function and to facilitate proper drainage (Gordon and others, 1997).

NURSE ALERT Carefully monitor the position of the system relative to the chest tube, especially during client transport.

d. Water seal for fluctuations with client's inspiration and expiration:	
(1) *Waterless system:* diagnostic indicator for fluctuations with client's inspirations and expirations.	In non–mechanically ventilated client, fluid should rise in water seal or diagnostic indicator with inspiration and fall with expiration. Opposite occurs in client who is mechanically ventilated. This indicates that system is functioning properly (Lewis and others, 2004).
(2) *Water-seal system:* bubbling in the water-seal chamber (see Table 12-2).	When system is initially connected to client, bubbles are expected from chamber. These are from air that was present in system and in client's intrapleural space.

Step	Rationale
	After short time, bubbling stops. Fluid continues to fluctuate in water seal on inspiration and expiration until lung is reexpanded or system becomes occluded.
(3) *Water-seal system:* bubbling in suction control chamber (when suction is being used) (see Table 12-2).	Suction control chamber has constant, gentle bubbling. Tubing to suction source should be free of obstruction, and suction source should be turned to appropriate setting.
e. *Waterless system:* bubbling in diagnostic indicator.	Mechanism to observe for presence of tidaling. Character of drainage indicates if normal or if infection or hemorrhage is developing.
f. *Type and amount of fluid drainage:* nurse should note color and amount of drainage, client's vital signs, and skin color. Look at fluid in collection tubing, not just fluid in collection chamber. Is drainage bright red, dark red, or pink? Is it opaque, or can you see through it?	
g. *Waterless system:* suction control (float ball) indicates amount of suction client's intrapleural space is receiving.	Suction float ball dictates amount of suction in system. Float ball allows no more suction than dictated by its setting. If suction source is set too low, suction float ball cannot reach prescribed setting. In this case, suction must be increased for float ball to reach prescribed setting.
25. After first 2 hours, assess client's physical and	Detects early signs and symptoms of complications:

Step	Rationale
psychological status at least every 4 hours or according to agency policy.	• *Apprehension*—increase in client anxiety, restlessness, and inability to concentrate. • *Respiratory distress*—alteration in rate and/or depth of respirations, difficulty breathing, and breath sounds. • *Subcutaneous emphysema*—air that is being trapped in subcutaneous tissue.

Recording and Reporting

- Record level of client comfort and baseline vital signs, including SpO$_2$. If postoperative client, record vital signs and SpO$_2$ every 15 minutes for at least 2 hours postoperatively. Record chest drainage output hourly for at least 2 hours, and then record as client status indicates. Document time, type, and amount of drainage. Record integrity of chest suction system (e.g., record amount of bubbling in water-seal suction control chamber, level of suction, intactness of system).
- Report client response to chest tube insertion or continuation, noting level of comfort, drainage, and intactness of the system.

Unexpected Outcomes	Related Interventions
1. Air leak unrelated to client's respirations occurs.	• Locate source (see Table 12-2). • Notify physician.
2. There is no chest tube drainage.	• Observe for kink or clot in chest drainage system. • Observe for possible clot in chest drainage system. • Observe for mediastinal shift or respiratory distress (medical emergency). • Notify physician.
3. Chest tube is dislodged.	• Immediately apply pressure over chest tube insertion site. • Have assistant apply gauze dressing and tape three sides. • Notify physician.

Cold Applications

Cold applications include cold compresses, chemical or cold packs, cooling pads, and immersion of a body part into a cold soak. Cold therapy treats localized inflammatory responses that lead to edema, hemorrhage, muscle spasm, or pain (Table 13-1). Cold reduces inflammation caused by injuries to the musculoskeletal system (Airaksinen and others, 2003; Poddar, 2003; Stitik and Nadler, 1998). Because reduction of inflammation is the primary goal, cryotherapy is the treatment of choice for the first 24 to 48 hours after an injury. When used appropriately, cold applications significantly lessen pain and immobility by reducing swelling of injured tissues (Airaksinen and others, 2003; Poddar, 2003; Stitik and Nadler, 1998). This is an important point for nurses to know when deciding on the choice of heat or cold for the treatment of acute injuries. Cold is also indicated as an adjunct analgesic for chronic pain and spasticity control. It also can be used as an analgesic after arthroscopic surgical procedures (Airaksinen and others, 2003).

Delegation Considerations

The skill of applying cold applications may be delegated to assistive personnel (AP) if, following assessment, there are no risks or complications.

- Caution AP to maintain proper temperature of the application throughout the treatment and to keep the application in place for only the length of time specified in the physician's order.
- Caution AP to check the client's skin for excessive redness or pain and to report immediately to the nurse if any adverse reactions occur.
- Instruct AP to report when treatment is complete so that the client's response can be evaluated.

Equipment

- Cold compress
- Absorbent gauze (clean or sterile) folded to desired size
- Clean or sterile basin with ice and water at desired temperature
- Bath towel or absorbent pad
- Two pairs of disposable or sterile gloves (according to agency policy)
- Cool water flow pad
- Cooling pad and electrical pump

TABLE 13-1   Therapeutic Effects of Warm and Cold Applications

Physiological Responses	Therapeutic Benefit	Examples of Conditions Treated
Warm application		
Vasodilation	Improves blood flow to injured body part, promotes delivery of nutrients and removal of wastes, decreases venous congestion in injured tissues.	Inflamed or edematous body part; new surgical wound; infected wound; arthritis, degenerative joint disease; localized joint pain, muscle strains; low back pain, menstrual cramping; hemorrhoidal, perianal, and vaginal inflammation; local abscesses.
Reduced blood viscosity	Improves delivery of leukocytes and antibodies to wound site.	
Reduced muscle tension	Promotes muscle relaxation and reduces pain from spasm or stiffness.	
Increased tissue metabolism	Increases blood flow; provides local warmth.	
Increased capillary permeability	Promotes movement of waste products and nutrients.	
Cold application		
Vasoconstriction	Reduces blood flow to injured body part, prevents edema formation, reduces inflammation.	Immediately after direct trauma such as sprains, strains, fractures, muscle spasms; after superficial lacerations or puncture wound; after minor burns; when malignancy is suspected in area of injury or pain; after injections; for arthritis, joint trauma.
Local anesthesia	Reduces localized pain by slowing or blocking peripheral nerve conduction.	
Reduced cell metabolism	Reduces enzyme function and oxygen needs of tissues.	
Increased blood viscosity	Promotes blood coagulation at injury site.	
Decreased muscle tension	Prevents muscle spasm by decreasing spasticity/tone and relieves pain.	

Data from Stitik T, Nadler S: I. When—and how—to use cold most effectively, *Consultant* 38(12):2881, 1998; Stitik T, Nadler S: II. When—and how—to apply the heat, *Consultant* 39(1):144, 1999.

- Tapes, ties, gauze roll, or elastic wrap bandage
- Ice bag or collar with water
- Chemical ice pack
- Towel or pillowcase
- Cloth ties or tape
- Disposable gloves (if blood or body fluids are present)

Step	Rationale
NURSE ALERT Keep the injured part immobilized and in alignment.	
1. Complete preprocedure protocol.	
2. Position client carefully, keeping body part in proper alignment and exposing only area to be treated.	Prevents further injury to body part. Avoids unnecessary exposure of body parts, maintaining client's comfort and privacy.
3. Place towel or absorbent pad under area to be treated.	Prevents soiling of bed linen.
4. ◤ Cold compress:	
a. Check temperature of solution, and submerge gauze into filled basin at bedside; wring out excess moisture.	Extreme temperature can cause tissue damage. Dripping gauze is uncomfortable to client.
b. Apply compress to affected area, molding it gently over site.	Ensures that cold is directed over site of injury.
5. Electric cooling pad:	
a. Wrap cool water flow pad around body part (Fig. 13-1).	Ensures even application of cold temperature.
b. Be sure correct temperature is set.	Ensures effective therapy.
c. Secure with elastic wrap bandage, gauze roll, or ties.	
6. Prepare ice bag or collar:	
a. Fill bag with water, secure cap, and invert.	Checks for leaks.
b. Empty water, and then fill bag two-thirds full with small ice chips.	Bag can be more easily molded over body part.

Step   **Rationale**

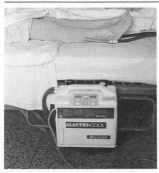

Fig. 13-1 Cooling pad.

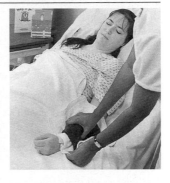

Fig. 13-2 Placement of ice bag (or pack) on extremity.

c. Release excess air from bag by squeezing its sides before securing cap.	Excess air interferes with cold conduction (Ruffolo, 2002).
d. Wipe bag dry.	Prevents skin maceration.
e. Apply snugly over area. Secure with tape as needed (Fig. 13-2).	Cold should be directly over injury to maximize therapeutic effect.
7. Prepare ice pack:	
a. Commercial packs are squeezed or kneaded.	Releases alcohol-based solution to create cold temperature.

NURSE ALERT Moisture may form on the outside of the bag if room temperature is warm. This does not indicate a leak

b. Apply pack directly over area. Wrap prepared bag or pack with towel or pillowcase.	Cold should be applied directly over injury. Protects client's tissue and absorbs condensation. Prevents direct exposure of cold against client's skin.

NURSE ALERT Do not reapply the ice pack to red or bluish areas; continual use of the pack creates ischemia.

Step	Rationale
8. Check condition of skin every 5 minutes for duration of application.	Determines if there are adverse reactions to cold. These include mottling, redness, burning, blistering, and numbness (Stitik and Nadler, 1998).
9. Complete postprocedure protocol.	
10. Next application, observe client perform procedure.	Measures level of learning.

Recording and Reporting

- Record procedure, including type, location, duration of application, and client's response, in nurses' notes.
- Describe any instruction given and client's success in demonstrating procedure.
- Report undesirable changes in condition of skin to nurse in charge or physician.

Unexpected Outcomes	Related Interventions
1. Skin takes on mottled, reddened, or bluish purple appearance as a result of prolonged exposure.	• Stop treatment. • Notify nurse in charge or physician. • Injury from prolonged exposure requires different therapy.
2. Client complains of burning type of pain and numbness.	• Stop treatment because these are signs of ischemia • Notify nurse in charge or physician.
3. Client cannot describe application or use compress correctly.	• Reinstruction and clarification are necessary.

Condom Catheter

The external application of a urinary drainage device is a convenient, safe method of draining urine in male clients. The condom catheter is suitable for incontinent or comatose clients who still have complete and spontaneous bladder emptying. The condom is a soft, pliable rubber sheath that slips over the penis and is kept in place with the use of an elastic adhesive strip.

The often-advised frequency for changing a condom catheter is every 24 hours. However, close monitoring every 4 hours to detect potential problems is necessary. With each catheter change, the nurse cleanses the urethral meatus and penis thoroughly and looks for signs of skin irritation.

Delegation Considerations

The skill of applying a condom catheter may be delegated to assistive personnel (AP). The nurse is responsible for determining that the procedure is appropriate and that the client is able to tolerate the procedure and for evaluating the client's response to the procedure.

- Instruct AP to ask whether the client has a latex allergy.
- Instruct AP to follow manufacturer's directions on how to apply the adhesive strip that secures the condom catheter because methods for applying the catheter differ from manufacturer to manufacturer.

Equipment

- Condom catheter kit (rubber condom sheath of appropriate size, strip of elastic adhesive, skin preparation)
- Urinary collection bag with drainage tubing or leg bag and straps
- Basin with warm water and soap
- Towels and washcloth(s)
- Bath blanket
- Nonsterile, disposable gloves
- Scissors and/or safety razor

Step	Rationale
1. Complete preprocedure protocol.	
2. Assess condition of penis.	Provides baseline to compare changes in condition of skin

Step	**Rationale**
	after condom catheter application.
3. Prepare urinary drainage collection bag and tubing. Clamp off drainage bag port. Secure collection bag to bed frame; bring drainage tubing up through side rails onto bed. *Optional:* Prepare leg bag for connection to condom.	Provides easy access to drainage equipment after condom catheter is in place.
4. ✋ Provide perineal care, and dry thoroughly.	Removes irritating secretions. Rubber sheath of condom rolls onto dry skin more easily.

NURSE ALERT Clip hair at the base of the penis. In some cases, shaving the hair at the base of the penis may be necessary. Hair adheres to the condom and is pulled during condom removal or may get caught in the rubber as the condom catheter is applied.

5. Apply skin preparation to penis, and allow to dry. If client is uncircumcised, return foreskin to normal position.	Skin preparation has alcohol base. Evaporation is necessary to prevent irritation.
6. With nondominant hand, grasp penis along shaft. With dominant hand, hold condom sheath at tip of penis and smoothly roll sheath onto penis (Fig. 14-1).	Prepares penis for easy condom placement.
7. Apply adhesive:	
a. Spiral-wrap penile shaft with strip of elastic adhesive. Strip should be spiral-wrapped and not overlap itself (Fig. 14-2). Do not use any tape except that provided by	Condom must be secured firmly so it is snug and stays on but not tight enough to cause constriction of blood flow. With some brands of catheters, adhesive strip is applied before condom is applied.

| **Step** | **Rationale** |

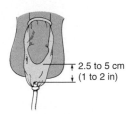

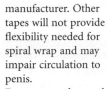

Fig. 14-1 Distance between end of penis and tip of condom.

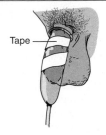

Fig. 14-2 Tape applied in spiral fashion.

manufacturer. Other tapes will not provide flexibility needed for spiral wrap and may impair circulation to penis.	
b. For newer catheters that are self-adhesive, apply catheter as in Steps 4 and 5 and then apply gentle pressure on penile shaft for 10 to 15 seconds to secure catheter.	
8. Connect drainage tubing to end of condom catheter. Be sure condom is not twisted. Catheter can be connected to large-volume bag or leg bag.	Allows urine to be collected and measured. Keeps client dry. Twisted condom obstructs urine flow.
9. Place excess coiling of tubing on bed, and secure to bottom sheet.	Prevents looping of tubing and promotes free drainage of urine.
10. Place client in safe, comfortable position. Lower bed, and place side rails accordingly.	Promotes safety and comfort.

Step	Rationale
11. Complete postprocedure protocol.	
12. Inspect penis with condom catheter in place within 30 minutes after application. Look for swelling and discoloration, and ask client if there is any discomfort.	Determines if catheter has been applied incorrectly.

Recording and Reporting

■ Report and record pertinent information: condom application; condition of penis, skin, and scrotum; and voiding pattern.

■ Monitor intake and output as indicated.

Unexpected Outcomes	Related Interventions
1. Skin around penis is reddened and excoriated. Results from pressure of adhesive or contact with urine.	• Check for allergy. • Remove condom, and notify physician. • Do not reapply until penis and surrounding tissue are free from irritation.
2. Penile swelling or discoloration occurs.	• Catheter has been improperly applied, or adhesive has been applied too snugly, resulting in impaired circulation. Remove catheter. Notify physician.

Continuous Passive Motion Machine

The continuous passive motion (CPM) machine exercises various joints such as the hip, ankle, knee, shoulder, and wrist. The CPM machine is most commonly used after knee surgery. The CPM machine is usually prescribed on the day of surgery or the first postoperative day, depending on the surgeon's preference and client's condition. The purpose of the CPM machine is to mobilize the joint to prevent contractures, muscle atrophy, venous stasis, and thromboembolism. The CPM machine can aid in alleviating pain, edema, stiffness, and dislocation and potentially can shorten a client's hospital stay (Babis and others, 2001; Hammesfahr and Serafino, 2002).

Delegation Considerations

The skill of using the CPM machine should not be delegated to assistive personnel (AP).

- Instruct AP to immediately report the client's increased pain, skin breakdown, or joint inflammation.

Equipment

- CPM machine
- Clean, nonsterile gloves

Step	Rationale
1. Complete preprocedure protocol.	
2. Assess CPM machine for electrical safety. Check setup of machine before placing on bed: check stability of frame, flexion/extension controls, padding of exposed metal parts or hard surfaces, and on/off switch.	All electrical equipment in health care settings is routinely checked for safety. Routine observation of electrical cord and functioning of equipment each time it is used further monitors safety. Ensures that all pieces of equipment are operational and will prevent damage to client's joint. Ensures that metal parts

Step	**Rationale**
	are padded to prevent skin breakdown or chafing of skin rubbing against metal or hard surfaces.
3. Provide analgesic 20 to 30 minutes before CPM machine is needed.	Assists client in tolerating exercise.
4. Apply gloves if wound drainage is present.	Reduce nurse's risk of exposure to blood-borne microorganisms.
5. Place elastic compression hose on client if ordered (see Skill 64).	Elastic hose promote venous return from lower extremities.
6. Place CPM machine on bed.	
7. Set limits of flexion and extension as prescribed by physician.	Prevents injury by setting machine at safe limits.
8. Set speed control to slow or moderate range.	
9. Put machine through one full cycle.	Ensures that CPM machine is working properly.
10. Stop CPM machine when in extension. Place sheepskin on CPM machine.	Ensures that all exposed hard surfaces are padded to prevent rubbing and chafing of client's skin.
11. Place client's extremity in CPM machine.	
12. Adjust CPM machine to client's extremity. Lengthen and shorten appropriate sections of frame.	
13. Center client's extremity on frame.	Avoids pressure areas on extremity.
14. Align client's joint with CPM's mechanical joint.	
15. Secure client's extremity on CPM machine with Velcro straps. Apply loosely.	
16. Start machine. When it reaches flexed position, stop machine and check degree of flexion.	Prevents possible complications and ensures correct settings.

Step	Rationale

Fig. 15-1   Client's extremity properly placed and secured on CPM machine.

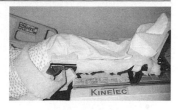

17. Start CPM machine, and observe for two full cycles.

Ensures that CPM machine is fully operational at preset extension and flexion modes.

18. Make sure client is comfortable.
19. Provide client with on/off switch.

Allows client to turn CPM machine on and off if it malfunctions.

20. Instruct client to turn CPM machine off if malfunctioning or if client experiencing pain. Instruct client to notify nurse immediately.
21. Check alignment and positioning every 2 hours, condition of skin, and ask client to rate pain on 0 to 10 scale.
22. Complete postprocedure protocol.

Recording and Reporting

- Record in nurses' notes client's tolerance for CPM machine, rate of cycles per minute, degree of flexion and extension used, condition of extremity and skin, condition of operative site if present, length of time CPM machine in use.
- Report immediately to nurse in charge or physician any resistance to range of motion; increased pain; swelling, heat, or redness in joint.

Unexpected Outcomes	Related Interventions
1. Client unable to tolerate increase in flexion or extension.	• Consult with physician and physical therapist to plan additional therapies to increase flexion and extension of joint. • Provide rest periods throughout day. • Consider need for additional analgesic before CPM machine is used.
2. Client develops reddened areas on bony prominences or extremity.	• Determine if hard surfaces on CPM machine are well padded. • Monitor client's alignment and positioning at least every 2 hours. • Provide skin care at least every 2 hours.

Continuous Subcutaneous Infusion

The continuous subcutaneous infusion (CSQI or CSCI) route of medication administration is used mainly for the administration of medications for pain management (e.g., opioids) and insulin. Box 16-1 summarizes benefits associated with the use of CSQI. The rate at which a medication can be absorbed subcutaneously determines the infusion rate of CSQI medications. Most clients can absorb 2 to 3 ml/hr of medication (Pasero, 2002). As the rate of infusion increases, absorption of the medication decreases.

Use a small-gauge (25 to 27), winged or butterfly intravenous (IV) needle to deliver CSQI. Alternatively, you may use a special commercially prepared Teflon cannula. Although Teflon needles generally are more expensive, they are more comfortable for the client, have lower rates of complications when compared with winged IV needles, and are associated with fewer needle-stick injuries (Dawkins and others, 2000; Torre, 2002). It is best to use a needle of the shortest length and the smallest gauge necessary to establish and maintain the infusion.

Anatomical sites for CSQI are the same as for subcutaneous injections (see Skill 68), as well as the upper chest. Site selection depends on the client's activity level and the type of medication delivered. For example, pain medications given to ambulatory clients are best delivered in the upper chest. This allows the client to move freely. Insulin is absorbed most consistently in the abdomen; thus a site in the abdomen away from the belt line is the preferred site for insulin administration. Sites should be free from irritation, away from bony prominences and the waistline, and rotated at least every 72 hours or whenever complications (e.g., infection, leaking) occur (MedTronic MiniMed, 2004).

Delegation Considerations

The skill of administering continuous subcutaneous medications should not be delegated to assistive personnel (AP).

- Instruct AP about potential medication side effects or drug reactions and to report to the nurse.
- Have AP report leaking, redness, discomfort at the insertion site.
- Instruct AP to report to the nurse any change in the client's status or vital signs.

BOX 16-1   Benefits Associated With Pain Management Delivered by Continuous Subcutaneous Infusion

- Can be used in clients with poor venous access.
- Provides pain relief to clients who are unable to tolerate oral pain medications.
- Allows client to be more mobile.
- Onset of action takes about 20 minutes.
- Provides better pain control than IM injections.
- Costs are almost half of costs associated with IV infusions.

Modified from Pasero C: Subcutaneous opioid infusion, *Am J Nurs* 102(7):61, 2002.

Equipment
Initiation of CSQI Therapy

- Clean gloves
- Alcohol swab
- Antibacterial skin prep such as chlorhexidine
- Small-gauge (25 to 27), winged IV catheter with attached tubing or catheter designed especially for CSQI (e.g., Sof-Set)
- Infusion pump
- Occlusive, transparent dressing
- Tape
- Medication in appropriate syringe or container

Discontinuing CSQI

- Clean, nonsterile gloves
- 2 × 2 gauze dressing and tape or adhesive bandage
- Alcohol swab and chlorhexidine (optional)

Step	Rationale
1. Complete preprocedure protocol.	
2. Check medication administration record or computer printout.	Verifies correct medication.
3. Check name of medication on label on syringe or container against medication administration record (MAR).	Ensures that client receives correct medication.

Step	Rationale
4. Check medication's expiration date.	Medications that have expired should not be used because potency of medications changes when medications become outdated.
5. Perform hand hygiene. Prepare correct medication dose from vial or ampule, or check dose on prefilled syringe, and prime tubing with medication. Check label of medication against MAR.	Prevents transmission of microorganisms. Ensures that medication is sterile and dose is accurate.
6. Obtain and program medication administration pump.	Promotes safe medication infusion.
7. Explain procedure to client.	Involves client in care and eases anxiety.
8. Identify client by checking identification bracelet and asking client's name. Compare with (MAR).	Ensures that correct client receives ordered drug. At least two client identifiers (neither to be client's room number) are to be used when administering medications (JCAHO, 2004).
9. **To initiate CSQI:**	
a. Select appropriate injection site. Most common sites used are subclavicular, abdomen, upper arms, or thighs.	Site must be free from irritation and not over bony prominences.
b. Assist client to comfortable position.	Eases pain associated with insertion of needle.
c. Cleanse injection site with alcohol using circular motion, followed by skin prep agent such as chlorhexidine using straight, cleansing strokes. Allow both agents to dry.	Reduces risk of infection at insertion site.

Step	Rationale
d. Hold needle in dominant hand, and remove needle guard.	Prepares needle for insertion.
e. Gently pinch or lift up skin with nondominant hand.	Ensures that needle will enter subcutaneous tissue.
f. Gently and firmly insert needle at 45- to 90-degree angle (Fig. 16-1).	Decreases pain related to insertion of needle.

NURSE ALERT Some prepackaged needles (e.g., Sof-Set, Sub-Q-Set) are inserted at a 90-degree angle. These needles are shorter than butterfly needles. Refer to the manufacturer's directions.

g. Release skin fold, and apply tape over "wings" of needle.	Secures needle.

NURSE ALERT Some cannulas have a sharp needle with a plastic catheter covering the needle. In this case, remove the needle and leave the plastic catheter in the skin.

h. Place occlusive, transparent dressing over insertion site (Fig. 16-2).	Protects site from infection and allows nurse to assess site during medication infusion.

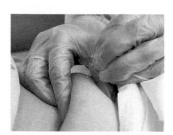

Fig. 16-1 Insertion of butterfly needle into subcutaneous tissue of abdomen.

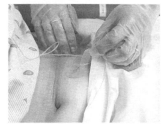

Fig. 16-2 Securing insertion site.

Step	Rationale
i. Attach tubing from needle to tubing from infusion pump.	Allows medication to be administered.
j. Turn infusion pump on.	Initiates medication therapy.
k. Dispose of any sharps in appropriate leak-proof, puncture-resistant container.	Prevents injury to client and health care personnel (OSHA, 2001).
10. To discontinue CSQI:	
a. Verify health care provider's order, and establish alternative method for medication administration if applicable.	If medication will be required after discontinuing CSQI, different medication and/or route may be necessary to continue to manage client's illness or pain.
b. Stop infusion pump.	Prevents spillage of medication.
c. 🔷 Remove dressing without dislodging or removing needle.	Exposes needle.
d. Remove tape from wings of needle, and pull needle out at same angle it was inserted.	Promotes comfort.
e. Apply pressure at site until no fluid leaks out of skin.	Dressing will stick to site if skin remains dry.
f. Apply 2 × 2 gauze dressing or adhesive bandage to site.	Prevents bacterial entry into puncture site.
11. Complete postprocedure protocol.	

NURSE ALERT If the medication is a narcotic, follow the institutional policy to document waste (Pasero, 2002).

Recording and Reporting

- Immediately after initiating CSQI, chart medication, dose, route, site, time, date, and type of medication pump in client's chart.
- Record client's response to medication and appearance of site every 4 hours or according to institutional policy.

■ Report to client's health care provider any adverse effects from medication or infection at insertion site, and document according to institutional policy. Client's condition may indicate need for additional medical therapy.

Unexpected Outcomes	Related Interventions
1. Client complains of localized pain or burning at needle's insertion site, or site appears red or swollen or is leaking.	• Symptoms indicate potential infection or needle is not securely in subcutaneous tissue. • Remove needle, and place new needle in different site.
2. Client displays signs of allergic reaction to medication.	• Follow institutional policy or guidelines for appropriate response to allergic reactions, and notify client's health care provider immediately.
3. CSQI becomes dislodged.	• Stop infusion, apply pressure at site until no fluid leaks out of skin, cover site with 2 × 2 gauze dressing or adhesive bandage, and initiate new site. • Assess client to determine effects of not receiving medication (e.g., assess pain level if client is receiving pain medication via CSQI).
4. Desired effect of medication not achieved.	• Follow established protocols for titration of medication, or notify client's health care provider for either change in dosage or medication.

Dressings: Dry and Wet-to-Dry

Wet-to-dry, moist-to-dry, and damp-to-dry dressings are gauze moistened with an appropriate solution such as normal saline. The primary purpose of these dressings is to mechanically debride a wound. The moistened contact layer of the dressing (primary dressing) increases the absorptive ability of the dressing to collect exudate and wound debris (Ovington, 2001). As the dressing dries, it adheres to the wound and debrides the wound of the tissue when the dressing is removed. One must *not apply a dressing so wet that it remains wet continuously.* A dressing that is too wet causes tissue maceration and bacterial growth. It also does not dry out and therefore does not remove the necrotic tissue when being removed from the wound. The moistened gauze must be covered with a secondary dressing layer that is dry. Disadvantages to wet-to-dry dressings are that the dressing needs to be changed every 4 to 6 hours and the removal of the dry dressing is likely to cause pain to the client (Nelson and Dilloway, 2002).

Delegation Considerations

The application of a wet-to-dry dressing should not be delegated to assistive personnel (AP). The skill of applying a dry dressing or changing a top dressing may be delegated to AP in uncomplicated wounds. A nurse must assess all wounds.

- Discuss with AP any unique modifications of the skill, such as the use of special tape or taping techniques to secure the dressing.
- Instruct AP about the signs of infection and poor wound healing and to immediately report the findings for further assessment.

Equipment

- Clean gloves
- Sterile gloves
- Sterile dressing set (scissors, forceps) (may be optional; check institution policy)
- Sterile drape (optional)
- Dressings: fine mesh gauze, sterile dressings, abdominal (ABD) pads
- Sterile basin (optional)

- Antiseptic ointment (as prescribed)
- Cleansing solution (as prescribed)
- Sterile normal saline or prescribed solution
- Tape, ties, or bandage as needed (include nonallergenic tape if necessary)
- Protective waterproof underpad
- Waterproof bag
- Adhesive remover (optional)
- Measurement device (optional): tape measure, camera (optional)
- Protective gown, mask, goggles used when spray from wound is a risk
- Additional lighting if needed (e.g., flashlight, treatment light)

Step	Rationale
1. Complete preprocedure protocol.	
2. Plan dressing change to occur 30 minutes after administration of analgesic.	Dressing change is better tolerated by client if analgesic has been administered at least 30 minutes before dressing change.
3. ⚡ Apply gown, goggles, and mask if risk of spray exists.	Reduces transmission of microorganisms.
4. Position client comfortably, and drape to expose only wound site. Instruct client not to touch wound or sterile supplies.	Draping provides access to wound yet minimizes unnecessary exposure.
5. Place disposable bag within reach of work area. Fold top of bag to make cuff.	Ensures easy disposal of soiled dressings. Prevents contamination of bag's outer surface.
6. Remove tape: pull parallel to skin, toward dressing, and hold down uninjured skin. If over hairy areas, remove in direction of hair growth. Remove remaining adhesive from skin.	Pulling tape toward dressing reduces stress on suture line or wound edges and reduces irritation and discomfort (Nelson and Dilloway, 2002).
7. With clean, gloved hand or forceps, remove dressings.	Primary dressing removes necrotic tissue and exudate.

Step	Rationale
Carefully remove outer secondary dressing first, and then remove inner primary dressing that is in contact with wound bed. If drains are present, slowly and carefully remove dressings one layer at a time.	Appearance of drainage may be upsetting to client. Avoids accidental removal of drain.

NURSE ALERT In wet-to-dry dressings, the inner primary dressing, if applied properly, will have dried and will adhere to underlying tissues; do not moisten it. It is incorrect technique and a common error by some clinicians to moisten the dried gauze before removing it. Moistening reduces the amount of debris the dressing will remove (Ramundo and Wells, 2000).

8. Inspect wound for color, edema, drains, exudate, and integrity (Fig. 17-1). Observe appearance of drainage on dressing. Assess for odor. Gently palpate wound edges for drainage, bogginess, or client report of increased pain. Measure wound size (length, width, and depth [if indicated])	Provides assessment of drainage and of wound's condition. Indicates status of healing. Presence of bleeding during this type of dressing change is indication that healthy tissue is being injured (Capasso and Munro, 2003).

Fig. 17-1 Abdominal wound with beefy red granulation tissue present and attached wound edges. (From Bryant RA: *Acute and chronic wounds: nursing management*, ed 2, St. Louis, 2000, Mosby.)

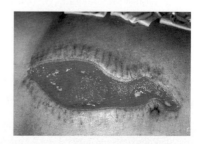

Step	Rationale

NURSE ALERT Dressings heavily saturated with exudate indicate a need to add more absorbent gauze.

9. Describe appearance of wound and any indicators of wound healing to client.

Wounds may appear unsettling and frightening to clients; it is helpful for client to know that wound appearance is as expected and what healing is taking place.

10. Dispose of soiled dressings in disposable bag. Remove gloves by pulling them inside out. Dispose of gloves in bag. Perform hand hygiene.

Reduces transmission of microorganisms to other persons.

11. Open sterile dressing tray or individually wrapped sterile supplies. Place on bedside table.

Sterile dressings remain sterile while on or within sterile surface. Preparation of all supplies prevents break in technique during dressing change.

12. Open prescribed cleansing solution, and pour over sterile gauze.

Keeps supplies sterile. Solution may be packaged to spray/pour directly on wound.

13. ⚡ Cleanse wound
    a. Use separate swab for each cleansing stroke, or spray wound surface.

    Prevents contaminating previously cleaned area.

    b. Clean from least contaminated area to most contaminated.

    Cleansing in this direction prevents introduction of organisms into wound.

    c. Cleanse around drain (if present), using circular stroke starting near drain and moving outward and away from insertion site.

    Correct aseptic technique in cleansing to prevent contamination.

14. Use dry gauze to blot away any moisture left in wound bed.

Drying reduces excess moisture, which could eventually harbor microorganisms.

15. Apply antiseptic ointment if ordered, using same

Helps reduce growth of microorganisms.

Step	Rationale

technique as for cleansing. Remove gloves.

16. Apply dressings to incision or wound site:

Dressing over wound can help clients gradually adjust to changes in body image (West and Gimbel, 2000).

   a. Don clean or sterile gloves depending on institution policy.

Research is insufficient to support either sterile or clean gloves as being more effective in decreasing infection and improving wound healing (Gray and Doughty, 2001).

   b. Dry dressing:

     (1) Apply loose woven gauze as contact layer.

Promotes proper absorption of drainage.

     (2) Cut 4 × 4 gauze flat to fit around drain if present, or use precut split-drain flat.

Secures drain and promotes drainage absorption at site.

     (3) Apply additional layers of gauze as needed.

Layering ensures proper coverage and optimal absorption.

     (4) Apply thicker woven pad (e.g., Surgipad, abdominal dressing).

This type of dressing is often used for postoperative wounds. Soft dressings over wounds protect wound from irritation and provide support (West and Gimbel, 2000).

   c. Wet-to-dry, damp-to-dry, moist-to-dry dressing:

     (1) Open or "fluff" woven gauze that will be placed directly against wound bed. Then place gauze or packing strip in container of sterile

Contact layer must be totally moistened to increase dressing's absorptive abilities (Ramundo and Wells, 2000).

Step	**Rationale**
solution. When using packing strip, cut amount of dressing anticipated to be used with sterile scissors.	
(2) Wring out excess fluid, and apply damp, fluffed woven-mesh gauze or packing strip directly onto wound surface without having gauze touch surrounding skin (Fig. 17-2, *A*).	Damp gauze absorbs drainage and adheres to debris (Hess, 2000). Inner gauze should be moist but not dripping wet. Damp gauze must be able to dry in wound. Having inner gauze too wet so it does not dry is common error in technique for this type of dressing.

NURSE ALERT If the wound is deep, gently lay damp woven gauze over the wound surface with forceps until all surfaces are in contact with gauze and the wound is loosely filled. Fill the wound, but avoid packing the wound too tightly or having the gauze extend beyond the top of the wound (see Fig. 17-2, *B*).

(3) Make sure any dead space from sinus tracts, undermining, or tunneling is loosely packed with gauze.	Do not overpack wound too tightly; it can cause wound trauma when dressing is removed (Ramundo and Wells, 2000).

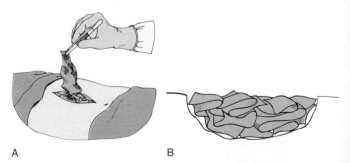

A   B

Fig. 17-2 A, Packing wound. B, Wound packed loosely.

Step	Rationale
(4) Apply dry sterile gauze over damp gauze.	Dry layer pulls moisture from wound.
(5) Cover packed wound with secondary dressing such as ABD pad, Surgipad, or gauze.	Protects wound from entrance of microorganisms.
17. Secure dressing with roll gauze (for circumferential dressings) (Fig. 17-3), tape, Montgomery ties or straps (which are applied perpendicular to the wound) (Fig. 17-4), or binder.	Supports wound and ensures placement and stability of dressing.

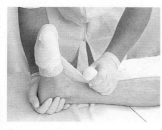

A

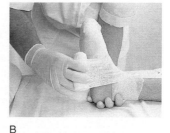

B

Fig. 17-3   Application of roll gauze.

Fig. 17-4   Securing Montgomery ties.

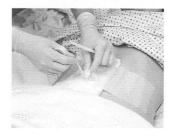

Step	Rationale
18. Routinely inspect condition of dressing and presence of any drainage.	Determines rate of healing.
19. Complete postprocedure protocol.	

Recording and Reporting

- Chart in nurses' notes appearance of wound; color, presence, and characteristics of exudate; change in wound characteristics, especially drainage amount, type, and amount of dressings applied; and tolerance of client to dressing change.
- Report to physician unexpected appearance of wound or drainage or accidental removal of drain.

Unexpected Outcomes	Related Interventions
1. Wound drainage increases.	• Increase frequency of dressing changes. • Notify physician, who may consider drain placement or alternate dressing method.
2. Client reports sensation that "something has given way under the dressing."	• Remove dressing, and inspect wound for dehiscence or evisceration. • Protect wound. Cover with sterile moist dressing. • Instruct client to lie still. • Remain with client to monitor vital signs. • Notify physician.
3. Skin around wound margins becomes red, macerated, or excoriated.	• Outer layer of wet-to-dry dressing is too moist. • Securing method for dressing is causing irritation. Change to paper tape.

Dressings: Hydrocolloid, Foam, or Absorption

Hydrocolloid dressings come in the form of granules, paste, or wafer dressings. Wound exudate is absorbed into the dressing, forming a jellylike substance next to the wound surface. The dressing maintains a moist, insulated environment that promotes rapid, effective healing. Hydrocolloid dressings are used to (1) maintain a moist wound environment for healing of clean, shallow to moderately deep wounds, (2) autolytically debride necrotic wounds, (3) protect high-friction areas on intact skin, (4) protect from contamination, and (5) provide absorption of minimal amount of exudates in superficial and shallow wounds (Cuzzell, 2002).

A foam dressing is a sponge-like polymer dressing that may or may not be adherent; it may be impregnated or coated with other materials and has some absorptive properties (AHCPR, 1994). These hydrophilic dressings are used in full-thickness wounds with minimal to moderate amounts of drainage. Foam dressings absorb moderate to heavy exudates in superficial or deep wounds, protect friable periwound skin, provide autolytic debridement, pad and protect high-trauma areas (e.g., pretibial area, forearms), and can be used with infected wounds following appropriate intervention and close monitoring of wound healing (Cuzzell, 2002).

Absorption dressings can contain large amounts of wound exudate. They may take the form of pastes, granules, sheeting, or rope. This group of dressings includes calcium alginate materials, which are manufactured from natural material (seaweed) and are known for their absorptive properties, forming a gel over the wound surface as exudate is contained. The exudate absorbers are nonadhesive, nonocclusive dressings that can be used in combination with other dressings. Generally, absorption and alginate dressings require a secondary dressing, and that dressing can be changed as needed (Cuzzell, 2002). The typical frequency of dressing changes is daily to once or twice a week.

Delegation Considerations

The skill of applying a hydrocolloid, hydrogel, foam, or absorption dressing should not be delegated to assistive personnel (AP).

- Instruct AP about the signs of infection or poor wound healing to report.

Equipment

- Sterile gloves (optional)
- Dressing set (optional)
- Sterile saline or other cleansing solution (as ordered)
- Clean gloves
- Waterproof bag for disposal
- Wound measurement devices (tape measure, tracing paper, camera)
- Dressing (size as needed) as prescribed (hydrocolloid, hydrogel, foam, absorption)
- Sterile gauze pads (4 × 4 inches)
- Secondary dressing of choice (if needed)
- Protective gown, mask, goggles (used when spray from wound is a risk)

Step	Rationale
1. Complete preprocedure protocol.	
2. Determine type of dressing. Do not use alginate or absorption dressings on nonexuding wounds. Most of these dressings are designed to absorb moderate to large amounts of wound drainage and therefore should not be used in wounds with minimal or no drainage (Cuzzell, 2002).	Dressing selection is based on type of wound, location of wound, amount and type of exudate (Nelson and Dilloway, 2002).
3. Expose wound site, and cover client.	Draping provides access to wound while minimizing client exposure.
4. Cuff top of disposable waterproof bag, and place within reach of work area.	Cuff prevents accidental contamination of top of outer bag. Nurse should not reach across sterile field.
5. ⬛ Apply moisture-proof gown, mask, and goggles when risk of spray exists.	Reduces transmission of infectious organisms.

Step	Rationale
6. Remove old dressing. For easier removal, pull back slowly across dressing in direction of hair growth. Check removal directions for specific brand of dressing being used.	Reduces irritation and possible injury to skin (Nelson and Dilloway, 2002).
7. Dispose of soiled dressings in waterproof bag. Remove disposable gloves by pulling them inside out, and dispose of them in waterproof bag. Avoid having client see old dressing because sight of wound drainage may be upsetting to client.	Reduces transmission of microorganisms.
8. Prepare sterile dressing supplies.	Reduces risk of break in sterile technique.
9. Pour saline or prescribed solution over 4 × 4 sterile gauze pads, or open spray wound cleanser.	Maintains sterility of dressing.
10. ✋ Don gloves, sterile if required by policy.	Allows nurse to handle dressings.
11. Cleanse area gently with moist 4 × 4 sterile gauze pads, swabbing exudate away from wound, or spray with wound cleanser.	Reduces introduction of organisms into wound. Cleansing effectively removes any residual dressing gel without injuring newly formed delicate granulation tissue in healing wound bed.
12. Thoroughly pat wound surface dry with dry 4 × 4 sterile gauze pads. Dry intact skin around wound.	Dressing will not adhere to damp surface. Periwound skin should be kept dry to prevent breakdown.
13. Inspect wound for tissue type, color, odor, and drainage. Measure wound size and depth.	Appearance and measurement indicate state of wound healing.

Step	Rationale

NURSE ALERT Hydrocolloid dressings interact with wound fluids and form a soft, whitish yellow gel, which is hard to remove and may have a faint odor. Normal discoloration may occur with some brands of foam dressings. A residual gel substance occurs in wound beds with some brands of absorption dressings (Cuzzell, 2002). These are normal findings; do not confuse with pus or purulent exudate.

14. Apply dressing according to manufacturer's directions:

    Ensures proper application of dressing. Different brands of dressings require different application techniques.

    a. Hydrocolloid dressings:
       (1) Apply hydrocolloid granules or paste before wafer dressing in deeper wounds.

       Dressing should not be stretched during application. Avoid wrinkles that would provide tunnel for exudate drainage. Hydrocolloid granules assist in absorbing drainage to increase wearing time of dressing (Rolstad and others, 2000).

       (2) Apply amorphous gels approximately 0.5- to 1.25-cm ($\frac{1}{4}$- to $\frac{1}{2}$-inch) thick across wound surface, or put hydrogel sheet over wound bed. For some brands of hydrocolloid wafers, size of dressing should be larger than wound size by a 2.5- to 3.75-cm (1- to 1$\frac{1}{2}$-inch) margin beyond wound edges. Cover with secondary dressing such as gauze, hydrocolloid, or foam.

       Fluid gels take form of cavity type of wounds. Secondary dressing must be used with hydrogel to hold it in place; it has no adhesive.

Step	Rationale

    (3) If necessary, apply tape around edges of hydrocolloid dressing to assist in keeping dressing in place.

  b. Foam dressings:

    (1) Apply foam smoothly; avoid wrinkles.

May be used with absorptive dressings to accommodate more highly draining wounds.

    (2) Make sure you know which side of foam dressing should be placed toward wound bed and which side should be facing away from wound bed.

Ensures proper absorption.

    (3) With some brands, dressings can be trimmed to fit wound size, whereas other brands of dressings cannot be cut.

Dressing should not overlap wound so as to avoid maceration of healthy skin.

    (4) Check with manufacturer as to which types of secondary dressings to avoid when covering foam dressing.

Could reduce effectiveness of foam dressing.

    (5) Some brands of foam dressings need slight tension on dressing while being applied. Some brands of foam dressings need to be

Step	Rationale

    covered with
    secondary dressing
    (Rolstad and others,
    2000).

  c. Absorption or alginate
     dressings:

     (1) Fill wound cavity   Allows for expansion with
         $^1/_2$ to $^2/_3$ full.   absorption.

     (2) For most brands of
         alginate dressings,
         dressing can be cut
         or folded to fit
         wound. For others,
         it is important not
         to completely fill
         wound bed with
         dressing but rather
         to allow space for
         alginate dressing to
         expand to fill
         wound bed. For
         some brands the
         alginate dressing
         should be applied
         moist, and for
         others it should be
         dry. Some brands
         need a secondary
         dressing that
         extends at least
         3 cm ($1^1/_4$ inches)
         beyond wound
         edges.

     (3) Apply secondary   Some secondary dressings may
         dressing, if   reduce effectiveness of alginate
         needed (check   or absorption dressing (Cuzzell,
         manufacturer's   2002).
         directions).

15. Complete postprocedure
    protocol.

Recording and Reporting

■ Chart in nurses' notes characteristics of wound tissue type: color, odor, viscosity, and amount of drainage; application of dressing; and client's tolerance to dressing change. Graph wound surface area or volume if wound is chronic wound.

■ Report unusual observations immediately.

Unexpected Outcomes	Related Interventions
1. Wound becomes infected.	• Dressing changes may need to be done more frequently. • Different type of dressing may be required. • May need to discontinue use of dressing.
2. Dressing does not stay in place.	• Evaluate size of dressing used for adequate margin (2.5 to 3.75 cm [1 to 1½ inches]), or dry skin more thoroughly before reapplication. • Consider custom shapes for difficult body parts. "Picture frame" edges of hydrocolloid dressing using tape. • Dressing may be secured with roll gauze, tape, transparent dressing, or dressing sheet.
3. Wound develops more necrotic tissue and increases in size.	• In rare instances, wounds do not tolerate hypoxia induced by hydrocolloid dressings. In these clients, use should be discontinued. • Evaluate appropriateness of wound care protocol. • Evaluate client for other impediments to wound healing.
4. Wound drainage is more than dressing can absorb.	• Change type of dressing to one that can absorb amount of wound drainage. • Foam dressings may be used over wound exudate absorbers.

Dressings: Transparent

A film or transparent dressing is a clear, adherent, nonabsorptive, polymer-based dressing that is permeable to oxygen and water vapor but not to water (AHCPR, 1994). Such dressings were developed to manage superficial wounds such as intravenous (IV) sites and wounds associated with laparoscopic surgery. Film dressings can also be used to prevent bruising or skin abrasions on high-risk intact skin and for autolytic debridement of small wounds with little or no exudate (Rolstad and others, 2000).

Pain and discomfort are diminished with the use of a transparent dressing, and the film conforms well to different body contours, making bodily movement less restricted compared with bulky gauze dressings. Transparent dressings may be used with or without adhesives. If used without adhesives, secure with hypoallergenic tape. For best results, these dressings should be used on clean, debrided wounds that are not actively bleeding. The film should be applied wrinkle free but not stretched over the skin. Should the fluid accumulation take on a white, opaque appearance with erythema of the surrounding tissue, one must assume that an infectious process is under way, and the dressing should be removed and a wound culture obtained.

Delegation Considerations

The skill of applying a transparent dressing to an uncomplicated wound may be delegated to assistive personnel (AP). AP cannot change IV site dressings. The care of acute new wounds and those that require sterile technique for dressing change should not be delegated. The assessment of the wound should not be delegated to AP even if the dressing change is delegated.

- Discuss with AP any modification of the skill such as removal or special taping needed.
- Instruct AP about the signs of infection or poor wound healing to report.

Equipment

- Sterile gloves (optional)
- Dressing set (optional)
- Sterile saline or other agent (as ordered)
- Cotton swabs

- Waterproof bag for disposal
- Mineral oil (optional)
- Transparent dressing (size as needed)
- Sterile gauze pads (4 × 4 inches)
- Skin preparation materials (optional)
- Protective gown, mask, goggles (used when spray from wound is a risk)

Step	Rationale
1. Complete preprocedure protocol.	
2. Position client to allow access to dressing site.	Facilitates application of dressing.
3. Keep sheet or gown draped over body parts not requiring exposure.	Provides privacy and decreases transfer of microorganisms.
4. Cuff top of disposable waterproof bag, and place within reach of work area.	Cuff prevents accidental contamination of rim of outer bag.
5. ▨ Moisture-proof gown, mask, and eye goggles are worn when risk of spray exists.	Reduces transmission of infectious organisms.
6. Remove old dressing. For easier removal, ease off using cotton swab soaked in mineral oil, or secure piece of tape to corner of dressing and pull back slowly in a direction parallel to the wound rather than upward.	Reduces excoriation or irritation of skin after dressing removal. The stretching action breaks the seal to increase ease of removal (Rolstad and others, 2000).
7. Dispose of soiled dressings in waterproof bag, remove disposable gloves by pulling them inside out, dispose of them in waterproof bag, and perform hand hygiene.	Reduces transmission of microorganisms.
8. Prepare sterile dressing supplies.	Reduces risk of break in sterile technique.

Step	Rationale
9. Pour saline or prescribed solution over 4 × 4 sterile gauze pads.	Maintains sterility of dressing.
10. ▰ Don clean or sterile gloves (check institution policy).	Allows nurse to handle dressings.
11. Cleanse area gently with moist 4 × 4 sterile gauze pads, or spray with wound cleanser. Cleanse from least contaminated to most contaminated area.	Reduces introduction of organisms into wound.
12. Pat skin dry around wound thoroughly with dry 4 × 4 sterile gauze pads.	Transparent dressing with adhesive backing does not adhere to damp surface (Rolstad and others, 2000).
13. Inspect wound for tissue type, color, odor, and drainage; measure wound if indicated.	Appearance indicates state of wound healing.

NURSE ALERT If the wound has a large amount of drainage, choose another dressing that is more absorptive.

14. Apply transparent dressing according to manufacturer's directions. Remove adherent backing. Apply one edge of dressing, then gently smooth remaining dressing over wound. *Film should not be stretched during application.* Avoid wrinkles in film. Label dressing with date and time changed (Fig. 19-1).	Wrinkles would provide tunnel for exudate drainage.
15. Complete postprocedure protocol.	

Fig. 19-1 Transparent dressing.

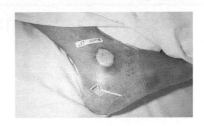

Recording and Reporting

- Chart in nurses' notes characteristics of wound: color, odor, viscosity, and amount of drainage; application of dressing; what was reported to physician.
- Report signs and symptoms of infection and poor wound healing to physician.

Unexpected Outcomes	Related Interventions
1. Wound becomes infected.	• Dressing changes may need to be done more frequently. • Different type of dressing may be required. • Obtain wound culture per agency policy.
2. Dressing does not stay in place.	• Evaluate size of dressing used for adequate wound margin (2.5 to 3.75 cm [1 to 1½ inches]). • Client's skin may be too dry or too moist.
3. Skin tears can occur with this type of dressing.	• Adhesive backing may be too strong for fragile skin. • Consider other dressing type.

Ear Drop Administration

When administering ear (otic) medications, be aware of certain safety precautions. Internal ear structures are very sensitive to temperature extremes. Failure to instill a solution at room temperature can cause vertigo (severe dizziness) or nausea and debilitate a client for several minutes. Although structures of the outer ear are not sterile, use sterile drops and solutions in case the eardrum is ruptured. Entrance of non-sterile solutions into the middle ear can cause serious infection. A final precaution is to avoid forcing any solution into the ear. Do not occlude the ear canal with a medicine dropper, because this can cause pressure within the canal during instillation and subsequent injury to the eardrum. If these precautions are followed, instillation of ear drops is a safe and effective therapy.

Delegation Considerations

The skill of administering ear medications should not be delegated to assistive personnel (AP).

- Instruct AP about potential side effects of medications and report their occurrence to nurse.
- Instruct AP to report any dizziness or light-headedness to the nurse for further assessment.

Equipment

- Medication bottle with dropper
- Cotton-tipped applicator
- Cotton ball (optional)
- Clean gloves (optional, only if client has drainage)
- Medication administration record (MAR)

Step	Rationale
1. Complete preprocedure protocol.	
2. Check accuracy and completeness of MAR with prescriber's written medication order. Check client's name, drug name and dosage, route of administration, and time for administration.	Order sheet is most reliable source and only legal record of drugs client is to receive. Ensures that right drug is administered.

Step	**Rationale**
Compare MAR with label of ear medication three times during drug preparation.	
3. Check client's identification bracelet, and ask name.	Ensures that correct client receives medication. At least two patient identifiers (neither to be patient's room number) are to be used whenever administering medications (JCAHO, 2004).
4. Explain each step of procedure to client, allowing for questions.	Reduces client anxiety; timing of instruction enhances learning.
5. ![] Don gloves (if drainage is present).	Reduces transmission of microorganisms.
6. Warm medication by running warm water over the bottle (without damaging the label directions or allowing water to get into the bottle).	Prevents nausea and vertigo that may occur if the medication is too cold.
7. Have client assume side-lying position (if not contraindicated by client's condition) with ear to be treated facing up, or client may sit in chair or on side of bed. Nurse should stabilize client's head with his or her hand.	Position provides easy access to ear for instillation of medication. Ear canal is in position to receive medication. Stabilizing head promotes safety during instillation with dropper.
8. For adults and children older than 3 years, gently pull pinna up and back; for children 3 years old or younger, pinna should be pulled down and back (Fig. 20-1) (Lilley and others, 2005).	Straightening of ear canal provides direct access to deeper external ear structures. Developmental differences in younger children and infants necessitate different methods of doing this.

Step	Rationale

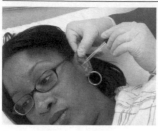
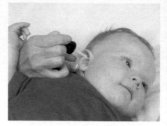

A   B

Fig. 20-1   **A,** Pull the pinna up and back for adults and children older than 3 years. **B,** Pull the pinna down and back for children 3 years old or younger.

9. If cerumen or drainage occludes outermost portion of ear canal, wipe out gently with cotton-tipped applicator.	Cerumen and drainage harbor microorganisms and can block distribution of medication.

NURSE ALERT Do not use the cotton-tipped applicator to force wax inward to block or occlude canal.

10. Instill prescribed drops, holding dropper 1 cm (½ inch) above ear canal.	Forceful instillation of drops into occluded canal can injure eardrum.
11. Ask client to remain in side-lying position for 5 to 10 minutes. Apply gentle massage or pressure to tragus of ear with finger. If medication is to be given in both ears, have client stay in the side-lying position for at least 5 minutes after the dose before turning to other side.	Allows complete distribution of medication. Pressure and massage move medication inward.
12. At times, prescriber orders insertion of portion of cotton ball into outermost	Inserting cotton into outer canal prevents escape of medication when client sits or stands. Cotton

Step	Rationale
part of canal. Do not press cotton into canal.	should not block canal to impair hearing.
13. Complete postprocedure protocol.	
14. Remove cotton after 15 minutes.	Time period promotes drug distribution and absorption.
15. Ask client to explain/ demonstrate technique for instilling ear drops and purpose of medication.	Evaluates degree of learning.

Recording and Reporting

- Immediately after administration, record on MAR the drug, concentration, number of drops, time administered, and ear (left, right, or both) into which drops were instilled. Do not chart medication administration until *after* it is given to client.
- If drug is withheld, record reason in nurses' notes. Circle on MAR the time drug normally would have been given (or follow institution's policy for noting withheld doses).
- Record condition of ear canal in nurses' notes.
- Report any sudden change in client's hearing acuity, adverse effects/client response, and/or withheld drugs to nurse in charge or physician.

Unexpected Outcomes	Related Interventions
1. Ear canal is inflamed, swollen, tender to palpation. Drainage is present.	• Symptoms of continuing ear infection are present; notify prescriber.
2. Client's hearing acuity continues to be reduced.	• Obstruction within ear canal is unrelieved. Notify prescriber.
3. Ear canal is occluded by cerumen.	• Wax has become impacted in canal. Ear irrigation may be necessary to remove wax impaction.
4. Client has difficulty self-administering ear drops.	• Reinstruction is needed. Have client demonstrate instillation of ear drops until performed correctly.

Ear Irrigations

Medications used to irrigate or wash out a body cavity such as the ear (otic) are delivered through a stream of solution. The common indications for irrigation of the external ear are presence of a foreign body, local inflammation of the canal, and accumulation of cerumen. Administer irrigations with liquid warmed to body temperature to avoid vertigo (dizziness) or nausea in clients (Phipps and others, 2003). The greatest danger during administration of ear irrigation is rupture of the tympanic membrane. Do not instill fluids under pressure or with the ear canal occluded by the irrigating device.

Delegation Considerations

The skill of ear irrigation should not be delegated to assistive personnel (AP).

- Instruct AP about the potential side effects of ear irrigation and to report their occurrence.
- Instruct AP to report any dizziness or light-headedness to the nurse for further assessment.

Equipment

- Clean gloves
- Otoscope (optional)
- Irrigation syringe
- Basin
- Towel
- Cotton balls
- Prescribed irrigation solution warmed to body temperature, mineral oil, or over-the-counter softener
- Medication administration record (MAR)

Step	Rationale
1. If client is found to have impacted cerumen, instill 1 to 2 drops of mineral oil or over-the-counter softener into ear twice a day for 2 to 3 days before irrigation.	Loosens cerumen and ensures easier removal during irrigation.

Step	**Rationale**
2. Complete preprocedure protocol.	
3. Check accuracy and completeness of MAR with prescriber's written medication or procedure order. Check client's name, drug name and dosage, route of administration, and time for administration. Compare MAR with label of ear irrigation solution.	Order sheet is most reliable source and only legal record of drugs or procedure client is to receive. Ensures that client receives correct medication.
4. Check client's identification by reading identification bracelet and asking name.	Ensures that correct client receives medication. At least two patient identifiers (neither to be patient's room number) are to be used whenever administering medications (JCAHO, 2004).
5. Explain procedure. Warn that irrigation may cause sensation of dizziness, ear fullness, and warmth.	Prepares client to anticipate effects of irrigation and promotes cooperation.
6. ⚡ Assist client to sitting or lying position with head turned toward affected ear. Place towel under client's head and shoulder, and have client, if able, hold basin under affected ear.	Position minimizes leakage of fluids around neck and facial area. Solution will flow from ear canal to basin.
7. Pour irrigating solution into basin.	
8. Gently clean auricle and outer ear canal with moistened cotton applicator. Do *not* force drainage or cerumen into ear canal.	Prevents infected material from reentering ear canal. Forceful instillation of solution into occluded canal can cause injury to eardrum.
9. Fill irrigating syringe with solution (approximately 50 ml).	Enough fluid is needed to provide steady irrigating stream.

Step	Rationale
10. For adults and children older than 3 years, gently pull pinna up and back; for children 3 years old or younger, pinna should be pulled down and back (Lilley and others, 2005).	Straightening of ear canal provides direct access to deeper external ear structures. Developmental differences in younger children and infants necessitate different techniques. Allows fluid to flow through length of canal.
11. Slowly instill irrigating solution by holding tip of syringe 1 cm (½ inch) above opening to ear canal. Fluid should be directed toward superior aspect of ear canal. Allow fluid to drain out into basin during instillation. Continue until canal is cleansed or solution is used (Fig. 21-1).	Slow instillation prevents buildup of pressure in ear canal and ensures contact of solution with all canal surfaces.
12. Do *not* occlude ear canal with tip of syringe.	Buildup of fluid in ear canal under forced pressure could cause rupture of tympanic membrane.
13. Dry outer ear canal with cotton ball. Leave cotton loosely in place for 5 to 10 minutes.	Maintains comfort. Absorbs excess moisture in ear canal.
14. Ask client to describe purpose of irrigation and demonstrate proper techniques for ear care.	Reflects client's understanding of procedure and proper hygiene.

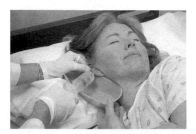

Fig. 21-1 Tip of syringe does not occlude ear canal during irrigation.

Step	Rationale

15. Complete postprocedure
    protocol.

Recording and Reporting

- Record appearance of external ear and client's hearing acuity, the
  procedure, amount of solution instilled, time of administration,
  ear receiving irrigation and client's response. Include initials or
  signature. Do not chart medication administration until *after* it is
  given to client.
- If drug is withheld, record reason in nurses' notes. On MAR, circle
  the time drug normally would have been given (or follow
  institution's policy for noting withheld doses).
- Report adverse effects/client response and/or withheld drugs to
  nurse in charge or physician.

Unexpected Outcomes	Related Interventions
1. Client experiences increased ear pain.	• Rupture of eardrum may have occurred. Stop irrigations immediately, and notify prescriber immediately.
2. Ear canal remains occluded with cerumen.	• Repeat irrigation is required.
3. Foreign body remains in ear canal.	• Refer client to otolaryngologist if foreign object remains after irrigation.
4. Client is unable to explain or demonstrate ear care practices.	• Reinstruction is necessary. • Include family members or caregivers if possible.

Enemas

An enema is the instillation of a solution into the rectum and sigmoid colon. The instillation of an enema solution promotes defecation by stimulating peristalsis. The volume or type of fluid breaks up the fecal mass, stretches the rectal wall, and initiates the defecation reflex.

Cleansing enemas promote complete evacuation of feces from the colon by stimulating peristalsis through infusion of large volumes of solution. Oil-retention enemas lubricate the rectum and colon. Feces absorb oil and become softer and easier to pass. Medicated enemas contain pharmacological agents and may be prescribed to reduce dangerously high serum potassium levels, as with use of a sodium polystyrene sulfonate (Kayexalate) enema, or to reduce bacteria in the colon before bowel surgery, as with use of a neomycin enema.

Delegation Considerations

The skill of administering an enema can be delegated to assistive personnel (AP).

- Inform and assist AP in positioning clients who have mobility restrictions.
- Instruct AP regarding positioning of clients with therapeutic equipment present, such as drains or intravenous (IV) catheters.
- Instruct AP regarding signs and symptoms of the client not tolerating the procedure, and when the enema must be stopped. These signs and symptoms may include abdominal pain more than a pressure sensation, abdominal cramping, abdominal distention, or rectal bleeding.
- Explain to AP the expected outcome of the enema and to immediately inform the nurse about the presence of blood in the stool or around the rectal area, any change in client vital signs, or new symptoms.

Equipment

- Clean gloves
- Water-soluble lubricant
- Waterproof, absorbent pads
- Toilet tissue
- Bedpan, bedside commode, or access to toilet
- Washbasin, washcloths, towel, and soap
- IV pole

Enema Bag Administration

- Disposable gloves
- Enema container
- Tubing and clamp (if not already attached to container)
- Appropriate-size rectal tube (adult: 22 to 30 Fr; child: 12 to 18 Fr)
- Correct volume of warmed solution (adult: 750 to 1000 ml; adolescent: 500 to 700 ml; school-age child: 300 to 500 ml; toddler: 250 to 350 ml; infant: 150 to 250 ml)

Prepackaged Enema

- Prepackaged enema container with rectal tip

Step	Rationale
1. Complete preprocedure protocol.	

NURSE ALERT An "enemas until clear" order means that enemas are repeated until the client passes fluid that is clear of fecal matter. Check agency policy, but usually the client should receive only three consecutive enemas to avoid disruption of fluid and electrolyte balance.

Step	Rationale
2. Assist client into left side-lying (Sims') position with right knee flexed. Children may also be placed in dorsal recumbent position.	Allows enema solution to flow downward by gravity along natural curve of sigmoid colon and rectum, thus improving retention of solution.

NURSE ALERT If the client is suspected of having poor sphincter control, position the client on the bedpan in comfortable dorsal recumbent position. Clients with poor sphincter control cannot retain all of the enema solution. Administering the enema with the client sitting on the toilet is unsafe because the curved rectal tubing can abrade the rectal wall.

Step	Rationale
3. Place waterproof pad under hips and buttocks.	Prevents soiling of linen.
4. Cover client with bath blanket, exposing only rectal area, clearly visualizing anus.	Provides warmth, reduces exposure of body parts, allows client to feel more relaxed and comfortable.
5. Separate buttocks, and examine perianal region for abnormalities, including hemorrhoids, anal fissure,	Findings will influence nurse's approach to insertion of enema tip. Prolapse contraindicates enema.

rectal prolapse (Moppett, 1999).

6. Place bedpan or commode in easily accessible position. If client will be expelling contents in toilet, ensure that toilet is unoccupied. (If client will be getting up to bathroom to expel enema, place client's slippers and bathrobe in easily accessible position.)

Used in case client is unable to retain enema solution.

7. Administer prepackaged disposable commercial (Fleet) enema:

a. Remove plastic cap from tip of container. Tip of nozzle is already lubricated, but more water-soluble jelly can be applied as needed.

Lubrication provides for smooth insertion of rectal tube without causing rectal irritation or trauma.

b. Gently separate buttocks, and locate rectum. Instruct client to relax by breathing out slowly through mouth.

Breathing out promotes relaxation of external rectal sphincter.

c. Expel any air from enema container.

Introducing air into colon can cause further distention and discomfort (Moppett, 1999).

d. Insert nozzle of container gently into anal canal, angling toward umbilicus (Fig. 22-1).
Adult: 7.5 to 10 cm (3 to 4 inches).
Adolescent: 7.5 to 10 cm (3 to 4 inches)
Child: 5 to 7.5 cm (2 to 3 inches)

Gentle insertion prevents trauma to rectal mucosa (Saltzstein and others, 1988).

Step	Rationale

Fig. 22-1 Tip of commercial enema is inserted into rectum. (From Sorrentino SA: *Mosby's textbook for nursing assistants,* ed 5, St. Louis, 2000, Mosby.)

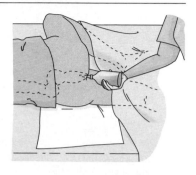

Infant: 2.5 to 3.75 cm (1 to 1^1/$_2$ inches)

NURSE ALERT If pain occurs or if resistance is felt at any time during the procedure, stop and confer with the physician.

e. Squeeze bottle until all of solution has entered rectum and colon. Instruct client to retain solution until urge to defecate occurs, usually 2 to 5 minutes.

Hypertonic solutions require only small volumes to stimulate defecation.

8. Administer enema using enema bag:

a. Add warmed solution to enema bag: warm tap water as it flows from faucet, place saline container in basin of hot water before adding saline to enema bag, and check temperature of solution by pouring small amount of solution over inner wrist.

Hot water can burn intestinal mucosa. Cold water can cause abdominal cramping and is difficult to retain.

Step	**Rationale**
b. Raise container, release clamp, and allow solution to flow long enough to fill tubing.	Removes air from tubing.
c. Reclamp tubing.	Prevents further loss of solution.
d. Lubricate 6 to 8 cm (2$^1/_2$ to 3 inches) of tip of rectal tube with lubricating jelly.	Allows smooth insertion of rectal tube without risk of irritation or trauma to mucosa.
e. Gently separate buttocks, and locate anus. Instruct client to relax by breathing out slowly through mouth.	Breathing out promotes relaxation of external anal sphincter.
f. Insert tip of rectal tube slowly by pointing tip in direction of client's umbilicus. Length of insertion varies: *Adult:* 7.5 to 10 cm (3 to 4 inches) *Adolescent:* 7.5 to 10 cm (3 to 4 inches) *Child:* 5 to 7.5 cm (2 to 3 inches) *Infant:* 2.5 to 3.75 cm (1 to 1$^1/_2$ inches)	Careful insertion prevents trauma to rectal mucosa from accidental lodging of tube against rectal wall. Insertion beyond proper limit can cause bowel perforation.

NURSE ALERT If the tube does not pass easily, do not force. Consider allowing a small amount of fluid to infuse, and then try to slowly reinsert the tube. The instillation of fluid may relax the sphincter and provide additional lubrication.

g. Hold tubing in rectum constantly until end of fluid instillation.	Bowel contraction can cause expulsion of rectal tube.
h. Open regulating clamp, and allow solution to enter slowly with container at client's hip level.	Rapid instillation can stimulate evacuation of rectal tube.

Step	Rationale
i. Raise height of enema container slowly to appropriate level above anus: 30 to 45 cm (12 to 18 inches) for high enema, 30 cm (12 inches) for regular enema, 7.5 cm (3 inches) for low enema. Instillation time varies with volume of solution administered (e.g., 1 L/10 min) (Fig. 22-2).	Allows for continuous, slow instillation of solution; raising container too high causes rapid instillation and possible painful distention of colon. High pressure can cause rupture of bowel in infant.
j. Lower container or clamp tubing if client complains of cramping or if fluid escapes around rectal tube.	Temporary cessation of instillation prevents cramping, which may prevent client from retaining all fluid, altering effectiveness of enema.
k. Clamp tubing after all solution is instilled.	Prevents entrance of air into rectum.
9. Place layers of toilet tissue around tube at anus, and gently withdraw rectal tube and tip.	Provides for client's comfort and cleanliness.

Fig. 22-2 Enema is given in Sims' position. IV pole is positioned so that enema bag is 12 inches above anus and approximately 18 inches above mattress (depending on client's size). (From Sorrentino SA: *Mosby's textbook for nursing assistants,* ed 5, St. Louis, 2000, Mosby.)

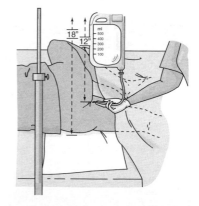

Step	Rationale
10. Explain to client that feeling of distention is normal, as well as some abdominal cramping. Ask client to retain solution as long as possible while lying quietly in bed. (For infant or young child, gently hold buttocks together for few minutes.)	Solution distends bowel. Length of retention varies with type of enema and client's ability to contract rectal sphincter. Longer retention promotes more effective stimulation of peristalsis and defecation.
11. Assist client to bathroom, or help to position client on bedpan.	Normal squatting position promotes defecation.
12. Observe character of feces and solution (caution client against flushing toilet before inspection).	Reveals result of enema.

NURSE ALERT When enemas are ordered "until clear," it is essential for nurse to observe the contents of solution passed. The enema return is considered "clear" when no solid fecal material exists, but the solution may be colored.

13. ✦ Assist client as needed with washing anal area with warm soap and water (if administering perineal care, use gloves).	Fecal contents can irritate skin. Hygiene promotes client's comfort.
14. Complete postprocedure protocol.	

Recording and Reporting

- Record type and volume of enema given, time administered, and characteristics of results.
- Report to physician failure of client to defecate and any adverse effects.

Unexpected Outcomes	Related Interventions
1. Abdomen becomes rigid and distended.	• Stop enema. • Obtain vital signs. • Notify prescriber.
2. Abdominal cramping or pain develops.	• Slow rate of instillation.
3. Bleeding occurs.	• Stop enema. • Notify prescriber. • Obtain vital signs, and assess abdomen and rectum.

Enteral Nutrition via a Gastrostomy or Jejunostomy Tube

When clients cannot tolerate nasoenteral feeding tubes, when they require permanent enteral feeding, or when nasoenteral feeding tubes interfere with rehabilitation, two options are available. One such option is gastric feeding. Gastric feedings permit the delivery of partially digested nutrients to the stomach or intestine at a normal physiological rate. Gastric feedings via a gastrostomy or jejunostomy feeding tube are relatively safe to administer, provided the client has normal gastric emptying and there is not excessive residual volume. A gastrostomy tube is surgically placed in the stomach and exits through an incision in the upper left quadrant of the abdomen, where it is sutured in place. A more current practice is insertion of a percutaneous endoscopic gastrostomy (PEG) tube by endoscopic visualization of the stomach (Fig. 23-1).

Jejunostomy tubes, like gastrostomy tubes, can be inserted during surgery or endoscopy. Endoscopic insertion is done through a PEG tube. After insertion of the large-bore PEG tube, the percutaneous endoscopic jejunostomy (PEJ) tube is passed through the PEG and advanced into the jejunum (Fig. 23-2).

Delegation Considerations

Administration of gastrostomy or jejunostomy tube feeding is a procedure that can be delegated to assistive personnel (AP). However, a nurse must first verify tube placement and patency.

- Instruct AP about the prescribed rate to infuse the feeding.
- Instruct AP to report any difficulty infusing the feeding or any discomfort voiced by the client.
- Have AP report any gagging, paroxysms of coughing, or choking.

Equipment

- Disposable feeding bag and tubing or ready-to-hang system
- 30-ml or larger Luer-Lok or catheter-tip syringe
- Stethoscope
- Infusion pump (required for continuous or intestinal feedings): use pump designed for tube feedings

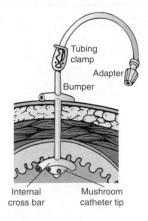

Fig. 23-1   Placement of PEG tube into stomach.

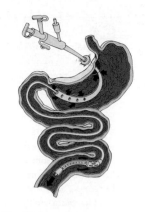

Fig. 23-2   Endoscopic insertion of jejunostomy tube.

- pH indicator strip (see Skill 43)
- Prescribed enteral feeding
- Clean gloves
- Equipment to obtain blood glucose by finger stick

Step	Rationale
1. Complete preprocedure protocol.	
2. Auscultate for bowel sounds. Consult physician if bowel sounds are absent.	Absent bowel sounds may indicate decreased ability of gastrointestinal (GI) tract to digest or absorb nutrients.
3. Prepare feeding container to administer formula continuously:	
a. Check expiration date on formula and integrity of container.	Ensures GI tolerance of formula. Prevents leakage of tube feeding.
b. Have tube feeding at room temperature.	Cold formula may cause gastric cramping and discomfort because liquid is not warmed by mouth and esophagus.

Step	Rationale

c. Connect tubing to container, or prepare ready-to-hang container. Use aseptic technique, and avoid handling feeding system.

Feeding system, including bag, connections, and tubing, must be free of contamination to prevent bacterial growth (Padula and others, 2004).

d. Shake formula container well, and fill container with formula. Open stopcock on tubing, and fill tubing with formula to remove air (prime tubing). Hang on pole.

Filling tubing with formula prevents excess air from entering GI tract once infusion begins.

4. For intermittent feeding, have syringe ready and be sure formula is at room temperature.

Cold formula causes gastric cramping.

5. Place client in high-Fowler's position, or elevate head of bed at least 30 degrees.

Elevated head helps prevent aspiration.

6. Determine tube placement (see Skill 43). Observe aspirate's appearance and note pH measurement.

Feedings instilled into misplaced tube may cause serious injury or death. On occasion, color alone may differentiate gastric from intestinal placement because most intestinal aspirates are stained by bile to distinct yellow color and most gastric aspirates are not (Metheny and others, 1999).

7. Check gastric residual volume.

a. *Gastrostomy tube:* Attach syringe, and aspirate gastric secretions. Return aspirated contents to stomach unless volume exceeds 100 ml. If

For adults, a volume in excess of 100 ml for gastrostomy tubes should raise concern about intolerance; however, feedings may continue while further examinations are conducted (ASPEN, 2002; McClave and

Step	Rationale
volume is more than 100 ml on several occasions, hold feeding and notify physician.	others, 1999; Murphy and Bickford, 1999). Fluids aspirated from the stomach contain electrolytes that, if withheld, may cause electrolyte imbalances. Notify physician if residual volume is excessive, and request order regarding whether residual fluid should be returned to client.

b. *Jejunostomy tube:* Aspirate intestinal secretions, observe volume, and return contents as above.

8. Irrigate tube with 30 ml water (see Skill 44).	Maintains patency after removal of aspirate.

9. Initiate feeding:

NURSE ALERT Do not add food coloring or dye to enteral nutrition to detect aspirated secretions. Dye may be systemically absorbed, may interfere with Hemoccult testing of stool, and has safety risks (Maloney and Metheny, 2002; McClave and others, 2002; Metheny and others, 2002). Use of dye may cause death.

a. *Syringe or intermittent feeding:*

(1) Pinch proximal end of gastrostomy/ jejunostomy feeding tube.	Prevents air from entering client's stomach.
(2) Remove plunger from syringe, and attach barrel of syringe to end of tube.	Barrel receives formula for instillation.
(3) Fill syringe with measured amount of formula. Release tube, elevate syringe to no more than	Height of syringe allows for safe, slow, gravity drainage of formula. Total delivery of bolus feedings may take several minutes, depending on amount

Step	Rationale
18 inches (45 cm) above insertion site, and allow it to empty gradually by gravity. Repeat Steps (1) through (3) until prescribed amount has been delivered to client.	of bolus. Administering feeding too quickly may cause abdominal discomfort to client or increase risk for aspiration.
(4) If feeding bag is used, prime tubing and attach gavage tubing to end of feeding tube. Set rate by adjusting roller clamp on tubing. Allow bag to empty gradually over 30 to 60 minutes (see Skill 24). Label bag with tube-feeding type, strength, and amount. Include date, time, and initials. Change bag every 24 hours.	Gradual emptying of formula by gravity from syringe or feeding bag reduces risk of abdominal discomfort, vomiting, or diarrhea induced by bolus or too-rapid infusion of tube feedings. Helps decrease bacterial colonization.
b. *Continuous drip method:*	
(1) Connect distal end of tubing to proximal end of feeding tube.	
(2) Connect tubing through infusion pump, and set rate (see Skill 24).	
10. Advance rate and concentration of tube	Helps prevent diarrhea and gastric intolerance to formula.

Step	Rationale
feeding gradually (see Box 24-1, Skill 24).	
11. Administer water via feeding tube as ordered or between feedings.	Provides client with source of water to help maintain fluid and electrolyte balance. Clears tubing of formula.
12. Flush tube with 30 ml of water every 4 to 6 hours around-the-clock and before and after administering medications via tube.	Maintains tube patency.
13. When tube feedings are not being administered, cap or clamp the proximal end of feeding tube.	Prevents air from entering stomach between feedings.
14. Rinse bag and tubing with warm water whenever feedings are interrupted. Use new administration set every 24 hours.	Rinsing bag and tubing with warm water clears old tube feedings and reduces bacterial growth.
15. Gastrostomy/jejunostomy exit site of tube is usually left open to air. However, if dressing is needed because of drainage, change dressing daily or as needed.	Leaking or gastric drainage may cause irritation and excoriation of skin. Skin around feeding tube should be cleansed daily with warm water and mild soap. Area must be dried completely before applying dressing.
16. Complete postprocedure protocol.	

Recording and Reporting

- Record amount and type of feeding, client's response to tube feeding, patency of tube.
- Record volume of formula and any additional water on intake and output form.
- Report type of feeding, status of feeding tube, client's tolerance, and adverse effects.

Unexpected Outcomes	Related Interventions
1. Feeding tube becomes clogged.	• Flush tube with water after checking residual volume (Edwards and Metheny, 2000).
2. Excessive gastric residual volume.	• Notify physician to determine if feedings need to be held. If feedings are held, reassess residual volume 1 hour after feeding is stopped to determine if volume has lessened or increased. If it has increased, make sure physician is aware.
	• Maintain client in high-Fowler's position or have head of bed elevated at least 45 degrees.
3. Client develops diarrhea three or more times in 24 hours; may indicate intolerance.	• Notify physician, and confer with dietitian to determine need to modify type of formula, concentration, or rate of infusion.
	• Consider other causes (e.g., bacterial contamination of feeding, client infection) (Eisenberg, 2002).
	• Determine if client is receiving antibiotics or medications (e.g., those containing sorbitol) that can induce diarrhea (Benya and others, 1991; Guenter and others, 1991).

Enteral Nutrition via a Nasogastric Feeding Tube

Gastric feedings are the most common type of enteral nutrition. Specially prepared formulas administered by way of small-bore nasogastric (NG) feeding tubes into the stomach pass gradually through the intestinal tract to ensure absorption. However, gastric ileus (decreased or absent peristalsis affecting the stomach but not the intestines), delayed gastric emptying, or gastric resection contraindicates gastric feedings.

Delegation Considerations

Administration of nasoenteral tube feeding can be delegated to assistive personnel (AP). However, a nurse must first verify tube placement and patency.

- Instruct AP about the prescribed rate to infuse the feeding.
- Instruct AP about any positioning restrictions for a specific client.
- Have AP report any difficulty infusing the feeding or any discomfort voiced by the client.
- Have AP report any gagging, paroxysms of coughing, or choking.

Equipment

- Disposable feeding bag and tubing or ready-to-hang system
- 60-ml Luer-Lok or catheter-tip syringe
- Stethoscope
- Infusion pump (required for continuous or intestinal feedings): use pump designed for tube feedings
- pH indicator strip
- Prescribed enteral feeding
- Clean gloves
- Equipment to obtain blood glucose by finger stick

Step	Rationale
1. Complete preprocedure protocol.	
2. Prepare feeding container to administer formula	

Step	Rationale
continuously (see Skill 23, step 3).	
3. For intermittent feeding, have syringe ready and be sure formula is at room temperature.	Cold formula causes gastric cramping.
4. Place client in high-Fowler's position, or elevate head of bed at least 30 degrees. For client forced to remain supine, place in reverse Trendelenburg position.	Elevated head helps prevent aspiration.
5. 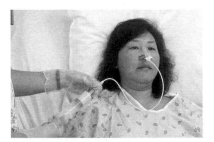 Determine tube placement (see Skill 43). Observe aspirate's appearance, and note pH measure.	Feedings instilled into a misplaced tube may cause serious injury or death. On occasion, color alone may differentiate gastric from intestinal placement because most intestinal aspirates are stained by bile to distinct yellow color, and most gastric aspirates are not (Metheny and others, 1999).
5. Check gastric residual volume (Fig. 24-1) before each feeding for intermittent feedings; every 4 to 12 hours.	For adults, a volume in excess of 200 ml for NG tubes should raise concern about intolerance; however, feedings may continue while further examinations are

Fig. 24-1 Check for gastric residual volume (small-bore tube).

Step	Rationale
	conducted (ASPEN, 2002; McClave and others, 1992, 1999; Murphy and Bickford, 1999).
a. Connect syringe to end of feeding tube, pull back slowly, and aspirate the total amount of gastric contents that may possibly be aspirated.	Fluids aspirated from stomach contain electrolytes that, if withheld, may cause electrolyte imbalances. Notify physician if residual volume is excessive, and request order regarding whether residual fluid should be returned to client.
b. Return aspirated contents to stomach unless volume is excessive (more than 100 ml). Verify with agency policy.	

7. Irrigate tube (see Skill 43).
8. Initiate feeding:

NURSE ALERT Do not add food coloring or dye to enteral nutrition to detect aspirated secretions. Dye may be systemically absorbed, interfere with Hemoccult testing of stool, and has safety risks (Maloney and Metheny, 2002; McClave and others, 2002; Metheny and others, 2002). Use of dye may cause death.

a. *Syringe or intermittent feeding:*	
(1) Pinch proximal end of feeding tube.	Prevents air from entering client's stomach.
(2) Remove plunger from syringe, and attach barrel of syringe to end of tube.	Barrel receives formula for instillation.
(3) Fill syringe with measured amount of formula. Release tube, and elevate syringe to no more than 45 cm	Height of syringe allows for safe, slow, gravity drainage of formula. Total delivery of bolus feedings may take several minutes, depending on amount of bolus. Administering feeding

Step	Rationale
(18 inches) above insertion site, and allow it to empty gradually by gravity. Repeat Steps (1) through (3) until prescribed amount has been delivered to client.	too quickly may cause abdominal discomfort to client or increase risk for aspiration.
(4) If a feeding bag is used, prime tubing and attach gavage tubing to end of feeding tube. Set rate by adjusting roller clamp on tubing. Allow bag to empty gradually over 30 to 60 minutes. Label bag with tube-feeding type, strength, and amount. Include date, time, and initials. Change bag every 24 hours.	Gradual emptying of tube feeding by gravity from syringe or feeding bag reduces risk of abdominal discomfort, vomiting, or diarrhea induced by bolus or too-rapid infusion of tube feedings. Helps decrease bacterial colonization.
b. *Continuous-drip method:*	
(1) Prime and hang feeding bag and tubing on feeding-pump pole.	Continuous feeding method is designed to deliver prescribed hourly rate of feeding. This method reduces risk of abdominal discomfort.
(2) Connect distal end of tubing to proximal end of feeding tube.	
(3) Connect tubing through infusion pump, and set rate.	Delivers continuous feeding at steady rate and pressure.

Step	Rationale

NURSE ALERT Maximum hang time for formula is 8 hours for an open system and 24 hours for a closed, ready-to-hang system (if it remains closed). Refer to manufacturer's guidelines.

Step	Rationale
9. Advance rate and concentration of tube feeding gradually (Box 24-1).	Helps prevent diarrhea and gastric intolerance to formula.
10. After intermittent infusion or at end of continuous infusion, irrigate nasogastric feeding tube (see Skill 43).	Provides client with source of water to maintain fluid and electrolyte balance. Clears tubing of formula.
11. When tube feedings are not being administered, cap or clamp proximal end of feeding tube.	Prevents air from entering stomach between feedings.
12. Rinse bag and tubing with warm water whenever feedings are interrupted. Use new administration set every 24 hours.	Rinsing bag and tubing with warm water clears old tube feedings and reduces bacterial growth.
13. Monitor finger-stick blood glucose (usually at least every 6 hours until maximum administration rate is reached and maintained for 24 hours).	Requires physician's order. Alerts nurse to client's tolerance of enteral nutrition. May require physician to revise type of formula administered.
14. Complete postprocedure protocol.	

Recording and Reporting

- Record amount and type of feeding, rate of infusion if continuous, client's response to tube feeding, patency of tube.
- Record volume of formula and any additional water on intake and output form.
- Report type of feeding, rate of infusion status of feeding tube, client's tolerance, and adverse effects.

BOX 24-1   Advancing the Rate of Tube Feeding

Intermittent

1. Start formula at full strength for isotonic formulas (300 to 400 mOsm) or at ordered concentration.

2. Infuse formula over at least 20 to 30 minutes via syringe or feeding container.

3. Begin feedings with no more than 150 to 250 ml at one time. Increase by 50 ml per feeding per day to achieve needed volume and calories in six to eight feedings. (NOTE: Concentrated formulas at full strength may be infused at slower rate until tolerance is achieved.)

Continuous

1. Start formula at full strength for isotonic formulas (300 to 400 mOsm) or at ordered concentration. Usually hypertonic formulas also are started at full strength but at a slower rate.

2. Begin infusion rate at designated rate.

3. Advance rate slowly (e.g., 10 to 20 ml/hr) per day to target rate if tolerated (tolerance indicated by absence of nausea and diarrhea, and low gastric residuals).

Unexpected Outcomes	Related Interventions
1. Gastric residual volume is excessive.	• Notify physician to determine if feedings need to be held. If feedings are held, reassess residual volume 1 hour after feeding is stopped to determine if volume has lessened or increased. If it has increased, make sure physician is aware. • Maintain client in Fowler's position; have head of bed elevated at least 45 degrees.
2. Client aspirates formula.	• Position on side with head down to promote drainage of food or fluid from mouth. • Suction airway (see Skills 70). • Anticipate chest x-ray to be ordered by doctor.
3. See Skill 23, Unexpected Outcomes.	

Epidural Analgesia

The term *intraspinal* refers to both the epidural space and intrathecal (subarachnoid) space that surround the spinal cord. It is safe to administer analgesics into these spaces. The epidural space is a potential space that extends from the foramen magnum to the sacral hiatus. Drugs administered in the epidural space can be distributed (1) by diffusion through the dura mater into the cerebrospinal fluid (CSF), where it acts directly on receptors in the dorsal horn of the spinal cord; (2) via blood vessels in the epidural space and delivered systemically; and/or (3) by means of absorption by fat in the epidural space, creating a depot where the drug is slowly released into the systemic circulation (Pasero, 2003).

Because opioids are delivered close to their site of action (central nervous system [CNS]), they have greater bioavailability and thus require much smaller doses to achieve adequate pain relief. Common opioids administered epidurally are morphine, hydromorphone (Dilaudid), fentanyl, and sufentanil. These opioids vary in their lipophilic (fat-loving) and hydrophilic (water-loving) properties, which alter absorption rate and duration of action.

A physician typically inserts an epidural catheter into the epidural space (Fig. 25-1) below the second lumbar vertebra, where the spinal cord ends; however, thoracic epidurals also may be inserted. When the catheter is intended for temporary or short-term use, it is usually not sutured in place and exits from the insertion site on the back (Fig. 25-2). By contrast, a catheter intended for permanent or long-term use is "tunneled" subcutaneously and exits on the side of the body or on the abdomen. Tunneling decreases the chance of infection or dislodging of the catheter. In both cases, the catheter is covered with a sterile occlusive dressing and secured to the client. The only way to ensure proper placement of an epidural catheter is radiologically.

Use of epidural opioids for pain control requires astute nursing observation and care. The catheter poses a threat to client safety because of its anatomical location, its potential for migration through the dura, and its proximity to spinal nerves and vessels. An epidural catheter migration into the subarachnoid space can produce medication levels too high for intrathecal use. You are responsible for assisting the client in obtaining pain control or relief, evaluating the analgesic effect, and intervening appropriately in the event of a complication or occurrence of side effects. Always question administering concurrent oral medications that are known to cause sedation and/or respiratory depression (e.g., muscle relaxants or anxiolytics). Obtain approval for

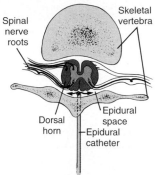

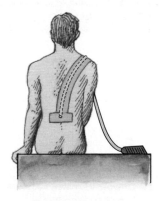

Fig. 25-1 Anatomical drawing of epidural space. (From Sinatra S: Spinal opioid analgesia: an overview. In Sinatra RS and others, editors: *Acute pain management*, St. Louis, 1992, Mosby.)

Fig. 25-2 Epidural catheter taped in place. (Courtesy AstraZeneca Pharmaceuticals, Wilmington, Del.)

their use from the health care professional managing the epidural analgesia.

Delegation Considerations

Administration of epidural anesthesia should not be delegated to assistive personnel (AP).

- Instruct AP to watch the insertion site when repositioning or ambulating clients, to prevent disruption of the catheter.
- Have AP report any catheter disconnection immediately.
- Instruct AP to immediately report any change in client status or comfort level.

Equipment

- Clean gloves
- Pre-diluted, preservative-free opioid or local anesthetic as prescribed by physician and prepared for use in intravenous (IV) infusion pump (usually prepared by pharmacy)
- 20-gauge needleless 3- to 5-ml syringe
- Infusion pump
- Infusion pump–compatible tubing without Y-ports; some infusion pumps have tubing color coded for intraspinal use

- Fitter needles
- Povidone-iodine swab
- Tape
- Label (for tubing)

Step	Rationale
1. Complete preprocedure protocol.	
2. ◤ See if catheter is secured to client's skin from back or front (Fig. 25-3). Check status of tubing and dressing.	Aids in preventing dislodging or migration of catheter.
3. Check physician's order for medication, dosage, and infusion method.	Medication administration is dependent nursing function and requires physician's prescription.
4. If continuous infusion, check infusion pump for proper calibration and operation, and check patency of tubing.	Ensures that client obtains prescribed analgesic dose. Kinked tubing will interrupt infusion.
5. Check client's identification bracelet and ask name.	Ensures that correct client receives ordered drug. At least two patient identifiers (neither to be patient's room number) are to be

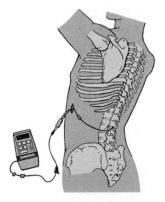

Fig. 25-3 External catheter connected to epidural catheter and an ambulatory infusion pump. (Courtesy Smiths Medical MD, Inc., St. Paul, Minn.)

Step	**Rationale**
	used whenever administering medications (JCAHO, 2004).
6. Attach "epidural line" label to infusion tubing.	Labeling helps ensure that medication is administered into correct line and into epidural space.
7. Select tubing *without* Y ports for continuous infusions.	Use of tubing without Y ports prevents accidental injection or infusion into epidural space of a medication meant for the vascular space.
8. Administer continuous infusion:	
a. Attach container of diluted, preservative-free medication to infusion pump tubing, and prime tubing (see Skill 52).	Tubing should be filled with solution and free of air bubbles to avoid air embolus.
b. Attach proximal end of tubing to pump and distal end to epidural catheter. Tape all connections. Start infusion.	Infusion pumps propel fluid through tubing. Taping maintains a secure, closed system to help prevent infection. A filter may be needed on tubing, depending on institutional policy.
c. Check infusion pump for proper calibration and operation. Many institutions have two nurses check settings.	Maintains patency and ensures that client is receiving proper dose and pain relief.
9. Administer bolus dose of medication:	
a. Draw up pre-diluted, preservative-free opioid solution through filter needle.	Preservative may be toxic to nerve tissue (Cosentino, 2000).
b. Change from filter needle to regular 20-gauge needleless adapter.	Prevents infusion of microscopic glass particles and allows medication to be injected.

Step	Rationale
c. Clean injection cap with povidone-iodine. (Do not use alcohol.)	Sterilizing injection port prevents inadvertent introduction of microorganisms into CNS. Alcohol causes pain and is toxic to neural tissue (Pasero, 2003).
d. Dry injection cap with sterile gauze.	Reduces possible injection of povidone-iodine.
e. Using a needleless system, attach syringe directly to injection cap. Aspirate.	Aspiration of more than 1 ml of clear fluid or bloody return means catheter may have migrated into subarachnoid space or into vessel (Pasero and others, 1999). Do not inject drug. Notify physician.
f. Inject opioid at rate of 1 ml over 30 seconds.	Slow injection prevents discomfort by lowering pressure exerted by fluid as it enters epidural space (Cox, 2001).
g. Remove syringe from injection cap. There is no need to flush with saline.	Catheter is in a space, not a blood vessel; thus flushing with saline is not required (McCaffery and Pasero, 1999).
h. Dispose of syringe in sharps container.	Prevents exposure to blood.
10. Observe for signs of adverse reactions to epidurally administered opioid or local analgesic.	Although pain is relieved with smaller doses and side effects are less severe with epidural opioid analgesic, side effects can still occur.
11. Observe respiratory rate, rhythm, depth, and pattern; and sedation level. Monitor respiratory rate and depth at least every 1 to 2 hours, depending on institutional policy.	Respiratory depression may result from epidural opioid use.
12. Complete postprocedure protocol.	

NURSE ALERT Be prepared to deliver an ampule of naloxone (Narcan), a strong opioid antagonist, 0.4 mg diluted in 9 ml of saline at 1 to 2 ml/min, if respirations fall below 8 breaths per minute and are shallow. Desired effect is to increase respirations, not reverse analgesia. Rapid reversal of opioids by Narcan could result in profound withdrawal, seizures, dysrhythmias, pulmonary edema, and severe pain (American Pain Society, 2003). Continue to assess respiratory status after Narcan administration because re-narcotization with resulting respiratory depression could occur (American Pain Society, 2003).

Recording and Reporting

- Record on appropriate medication record the drug, dose, and time begun and ended. Specify concentration and diluent.
- Record any supplemental analgesic requirements.
- Review pump settings and usage with personnel on the next shift.
- Record regular, periodic assessment of client's status in nurses' notes or flowsheets. Indicate vital signs, intake and output, sedation level, pain status, neurological status, status of epidural site, presence or absence of adverse reactions to medication, and presence or absence of complications resulting from placement and maintenance of epidural catheter.
- Report any adverse reactions or complications to physician.

Unexpected Outcomes	Related Interventions
1. Client states pain is still present.	• Check all tubing, connections, medication doses, and pump settings.
2. Client is sedated or not easily aroused.	• Stop epidural infusion. • Administer opioid reversing agent per physician order. • Monitor continuously until client is easily aroused.
3. Client experiences periods of apnea, or respirations are fewer than 8 breaths per minute, shallow, or irregular.	• Instruct client to take deep breaths. • Stop or reduce rate of infusion. • Notify physician. • Prepare to administer opioid reversing agent per physician order. • Monitor every 30 minutes until

Unexpected Outcomes	Related Interventions
	respirations are 8 or more and of adequate depth.
4. Client reports sudden headache. Clear drainage is present on epidural dressing or more than 1 ml of fluid can be aspirated from catheter.	• Stop infusion. • If receiving bolus doses, do not administer. • Notify physician.
5. Blood is present on epidural dressing or can be aspirated from catheter.	• Stop infusion. • Notify physician.

Eye Irrigation

Eye irrigation flushes out exudates, irritating solutions, or foreign particles. It is often performed in an emergency attempt to preserve vision. When a chemical or irritating substance contaminates the eyes, irrigate immediately with copious amounts of cool water for at least 15 minutes to minimize corneal damage (U.S. National Library of Medicine, 2003). Users of contact lenses or artificial eyes may need eye irrigation to flush out particles of dust or fibers from the eye or socket.

Delegation Considerations

The skill of eye irrigation may not be delegated to assistive personnel (AP).

Equipment

- Bath towel or waterproof pad
- Prescribed irrigation solution, usually 30 to 180 ml at 90° to 100° F (about 32° to 38° C)
- Sterile basin or bag for solution
- Soft bulb syringe, eyedropper, or intravenous (IV) tubing
- Emesis basin
- 4 × 4 inch gauze pads
- Disposable gloves

Step	Rationale
1. Complete preprocedure protocol.	
2. Observe eye for redness, tearing, discharge, and swelling.	Establishes baseline signs and symptoms.

NURSE ALERT Spasm of the eyelid or pain may make opening the eye difficult. Topical anesthetic eye drops or additional assistance may be necessary (Kuchelkorn and others, 2002).

3. Assist client to side-lying position on side of affected eye or supine position for simultaneous irrigation of both eyes.	Position facilitates flow of solution from inner to outer canthus, preventing contamination of unaffected eye and nasolacrimal duct.

Step	Rationale
4. [image] Remove any contact lens if possible.	Contact lens may have absorbed irritant, or it may prevent thorough irrigation. Lens may be lost if flushed out by irrigation.

NURSE ALERT In an emergency, such as first aid for a chemical burn, do not delay by removing the client's contact lens before irrigation (U.S. National Library of Medicine, 2003). Advise the client to consult physician before continuing to use contact lens.

5. Place towel just below client's face, and place emesis basin just below client's cheek.	Catches irrigation fluid.
6. Clean visible secretions or foreign material from eyelids and lashes, wiping from inner to outer canthus.	Minimizes transfer of material into eye during irrigation. Prevents secretions from entering nasolacrimal duct.
7. Gently retract eyelids. Hold open by applying pressure to orbit, not to eyeball.	Exposes eye and minimizes blinking.
8. Hold solution-filled bulb, dropper, or tubing approximately 1 inch (2.5 cm) from inner canthus.	Eye may be injured by direct contact with irrigation equipment.
9. Ask client to look toward brow. Gently irrigate with steady stream toward lower conjunctival sac (Fig. 26-1).	Minimizes force of stream on cornea. Flushes irritant out of eye and away from other eye and nasolacrimal duct.
10. Reinforce importance of procedure, and encourage client using calm, confident, soft voice.	Reduces anxiety.
11. Allow client to blink periodically.	Moves irritant from upper conjunctival sac.
12. Continue for prescribed volume and/or time or until secretions have been cleared.	Ensures complete removal of irritant.

Step	Rationale

Fig. 26-1 Irrigation of eye from inner to outer canthus.

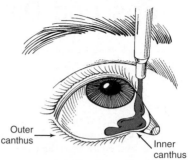

Outer canthus

Inner canthus

13. Blot excess moisture from eyelids and face with gauze or towel.

Removes moisture that may contain microbes or irritant. Promotes client comfort.

14. Inspect eye for reaction to light, accommodation, and eye movement.

Impaired reaction to light, accommodation, or movement may indicate injury.

15. Complete postprocedure protocol.

Recording and Reporting

- Record in nurses' notes condition of eye, type and amount of irrigation solution, duration of irrigation, and client's report of pain and visual symptoms.
- Report continuing symptoms of pain or blurred vision.

Unexpected Outcomes	Related Interventions
1. Anxiety	• Reinforce rationale for irrigation. • Allow client to close eye periodically during irrigation. • Seek extra assistance as needed to prevent injury.
2. Pain or foreign body sensation	• Advise client to close eye and avoid eye movement. • Immediately notify physician or eye care practitioner.

Eye Medications: Drops and Ointment

The eye is the most sensitive organ to which you apply medications. The cornea is richly supplied with sensitive nerve fibers. Use caution to prevent instilling medication directly onto the cornea. The conjunctival sac is much less sensitive and thus a more appropriate site for medication instillation. Eye medications come in a variety of concentrations. Instilling the wrong concentration may cause local irritation of eyes, as well as systemic effects. Certain eye medications, such as mydriatics and cycloplegics, temporarily blur a client's vision. Use of the wrong drug concentration can prolong these undesirable effects.

Delegation Considerations

The skill of administering eye medications should not be delegated to assistive personnel (AP).

- Instruct AP about potential side effects of medications to report.
- Instruct care providers in the potential for temporary visual impairment after administration of eye medications.

Equipment

- Medication bottle with sterile eye dropper, ointment tube, or medicated intraocular disk
- Cotton ball or tissue
- Washbasin filled with warm water and washcloth
- Eye patch and tape (optional)
- Clean gloves
- Medication administration record (MAR)

Step	Rationale
1. Complete preprocedure protocol.	
2. Check accuracy and completeness of each MAR with prescriber's written medication order. Check client's name, drug name and dosage, route of	Order sheet is most reliable source and only legal record of drugs client is to receive. Ensures that right drug is administered.

Step	Rationale
administration, and time for administration. Compare MAR with label of eye medication three times during preparation of medication.	
3. Check client's identification bracelet, and ask name.	Ensures that correct client receives medication. At least two patient identifiers (neither to be patient's room number) are to be used whenever administering medications (JCAHO, 2004).
4. ![icon] If eye drops are stored in refrigerator, rewarm to room temperature before administering.	Reduces irritation to eye caused by cold temperature of solution.
5. Ask client to lie supine or sit back in chair with head slightly hyperextended.	Position provides easy access to eye for medication instillation and minimizes drainage of medication through tear duct.

NURSE ALERT Do not hyperextend the neck of a client with cervical spine injury.

Step	Rationale
6. If crusts or drainage is present along eyelid margins or inner canthus, gently wash away. Soak any crusts that are dried and difficult to remove by applying damp washcloth or cotton ball over eye for few minutes. Always wipe clean from inner to outer canthus (Fig. 27-1).	Crusts or drainage harbor microorganisms. Soaking allows easy removal and prevents pressure from being applied directly over eye. Cleansing from inner to outer canthus avoids entrance of microorganisms into lacrimal duct.
7. Hold cotton ball or clean tissue in nondominant hand on client's cheekbone just below lower eyelid.	Cotton or tissue absorbs medication that escapes eye.

Step	**Rationale**

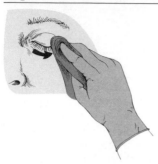

Fig. 27-1 Cleanse eye, washing from inner to outer canthus before administering drops or ointment.

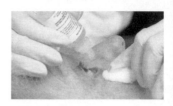

Fig. 27-2 Eye dropper held above conjunctival sac.

Step	Rationale
8. With tissue or cotton resting below lower lid, gently press downward with thumb or forefinger against bony orbit. Never press directly against client's eyeball.	Technique exposes lower conjunctival sac. Retraction against bony orbit prevents pressure and trauma to eyeball and prevents fingers from touching eye. Pressure to the eyeball may cause damage.
9. Ask client to look at ceiling, and explain steps to client.	Action moves sensitive cornea up and away from conjunctival sac and reduces stimulation of blink reflex. Explanation promotes client's cooperation.
10. Instill eye drops: a. With dominant hand resting on client's forehead, hold filled medication eye dropper approximately 1 to 2 cm ($\frac{1}{2}$ to $\frac{3}{4}$ inch) above conjunctival sac (Fig. 27-2).	Helps prevent accidental contact of eye dropper with eye structures, thus reducing risk of injury to eye and transfer of infection to dropper. Ophthalmic medications are sterile.
b. Drop prescribed number of medication drops into conjunctival sac.	Conjunctival sac normally holds 1 or 2 drops. Provides even distribution of medication across eye.

Step	Rationale
c. If client blinks or closes eye or if drops fall on outer lid margins, repeat procedure.	Therapeutic effect of drug is obtained only when drops enter conjunctival sac.
d. After instilling drops, ask client to close eye gently.	Distributes medication. Squinting eyelids forces medication from conjunctival sac.
e. When administering drugs that cause systemic effects, apply gentle pressure with clean tissue to client's nasolacrimal duct for 30 to 60 seconds.	Prevents overflow of medication into nasal and pharyngeal passages. Prevents absorption into systemic circulation.

11. Instill eye ointment:

a. Holding applicator above lower lid margin, apply thin ribbon of ointment evenly along inner edge of lower eyelid on conjunctiva (Fig. 27-3) from the inner canthus to outer canthus.	Distributes medication evenly across eye and lid margin.
b. Have client close eye and rub lid lightly in circular motion with cotton ball, if rubbing is not contraindicated.	Further distributes medication without traumatizing eye.

12. Intraocular disk:
    a. Application:

Fig. 27-3 Nurse applies ointment along the lower eyelid from the inner to outer canthus.

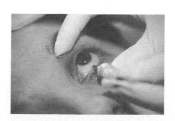

Step	Rationale
(1) Open package containing disk. Gently press your fingertip against disk so that it adheres to your finger. (NOTE: It may be necessary to moisten gloved finger with sterile saline.) Position convex side of disk on your fingertip.	Allows nurse to inspect disk for damage or deformity. Prepares disk for proper administration.
(2) With your other hand, gently pull client's lower eyelid away from clinet's eye. Ask client to look up.	Prepares conjunctival sac for receiving medicated disk.
(3) Place disk in conjunctival sac, so that it floats on sclera between iris and lower eyelid (Fig. 27-4).	Ensures delivery of medication.
(4) Pull client's lower eyelid out and over disk (Fig. 27-5).	Ensures accurate medication delivery.

NURSE ALERT You should not be able to see the disk at this time. Repeat Step (e) if you can see the disk.

   b. Removal:
      (1) Gently pull on client's lower eyelid to expose disk.
      (2) Using your forefinger and

Step	**Rationale**

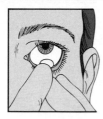

Fig. 27-4   Place intraocular disk in the conjunctival sac between the iris and the lower eyelid.

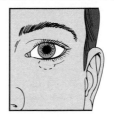

Fig. 27-5   Gently pull the client's lower eyelid over the disk.

thumb of your opposite hand, pinch disk and lift it out of client's eye (Fig. 27-6).	
13. If excess medication is on eyelid, gently wipe it from inner to outer canthus.	Promotes comfort and prevents trauma to eye.
14. If client had eye patch, apply clean one by placing it over affected eye so entire eye is covered. Tape securely without applying pressure to eye.	Clean eye patch reduces chance of infection.
15. Clients experienced in self-instillation may be allowed to give drops under nurse's supervision (check agency policy).	Retains client's independence.

Fig. 27-6   Carefully pinch the disk to remove it from the client's eye.

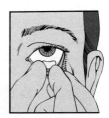

Step	Rationale
16. Complete postprocedure protocol.	
17. Ask client to discuss purpose, action, side effects, and technique of administration and have client demonstrate self-administration of next dose.	Determines client's level of understanding. Provides feedback regarding competency with skill.

Recording and Reporting

- Immediately after administration, record on MAR the drug, concentration, number of drops, time of administration, and eye (left, right, or both) that received medication. Do not chart medication administration until *after* it is given to client.
- If drug is withheld, record reason in nurses' notes. Circle time drug normally would have been given on MAR (or follow institution's policy for noting withheld doses).
- Record appearance of eye in nurses' notes.
- Report adverse effects/client response and/or withheld drugs to nurse in charge or physician.

Unexpected Outcomes	Related Interventions
1. Client complains of burning or pain or experiences local side effects (e.g., headache, bloodshot eyes, local eye irritation).	• Notify prescriber for possible adjustment in medication type and dosage.
2. Client experiences systemic effects from drops (e.g., increased heart rate and blood pressure from epinephrine, decreased heart rate and blood pressure from timolol).	• Notify prescriber immediately. • Remain with client. • Withhold further doses. • Ophthalmic anesthetics and antibiotics may cause the same type of adverse reactions as systemically administered drugs (e.g., anaphylaxis).

Fall Prevention in a Health Care Facility

Falls are a common cause of injury in hospitalized clients. In 2001 more than 1.6 million older adults were treated in emergency departments for fall-related injuries, and nearly 388,000 were hospitalized (CDC, 2003). The injuries that result from falls reduce a person's mobility and independence (Sterling and others, 2001). Frail older adults with impaired strength, mobility, balance, and endurance are twice as likely to fall as healthier persons of the same age (CDC, 2003). Because of the frequency of falls in health care facilities, the Joint Commission on Accreditation of Healthcare Organizations (JCAHO) (2004) has established patient safety goals for fall prevention.

Accurately assess clients and their environment for fall risk factors. In this way, you may institute measures to reduce and/or eliminate hazards before client injury occurs. In the hospital setting, risk assessment tools (Box 28-1) are useful in identifying clients at risk for falling. Assess the client's physical status, mental status, medications, and devices used to ambulate to determine the degree of risk.

Routine safety measures include explaining the call light/intercom system to the client and family. Be sure to use side rails appropriately. A full set of raised side rails (two to a bed or four to a bed) may be considered a physical restraint. Raising only one of two or three of four side rails gives clients room to exit a bed safely and to maneuver within the bed. Always lock beds and wheelchairs, and keep beds in the low position after providing client care. Only use wheelchairs to transport clients. For clients who attempt to ambulate without assistance, use an electronic bed or chair alarm device. These devices warn nursing staff that a client is attempting to leave the bed or a chair unassisted.

Delegation Considerations

Assessment of a client's risk for falling should not be delegated to assistive personnel (AP). However, the skills necessary to prevent falls can be delegated.

- Inform AP about a client's mobility limitations and any specific measures to minimize risks.
- Instruct AP on any specific environmental safety precautions.

BOX 28-1 Risk for Falls Assessment Tools

Tool 1: Risk Assessment Tool for Falls

DIRECTIONS: Place a check mark in front of elements that apply to your client. The decision as to whether a client is at risk for falls is based on your nursing judgment.

GUIDELINE: A client who has a check mark in front of an element with an asterisk (*) or four or more of the other elements would be identified as at risk for falls.

General data

- Age over 60
- History of falls before admission*
- Postoperative/admitted for surgery
- Smoker

Physical condition

- Dizziness/imbalance
- Unsteady gait
- Diseases/other problems affecting weight-bearing joints
- Weakness
- Paresis
- Seizure disorder
- Impairment of vision
- Impairment of hearing
- Diarrhea
- Urinary frequency

Mental status

- Confusion/disorientation*
- Impaired memory or judgment
- Inability to understand or follow directions

Medications

- Diuretics or diuretic effects
- Hypotensive or central nervous system suppressants (e.g., narcotic, sedative, psychotropic, hypnotic, tranquilizer, antihypertensive, antidepressant)
- Medication that increases gastrointestinal motility (e.g., laxative, enema)

BOX 28-1   Risk for Falls Assessment Tools—cont'd

Ambulatory devices used
- Cane
- Crutches
- Walker
- Wheelchair
- Geriatric (Geri) chair
- Braces

Tool 2: Reassessment Is Safe "Kare" (RISK) Tool

DIRECTIONS: Place a check mark in front of any element that applies to your client. A client who has a check mark in front of any of the first four elements would be identified as at risk for falls. In addition, when a high-risk client has a check mark in front of the element "Use of a wheelchair," the client is considered to be at greater risk for falls.
- Unsteady gait/dizziness/imbalance
- Impaired memory or judgment
- Weakness
- History of falls
- Use of a wheelchair

From *Rehabilitation Nursing*, 16(2), 68. Used with permission of Association of Rehabilitation Nurses, 4700 W. Lake Arenue, Glenview, IL 60065-1485. Copyright ©1991.

Equipment

- A risk assessment tool for falls
- Hospital bed with side rails
- Call light

Step	Rationale
1. Assess older adult directly, and review medical history for physiological alterations that increase risk of falling (e.g., impaired memory and cognition, osteoporosis, osteoarthritis, decreased hearing, decreased night vision, cataracts or	Physiological alterations predispose client to falls (e.g., postmenopausal woman is prone to osteoporosis and therefore at risk of breaking hip or ankle when walking: fall results from stress fracture; fracture is not caused by fall).

Step	Rationale
glaucoma, or orthostatic) hypotension.	
2. Review client's medication history (including over-the-counter medications) for use of diuretics, antihypertensives, psychotropics, and polypharmacy (use of multiple medications).	Medications may cause physical or cognitive effects that lead to falls.
3. Assess risk factors in health care facility that pose threat to client's safety (e.g., improperly lighted room, obstructed walkway, clutter of supplies and equipment).	Provides opportunity to decrease risk of accidents.
4. Perform timed "Get Up and Go" test, which involves looking for unsteadiness as client gets up from chair without using his or her arms, walks few feet, and returns.	Examination easily incorporated into clinical care is useful in screening client for altered balance and gait (Tinetti, 2003).
5. Determine if client has had history of falls or other injuries within home. Assess the acronym *SPLATT* (Lueckenotte, 2000): **S**ymptoms at time of fall **P**revious fall **L**ocation of fall **A**ctivity at time of fall **T**ime of fall **T**rauma postfall	Key symptoms can be helpful in identifying cause of fall. Onset, location, and activity associated with fall provide further details on causative factors and how future falls might be prevented.
6. Determine what client knows about risks for falling and steps he or she takes to prevent falls.	Client's own knowledge of risks influences ability to take necessary precautions in reducing falls.
7. Complete preprocedure protocol.	

Step	**Rationale**
8. Adjust bed to proper height, and lower side rail on side of client contact.	Allows for proper body mechanics and prevents injury. Proper height of bed allows ambulatory client to get in and out of bed easily and safely.
9. Call light/intercom system:	
a. Explain and demonstrate how to turn call light/intercom system on and off at bedside and in bathroom.	Knowledge of location and use of call light is essential to client safety.
b. Consistently secure call light/intercom system to accessible location.	Ensures that client can reach immediately when needed.
10. Side rails:	
a. Explain to client and family two main reasons for using side rails: preventing falls and turning self in bed.	Promotes client and family cooperation.
b. Check agency policies regarding side rail use.	Side rails are a restraint device when used to prevent ambulatory client from getting out of bed (Centers for Medicaid and Medicare Services [CMS], 2004).
c. Keep top two side rails up and two lower side rails down, and bed in low position with bed wheels locked when client care is not being administered and client is older adult, weak, confused, sedated, or sleeping.	Prevents client from falling out of bed. With bed in low position, if client climbs out of bed and falls, trauma may be reduced.
d. Leave one side rail up and one down on side where oriented and ambulatory client gets out of bed.	Getting into bed is easier; client can use side rail to position self once in bed.

Step	Rationale
11. Provide clear instructions to client and family regarding any mobility restrictions, ambulation and transfer techniques.	Promotes client independence and understanding of treatment plan.
12. Explain to client specific safety measures to prevent falls (e.g., wear well-fitting, flat footwear with nonskid soles; dangle feet for a few minutes before standing; walk slowly; ask for help if dizzy or weak).	Promotes client understanding and cooperation. Dangling provides adjustment to orthostatic hypotension, allowing blood pressure to stabilize before ambulating (see Skill 9).
13. Make sure ambulatory client's pathway to bathroom facilities is clear.	Eliminates potential hazards and promotes client independence.
14. Provide adequate, non-glare lighting throughout room.	Reduces likelihood of falling over objects or bumping into them. Glare is major problem for older adults.
15. Remove unnecessary objects from rooms (e.g., suction machines, extra intravenous [IV] poles).	Eliminates potential hazards when client gets out of bed or ambulates.
16. Arrange necessary objects in logical way, placing them consistently in easy-to-reach locations.	Placing items such as eyeglasses, dentures, hearing aid, and telephone within client's reach allows client to carry out self-care activities safely.
17. Confer with physical therapy personnel on feasibility of gait training and muscle-strengthening exercise.	Single intervention strategies that have proved effective among older adults at risk for falling include gait and exercise training (Tinetti, 2003).
18. Confer with physician or primary care provider about possibility of adjusting number of medications client receives to reduce side effects and interactions.	Number of medications client receives can be reduced safely if balance is achieved between benefits of medications and risk of adverse events (Tinetti, 2003).

Step	Rationale
19. Observe client's immediate environment for presence of hazards.	Ensures that there are no obstacles or barriers to client's freedom of movement.
20. Evaluate need for assistive devices such as walker, cane, or bedside commode (see Skill 5).	Assistive device may provide more stability and help client assume a more active role.
21. Ask client or family member to identify safety risks.	Ensures that client is able to identify risks to safety.

Recording and Reporting

- On risk assessment tool or nurses' notes, record specific risks to client safety and interventions to reduce them.
- Report to all health care personnel specific risks to client's safety and measures taken to minimize risks.
- Document relevant information related to instructions given to client and family and other safety measures employed (e.g., side rails, call light, electronic monitoring device).
- If client suffers a fall, inform physician. Document what occurred, including description of fall as given by client or witness. Be sure to include any injuries noted, tests or treatments given, follow-up care, and additional safety precautions taken after fall.

Unexpected Outcomes	Related Interventions
1. Client is unable to identify safety risks.	• Reinforce identified risks with client, or involve family member/friend and review safety measures needed to prevent fall.
2. Client suffers fall despite all measures taken. Safety measures were unsuccessful.	• Nurse must attend to client's immediate physical needs, inform physician of fall and any apparent injury, reassess client's environment to ensure that environment is free of safety hazards, complete incident report, and communicate to other care providers that client is at risk for falls.

Fecal Impaction: Removing Digitally

Fecal impaction, the inability to pass a hard collection of stool, occurs in all age groups. Physically and mentally incapacitated persons and institutionalized older adult clients are at greatest risk. Symptoms of fecal impaction include constipation, rectal discomfort, anorexia, nausea, vomiting, abdominal pain, diarrhea (around the impacted stool), and urinary frequency. This procedure can be very uncomfortable and embarrassing for the client. Excessive rectal manipulation may cause irritation to the mucosa, bleeding, and stimulation of the vagus nerve, which can cause a reflex slowing of the heart rate.

Delegation Considerations

This skill should not be delegated to assistive personnel (AP). In some institutions only physicians perform this procedure.

- Instruct AP to observe any evacuated stool for color and consistency.
- Instruct AP to immediately report any signs of blood or bloody mucous discharge to the nurse for further assessment.

Equipment

- Clean gloves
- Water-soluble local anesthetic lubricant (NOTE: Some institutions require use of water-soluble lubricant without anesthetic when nurse performs procedure.)
- Waterproof, absorbent pads
- Bedpan
- Bedpan cover
- Bath blanket
- Washbasin, washcloths, towels, and soap

NURSE ALERT Because of the potential to stimulate the sacral branch of the vagus nerve, clients with a history of dysrhythmia or heart disease have a greater risk of changes in heart rhythm. Be sure to monitor client's pulse before and during procedure. This procedure may be contraindicated in cardiac clients; if in doubt, verify with physician.

Step	Rationale
1. Complete preprocedure protocol.	Distention can contribute to constipation.
2. Check client's record to determine if physician's order exists to remove stool manually.	Because this procedure may involve excessive stimulation of vagus nerve, physician's order must be written in client's record before nurse can perform procedure.
3. Obtain assistance to help change client's position, if necessary. Raise bed horizontally to comfortable working height.	Promotes client safety and use of good body mechanics by nurse.
4. Keeping far side rail raised, assist client to left side-lying position with knees flexed and back toward nurse.	Promotes client safety. Provides access to rectum.
5. With near side rail lowered, drape client's trunk and lower extremities with bath blanket and place waterproof pad under client's buttocks.	Prevents unnecessary exposure.
6. Place bedpan next to client.	Bedpan is receptacle for stool.
7. ⚡ Lubricate gloved index finger and middle finger of dominant hand with anesthetic lubricant.	Permits smooth insertion of finger into anus and rectum.

NURSE ALERT Observe for the presence of perianal skin irritation. Presence of such indicates the need for postprocedure skin care to the perianal region to reduce pain during subsequent bowel elimination.

8. Instruct client to take slow, deep breaths, and gradually and gently insert gloved index finger and feel anus relax around finger. Then insert middle finger.	Slow, deep breaths may help relax client. Gradual insertion of index finger helps dilate anal sphincter.

Step	Rationale
9. Gradually advance fingers slowly along rectal wall toward umbilicus.	Allows nurse to reach impacted stool high in rectum.
10. Gently loosen fecal mass by moving fingers in scissors motion to fragment fecal mass. Work fingers into hardened mass.	Loosening and penetrating mass allows nurse to remove it in small pieces, resulting in less discomfort to client.
11. Work stool downward toward end of rectum. Remove small sections of feces, and discard into bedpan.	Prevents need to force finger up into rectum and minimizes trauma to mucosa.
12. Periodically assess heart rate, and look for signs of fatigue.	Vagal stimulation slows heart rate and may cause dysrhythmia. Procedure may exhaust client.

NURSE ALERT   Stop the procedure if heart rate drops or rhythm changes from the client's baseline.

Step	Rationale
13. Continue to clear rectum of feces, and allow client to rest at intervals.	Rest improves client's tolerance of procedure, allowing heart rate to slow.
14. Remove bedpan, and inspect feces for color and consistency. Dispose of feces. Remove gloves by turning inside out and discarding in proper receptacle.	Determines charactor of stool.
15. Assist client to toilet or clean bedpan. (Procedure may be followed by enema or cathartic.)	Disimpaction may stimulate defecation reflex.
16. Complete postprocedure protocol.	
17. Reassess vital signs and monitor client for 1 hour for bradycardia.	Determines extent of vagal stimulation.

Recording and Reporting

- Record client's tolerance to procedure, amount and consistency of stool removed, and adverse effects.
- Report any adverse effects to nurse in charge or physician.

Unexpected Outcomes	Related Interventions
1. Client experiences bleeding from rectum.	• Assess anal and perianal region for source of bleeding. • Stop if bleeding is excessive.
2. Changes from baseline vital signs occur.	• Stop procedure, and retake vital signs. • Notify prescriber if vital signs remain altered.
3. Diarrheal stool is present.	• Assess client for continuing impaction. • Administer suppositories or enemas as ordered.

Hypothermia and Hyperthermia Blankets

Clients can have high, prolonged fevers from infectious and neurological diseases and as side effects from anesthesia. When the client presents with hyperthermia from injury to the anterior hypothalamus or as a side effect of anesthesia, the application of a hypothermia (cooling) blanket is recommended (Nicoll, 2002). Hypothermia blankets are fluid-filled, rubberized blankets that circulate cooled solution (usually distilled water) through the blanket. When placed on top of the client, the cooling blanket reduces the client's body temperature. A hypothermia (cooling) blanket is not recommended in caring for the client with an infectious fever (Nicoll, 2002).

Conversely, clients whose body temperature is abnormally low because of extreme exposure to cold or because of hypothermia induced for neurological or cardiac surgery require a hyperthermia (warming) blanket to return the body to near-normal temperature (Nicoll, 2002). In the case of hyperthermia or rewarming therapy, a warmed solution is circulated through the blanket to help return the client's body temperature to normal.

Delegation Considerations

This skill may be delegated to assistive personnel (AP). Initially assess the client and explain the purpose of the treatment. If there are no risks or complications, this skill can be delegated.

- Caution AP to maintain proper temperature of the application throughout the treatment and to discontinue the application as specified in the physician's order.
- Caution AP to inform the nurse if client develops shivering or redness to the skin.
- Instruct AP to report when treatment is complete so that the client's response can be evaluated.

Equipment

- Hypothermia or hyperthermia blanket with control panel and rectal probe
- Sheet or thin bath blanket
- Distilled water to fill the units if necessary

- Disposable gloves
- Rectal thermometer

Step	Rationale
1. Complete preprocedure protocol.	
2. Prepare blanket according to agency policy and manufacturer's instructions.	Agencies have specific policies as to who should maintain equipment in functional order. Each type of blanket varies from one manufacturer to another. Manufacturer's instructions are located on machine. Read before using.
3. ✋ Measure temperature, pulse, respirations, and blood pressure.	Provides baseline for determining response to therapy.
4. Apply lanolin or mixture of lanolin and cold cream to client's skin where it will touch blanket.	Helps protect skin from heat and cold sensations.
5. Turn on blanket, and observe that cool or warm light is on. Precool or prewarm blanket, setting pad temperature to desired level.	Verifies that blanket is correctly set to assist in reducing (cool) or increasing (warm) client's body temperature. Prepares blanket for prescribed therapy.
6. Verify that pad temperature limits are set at desired safety ranges.	Safety ranges prevent excessive cooling or warming. Blanket automatically shuts off when preset body temperature is achieved.
7. Cover hypothermia or hyperthermia blanket with thin sheet or bath blanket.	Protects client's skin from direct contact with blanket, thus reducing risk of injury to skin. Sheet or blanket covers plastic and provides insulation between client and appliance.
8. Position hypothermia or hyperthermia blanket on top of client.	Provides wide distribution of blanket against client's skin.

Step	Rationale

NURSE ALERT When using a blanket for hypothermia, the client has the potential to develop pressure ulcers because of decreased blood flow in the skin.

a. Wrap client's hands and feet in gauze.	Reduces risk of thermal injury to body's distal areas.
b. Wrap scrotum with towels.	Protects sensitive tissue from direct contact with cold.
9. Lubricate rectal probe, and insert into client's rectum.	When using hypothermia or hyperthermia blanket, it is imperative that nurse continuously monitor client's core interior (rectal) temperature.
10. Turn and position client regularly to protect from pressure ulcer development and impaired body alignment (see Skill 57). Keep linens free of perspiration and condensation.	Client has increased risk of pressure ulcer development because of skin moisture created by blanket and client's body temperature.
11. Double-check fluid thermometer on control panel of blanket before leaving room.	Verifies that pad temperature is maintained at desired level.
12. Complete postprocedure protocol.	

NURSE ALERT It is generally accepted to discontinue hypothermia treatment when the client's core temperature is 1° F above desired temperature.

Recording and Reporting

- Record baseline data: vital signs, neurological and mental status, status of peripheral circulation and skin integrity when therapy was initiated.
- Note type of hyperthermia-hypothermia unit used; control settings (manual or automatic, and temperature settings); date, time, duration, and client's tolerance of treatment.

Step	Rationale

- Chart on temperature graph repeated measurements of vital signs to document response to therapy.
- Report any unexpected outcome to physician.

Unexpected Outcomes	Related Interventions
1. Client's core body temperature decreases or rises rapidly.	• Adjust blanket temperature no more than 1° F every 15 minutes to avoid complications.
2. Client's core temperature remains unchanged.	• Client may need hypothermic or hyperthermic treatment of additional sites, such as axilla, groin, and neck, in addition to those covered by blanket. • Discuss use of an antipyretic with physician.
3. Client begins to shiver.	• Adjust temperature to more comfortable range, and assess if shivering decreases. • If shivering continues, stop treatment and notify physician.
4. Skin breaks down from frostbite or burn from blanket.	• Stop treatment. • Notify physician.

Incentive Spirometry

Incentive spirometry assists the client in deep breathing. As a nurse, you use an incentive spirometer (IS) for clients after abdominal or thoracic surgery to reduce the incidence of postoperative pulmonary atelectasis. The use of IS is especially important in clients with underlying pulmonary diseases because of their risk for postoperative pneumonia (Snow and others, 2001).

Delegation Considerations

This skill may be delegated to assistive personnel (AP).

- Inform AP of the client's target goal for spirometry.
- Instruct AP to immediately inform the nurse if client develops chest pain, excessive sputum production, and fever.

Equipment

- Flow-oriented IS or volume-oriented IS

Step	Rationale

NURSE ALERT Incentive spirometry is usually contraindicated in clients with flail chest. These clients require other respiratory maneuvers to correct asymmetrical chest wall motion. Clients who may experience difficulty with incentive spirometry include those who are confused, malnourished, or cognitively impaired and those who lack necessary motor skills.

Step	Rationale
1. Complete preprocedure protocol.	
2. Indicate to client where on spirometer is target volume.	Clients are encouraged to "do better" with each breath and to meet or exceed target volume. When clients have visual target, they can gauge their improvement.
3. Position client in semi-Fowler's or high-Fowler's position.	Promotes optimal lung expansion during respiratory maneuver.
4. Instruct client to place lips completely over mouthpiece.	Showing client to correctly place mouthpiece is reliable technique for teaching psychomotor skill and enables client to ask questions.

Step	Rationale
5. Instruct client to take slow, deep breath and maintain constant flow, like pulling through straw. When maximal inspiration is reached, client should hold breath for 2 to 5 seconds and then exhale slowly.	Maintains maximal inspiration; reduces risk of progressive collapse of individual alveoli.

NURSE ALERT Clients with chronic obstructive pulmonary disease (COPD) may be able to hold their breath for only 2 to 3 seconds. Encourage clients to do their best and to try to extend the duration of breath holding. Allow clients to rest between incentive spirometry breaths to prevent hyperventilation and fatigue.

Step	Rationale
6. Have client repeat maneuver until goals are achieved.	Ensures correct use of spirometer and client's understanding of use.
7. Complete postprocedure protocol.	

Recording and Reporting

- Record lung sounds before and after incentive spirometry, frequency of incentive spirometry use, volumes achieved, and any adverse effects.
- Report any changes in respiratory assessment or client's inability to use incentive spirometry.

Unexpected Outcomes	Related Interventions
1. Client is unable to achieve incentive spirometry target volume.	• Encourage client to attempt incentive spirometry more frequently, followed by rest periods. • Teach client how to splint and protect incision sites during deep breathing.
2. Client has decreased lung expansion and/or abnormal breath sounds.	• Teach client cough-control exercises. • Provide assistance with suctioning if client cannot effectively cough up secretions.

Intradermal Injections

Intradermal injections are for skin testing, for example, in tuberculin screening and allergy tests. Because these medications are potent, they are injected into the dermis, where blood supply is reduced and drug absorption occurs slowly. A client may have an anaphylactic reaction if the medications enter the client's circulation too rapidly. Intradermal sites should be free of lesions and injuries and should be relatively hairless. The inner forearm and upper back are ideal locations. To administer an injection intradermally, use a tuberculin (TB) or small syringe with a short (⅜- to ⅝-inch), fine gauge (25 to 27) needle. The angle of insertion for an intradermal injection is 5 to 15 degrees (Fig. 32-1). Inject only small amounts of medication (0.01 to 0.1 ml) intradermally.

Delegation Considerations

Administering intradermal injections should not be delegated to assistive personnel (AP).

- Instruct AP about potential medication side effects and to report their occurrence to the nurse.
- Instruct AP about informing the nurse of any change in client's condition, including change in vital signs or level of consciousness.

Equipment

- 1-ml tuberculin syringe with preattached 25- or 27-gauge needle
- Small gauze pad and/or alcohol swab
- Vial or ampule of skin test solution
- Clean gloves
- Medication administration record (MAR) or computer printout
- Skin pencil (optional)

Step	Rationale
1. Complete preprocedure protocol.	
2. Assemble supplies in medication room.	Reduces transfer of microorganisms.
3. Check accuracy and completeness of MAR with prescriber's written medication order. Check client's name, drug name and dosage, route of	Verifies correct medication.

Step	**Rationale**

Fig. 32-1
Intradermal needle
tip inserted into
dermis.

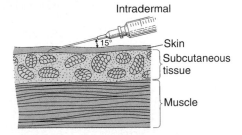

Intradermal

Skin
Subcutaneous
tissue
Muscle

administration, and time of administration. Check MAR or computer printout.	
4. Check name of medication on vial/ampule label against MAR.	First check of label ensures that client receives correct medication.
5. Check medication's expiration date.	Medications that have expired should not be used because potency of medications changes when medications become outdated.
6. Prepare correct dose from vial or ampule (see Skill 51). Check dose carefully and compare MAR with prepared drug label.	Ensures that medication is sterile. Second check of label ensures that dose is accurate and client receives correct medication.
7. Identify client by checking identification bracelet and asking client's name. Compare with MAR.	Ensures that correct client receives ordered drug. At least two patient identifiers (neither to be patient's room number) are to be used when administering medications (JCAHO, 2004).
8. Explain steps of procedure, and tell client that injection will cause a slight burning or sting.	Helps minimize client's anxiety.
9. ⬛ Select appropriate injection site. Inspect skin surface over sites for	Injection sites should be free of abnormalities that may interfere with drug absorption.

Step	Rationale
bruises, inflammation, or edema. Note lesions or discolorations of skin. If possible, select a site three to four finger widths below antecubital space and one hand width above wrist (CDC, 2004). If forearm cannot be used, inspect upper back. If necessary, sites appropriate for subcutaneous injections (see Skill 68) can be used.	Intradermal site should be clear so that results of skin test can be seen and interpreted correctly.
10. Assist client to comfortable position. Extend and support elbow and forearm on flat surface if using arm.	Stabilizes injection site for easiest accessibility.
11. Cleanse site with antiseptic swab. Apply swab at center of site, and rotate outward in circular direction for about 5 cm (2 inches).	Mechanical action of swab removes secretions containing microorganisms.
12. Hold swab or square of sterile gauze between third and fourth fingers of nondominant hand.	Gauze or swab remains readily accessible when needle is withdrawn.
13. Remove needle cap or sheath from needle by pulling it straight off.	Keeping needle from touching sides of cap prevents contamination.
14. Hold syringe between thumb and forefinger of dominant hand with bevel of needle pointing up.	Smooth injection requires proper manipulation of syringe parts. With bevel up, medication is less likely to be deposited into tissues below dermis.
15. With nondominant hand, stretch skin over site with forefinger or thumb.	Needle pierces tight skin more easily.
16. With needle almost against client's skin, insert it slowly at 5- to 15-degree angle	Ensures that needle tip is in dermis. Inaccurate results will be obtained if solution is not

Step	Rationale

until resistance is felt. Then advance needle through epidermis to approximately 3 mm (⅛ inch) below skin surface. Needle tip can be seen through skin.

injected at correct angle and depth (CDC, 2004).

17. Inject medication slowly. Normally, resistance is felt. If not, needle is too deep; remove and begin again.

Slow injection minimizes discomfort at site. Dermal layer is tight and does not expand easily when solution is injected.

NURSE ALERT It is not necessary to aspirate because dermis is relatively avascular.

18. While injecting medication, notice that small bleb approximately 6 mm (¼ inch) in diameter (resembling mosquito bite) appears on skin's surface (Fig. 32-2).

Bleb indicates that medication is deposited in dermis.

19. Withdraw needle while applying alcohol swab or gauze gently over site.

Support of tissue around injection site minimizes discomfort during needle withdrawal.

20. Do not massage site or apply bandage to site.

Massage or pressure to site may disperse medication into underlying tissue layers and alter test results.

21. Use skin pencil, and draw circle around perimeter of injection site. Read site within appropriate amount

Results of skin testing are determined at various times, based on type of medication used or type of skin testing.

Fig. 32-2 Injection creates small bleb.

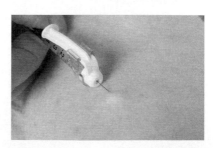

Step	Rationale
of time, designated by type of medication or skin test given.	Refer to manufacturer's directions to determine when to read test's results.
22. Complete postprocedure protocol.	

NURSE ALERT Read TB test at 48 to 72 hours. Positive TB reaction is indicated by induration (hard, dense, raised area) of skin around injection site of:

- 15 mm or more in clients with no known risk factors for TB
- 10 mm or more in clients who are recent immigrants; injection drug users; residents and employees of high-risk settings; clients with certain chronic illnesses; children younger than 4 years; and infants, children, and adolescents exposed to high-risk adults
- 5 mm or more in clients who are human immunodeficiency virus (HIV) positive, immunocompromised clients, or clients recently exposed to TB (CDC, 2004)

Recording and Reporting

- Record on MAR the amount and type of testing substance and date and time.
- Record in nurses' notes the area of injection and appearance of skin.
- Report any undesirable effects from medication to client's health care provider, and document adverse effects.

Unexpected Outcomes	Related Interventions
1. Raised, reddened, or hard zone forms around test site (induration), indicating sensitivity to injected allergen (positive TB test).	• Document results, and notify client's health care provider.
2. Onset of allergic reaction develops within minutes.	• Follow institutional policy or guidelines for appropriate response to allergic reactions, and notify client's health care provider.

Intramuscular Injections

An intramuscular (IM) injection deposits medication into deep muscle tissue. Because muscles have a rich blood supply, injections given IM absorb faster when compared with the subcutaneous (Sub-Q) route, which has a poor vascular supply (McKenry and Salerno, 2003).

The injection site used for IM injections is the most predictive factor associated with complications (Nicoll and Hesby, 2002). To avoid these complications, assess the client's age, the medication type, and the medication volume when selecting the appropriate injection site. The ventrogluteal site has been shown to be the safe site for infants, children, and adults (Nicoll and Hesby, 2002; Hockenberry and others, 2003). The dorsogluteal site has been a traditional site for IM injection. However, studies have demonstrated that the exact location of the sciatic nerve varies from one person to another. If a needle hits the sciatic nerve, the client may experience permanent or partial paralysis of the involved leg. Therefore, **do not** use the dorsogluteal site for IM injections (Nicoll and Hesby, 2002).

You can administer most immunizations and parenteral medications mixed in aqueous solutions using a 22- to 27-gauge 1- to $1^1/_2$-inch needle. However, if medications are oil-based or more viscous, use an 18- to 25-gauge needle (Nicoll and Hesby, 2002). An older adult or cachectic client may require a shorter, smaller-gauge 1- to $1^1/_2$-inch needle because of muscle atrophy. Infants younger than 4 months require a $^5/_8$-inch needle. For infants older than 4 months, a 1-inch needle is acceptable. For well-developed children through adolescence, use a $^5/_8$-inch needle for deltoid injections and a 1-inch needle for ventrogluteal injections (Hockenberry and others, 2003).

Delegation Considerations

The skill of administering IM medications should not be delegated to assistive personnel (AP).

- Instruct AP about potential medication side effects to report or client's report of pain at the injection site.
- Have AP report to the nurse any changes in the client's condition including change in vital signs or level of consciousness.

Equipment

- Syringe with vial access device or filter needle: 2 to 3 ml for adult; 0.5 to 1 ml for infants and small children

- Needle, length corresponding to site of injection and age of client according to the following guidelines (Nicoll and Hesby, 2002):
  - Infants and children: $\frac{5}{8}$ to 1 inch (based on size of child)
  - Vastus lateralis (adults): 1 to $1\frac{1}{2}$ inch
  - Deltoid (adults): 1 to $1\frac{1}{2}$ inch
  - Ventrogluteal (adults): $1\frac{1}{2}$ inch
- Alcohol swab
- 2 × 2 gauze pad (optional)
- Medication ampule or vial
- Clean gloves
- Medication administration record (MAR) or computer printout

Step	Rationale
1. Complete preprocedure protocol.	
2. Assemble supplies in medication room.	
3. Check accuracy and completeness of MAR with preseriber's written medication order. Check client's name, drug name and dosage, route of administration, and time of administration.	Verifies correct medication.
4. Check name of medication on vial/ampule label against MAR.	First check of label ensures that client receives correct medication.
5. Check medication's expiration date.	Medications that have expired should not be used because potency of medications changes when medications become outdated.
6. Prepare correct dose from ampule or vial (see Skill 49). Check dose carefully and compare MAR with prepared drug label.	Ensures that medication is sterile. Second check of label ensures that dose is accurate and that client receives correct medication.
7. Remove vial access device or filter needle on syringe, and replace with needle for injection.	Vial access devices and filter needles cannot be used for IM injection.

Step	**Rationale**
8. For adults, select a 1- to 1½-inch, 22- to 27-gauge needle for medications prepared in aqueous solutions. If medications are viscous or in oil-based solutions, select an 18- to 25-gauge, 1- to 1½-inch needle. For children, select a ⅝- to 1-inch needle.	Needle must be long enough to reach muscle. Needles less than 1½ inches in length may not reach the muscle, especially in women (Engstrom and others, 2000; Katsma and Katsma, 2000).
9. Identify client by checking identification bracelet and asking client's name. Compare with MAR.	Ensures that correct client is receiving medication. At least two patient identifiers (neither to be the patient's room number) are to be used when administering medications (JCAHO, 2004).
10. Explain procedure, location of injection site, and how positioning lessens discomfort. Proceed in calm manner.	Allows client to anticipate injection so as to lessen anxiety.
11. Close room curtains and/or door.	Provides client privacy.
12. Keep sheet or gown draped over body parts not requiring exposure.	Maintains client's dignity.
13. ⚡ Select appropriate injection site by assessing size and integrity of muscle. Palpate for areas of tenderness or hardness. Note presence of bruising or area of infection.	The ventrogluteal site is the preferred site for all infants, children, and adults unless there are contraindications to this site.

NURSE ALERT When choosing an injection site, do not use an area that is bruised, has indurations, has muscular atrophy, has reduced blood flow, or has signs associated with infection.

Step	Rationale
14. Assist client to comfortable position depending on site chosen. For ventrogluteal: client lies on side or back, flexes knee and hip on side to be injected (Fig. 33-1, *A*); for vastus lateralis: client lies flat, supine, with knee slightly flexed (see Fig. 33-1, *B*); for deltoid: client may sit or lie flat with hand on hip or lower arm flexed but relaxed across abdomen or lap (see Fig. 33-1, *C*).	Position that reduces strain on muscle minimizes discomfort of injection.
15. Relocate site using anatomical landmarks.	Injection into correct anatomical site prevents injury to nerves, bones, and blood vessels.
16. Cleanse site with antiseptic swab. Apply swab to center of site, and rotate outward in circular direction for about 5 cm (2 inches).	Mechanical action of swab removes secretions containing microorganisms.
17. Hold swab or square of sterile gauze between third and fourth fingers of nondominant hand.	Swab or gauze remains readily accessible when needle is withdrawn.
18. Position nondominant hand just below site, and pull the skin approximately 2.5 to 3.5 cm (1 to $1^{1}/_{2}$ inches) down or laterally with ulnar side of hand to administer in a Z-track (Fig. 33-2). Hold this position until medication is injected and needle is withdrawn.	Reduces discomfort and incidence of leaking of medication.

NURSE ALERT If the client's muscle mass is small, as in the case of a child, grasp the body of the muscle between the thumb and fingers. This ensures that

Step	Rationale

Fig. 33-1
A, Anatomical site for ventrogluteal injection.
B, Anatomical site for vastus lateralis injection.
C, Anatomical site for deltoid injection.

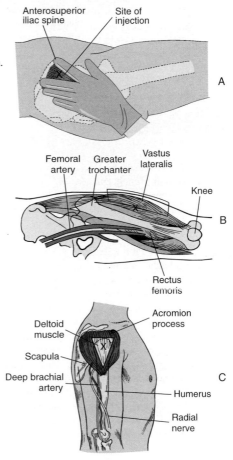

the medication reaches the muscle mass (Hockenberry and others, 2003; Nicoll and Hesby, 2002).

19. Place needle cap or sheath from needle between thumb and index finger of nondominant hand. Hold	Preventing needle from touching sides of cap prevents contamination.

Step	Rationale

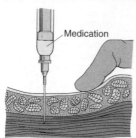

During Injection

Fig. 33-2 Pulling on overlying skin during IM injection moves tissue to prevent later tracking.

   barrel in dominant hand,
   and pull cap straight off.

20. Hold syringe between
    thumb and forefinger of
    dominant hand as if
    holding dart. Hold it with
    palm down with needle
    perpendicular to client's
    body.

   Quick, smooth injection requires proper manipulation of syringe.

21. Administer injection:
    a. Inject needle quickly,
       perpendicular to client's
       body, as close to
       90-degree angle as
       possible.

   Smooth, quick injection lessens pain. Angle ensures that medication reaches muscle mass (Katsma and Katsma, 2000; Nicoll and Hesby, 2002).

    b. After needle enters site,
       grasp lower end of
       syringe barrel with
       nondominant hand
       (while still holding skin
       back) to stabilize
       syringe. Continue to
       hold skin tightly with
       nondominant hand.
       Move dominant hand
       to end of plunger. Avoid
       moving syringe.

   Smooth manipulation of syringe parts reduces discomfort from needle movement. Skin must remain pulled until after drug is injected to ensure Z-track administration.

    c. Pull back on plunger 5
       to 10 seconds. If no
       blood appears, inject

   Aspiration of blood into syringe indicates accidental intravenous (IV) placement of needle.

Step	Rationale
medication slowly at rate of 1 ml/10 sec.	Intramuscular medications are not for IV use. Slow injection allows the muscle fibers to stretch and accommodate to injected volume, which reduces pain and tissue trauma (Nicoll and Hesby, 2002).

NURSE ALERT If blood appears in syringe, remove needle and dispose of medication and syringe properly. Repeat preparation procedure.

d. Wait 10 seconds, and then smoothly and steadily withdraw needle and release skin while placing antiseptic swab or dry gauze gently above or over injection (Fig. 33-3).	Support of tissues around injection site minimizes discomfort during needle withdrawal. Dry gauze may minimize client discomfort associated with alcohol on nonintact skin.
22. Apply gentle pressure. *Do not massage site.*	Massage can damage underlying tissue.
23. For ventrogluteal and vastus lateralis sites, encourage leg exercises.	Promotes drug absorption.
24. Discard uncapped needle or needle enclosed in safety shield and attached syringe into sharps container.	Prevents injury to client and health care personnel. Recapping needles increases risk of needle-stick injury (OSHA, 2001).

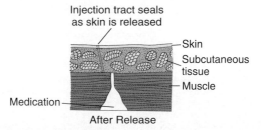

Fig. 33-3 The Z-track left after injection prevents the deposit of medication from leaking through sensitive tissue.

Step	Rationale
25. Complete postprocedure protocol.	
26. Return to room, and ask if client feels any acute pain, burning, numbness, or tingling at injection site.	Continued discomfort may indicate injury to underlying bones or nerves.

Recording and Reporting

- Immediately chart on MAR the medication, dose, route, site, time, and date administered. Correctly sign MAR according to institutional policy.
- Record client's response to medication if indicated (e.g., response to pain medication).
- Document and report any undesirable effects from medication to client's health care provider. Be aware that possible allergic reactions may not appear for several hours after a medication is given, especially when the client is receiving the medication for the first time.

Unexpected Outcomes	Related Interventions
1. While administering injection, it feels as though the needle has hit bone.	• Pull back on syringe about $\frac{1}{4}$ inch, being careful not to pull needle out of skin. Continue with medication administration (Gilsenan, 2000).
2. Client complains of localized pain or continued burning at injection site.	• Assess injection site for abscess formation. Monitor client's heart rate, respirations, blood pressure, and temperature. Notify client's health care provider, and do not reuse site (Gilsenan, 2000).
3. Client displays signs of adverse reaction, including urticaria, eczema, pruritus, wheezing, and dyspnea.	• Follow institutional policy or guidelines for appropriate response to allergic reactions, and notify client's health care provider immediately.

Intravenous Medications: Adding Medications to Intravenous Fluid Containers

The safest method for administering intravenous (IV) medications is to add the drugs to large-volume fluid containers. Then the medication infuses slowly, the risk of side effects is minimal, and therapeutic blood levels are maintained. The nurse or pharmacist dilutes IV medications in volumes of 50 to 1000 ml of compatible IV fluids such as normal saline, dextrose and water, or lactated Ringer's solution. In many hospital settings, the pharmacist adds drugs to primary containers of IV solutions to ensure asepsis and minimize medication errors. The pharmacist may use special plastic caps to seal containers previously mixed.

Delegation Considerations

The skill of adding medications to IV fluid containers should not be delegated to assistive personnel (AP).

- Instruct AP about expected actions of the medications to report.
- Instruct AP to report any changes in the client's status, vital signs, or level of comfort.
- Instruct AP to report any client complaints of moisture or discomfort around IV insertion site.

Equipment

- Vial or ampule of prescribed medication
- Syringe of appropriate size (1 to 20 ml)
- Sterile needle (1 to 1½ inch, 19 to 21 gauge) with special filters if indicated
- Correct diluent if indicated (e.g., sterile water, normal saline)
- Sterile IV fluid container (bag or bottle, 50 to 1000 ml in volume)
- Alcohol or antiseptic swab
- Label to attach to IV bag or bottle

- Medication administration record (MAR) or computer printout
- Clean gloves

Step	Rationale
1. Complete preprocedure protocol.	
2. Assess IV insertion site for signs of infiltration or phlebitis (see Skill 53). Discard gloves and perform hand hygiene.	An intact, properly functioning site ensures that medication is given safely.
3. Assemble supplies in medication area.	Ensures orderly procedure with less chance of supply contamination.
4. Check accuracy and completeness of MAR with prescriber's written medication order. Check client's name, drug name and dose, route, and IV solution.	Verifies correct medication.
5. Check name of medication on vial/ampule label against MAR.	Ensures that client receives correct medication.
6. Check medication's expiration date.	Medications that have expired should not be used because the potency of the medications changes when medications become outdated.
7. Prepare prescribed medication from vial or ampule (see Skill 49). (If filter needle is used, replace it with regular needle before injecting medication into IV fluid container.) Check dose carefully and compare MAR with prepared drug label.	Different techniques are used for each type of container. Ensures that correct medication given to client.
8. Identify client by reading identification band and	Ensures that correct client receives ordered medication. At least two

Step	**Rationale**
asking name. Compare with MAR.	patient identifiers (neither to be the patient's room number) are to be used when administering medications (JCAHO, 2004).
9. Prepare client by explaining that medication is to be given through existing IV line or one to be started. Explain that no discomfort should be felt during drug infusion. Encourage client to report symptoms of discomfort.	Most IV medications do not cause discomfort when diluted. However, some medications, such as potassium chloride, can be irritating. Pain at insertion site may be early indication of infiltration.
10. **To add medication to new container:**	
a. *Solution in bag:* Locate medication injection port on plastic IV solution bag. Port has small rubber stopper at end. Do not select port for IV tubing insertion or air vent.	Medication injection port is self-sealing to prevent introduction of microorganisms after repeated use.
b. *Solution in bottle:* Locate injection site on IV solution bottle, which is often covered by metal or plastic cap.	Accidental injection of medication through main tubing port or air vent can alter pressure within bottle and cause fluid leaks through air vent. Cap seals bottle to maintain its sterility.
c. Wipe port or injection site with alcohol or antiseptic swab.	Reduces risk of introducing microorganisms into bag during needle insertion.
d. Remove needle cap or sheath from syringe, and insert needle or needleless adapter of syringe through center of injection port or site; inject medication.	Injection of needle into sides of port may produce leak and lead to fluid contamination.
e. Withdraw syringe from bag or bottle.	Open tubing port in bottle provides direct route for

Step	Rationale
	microorganisms to enter solution. Bags have self-sealing port.
f. Mix medication and IV solution by holding bag or bottle and turning it gently end to end.	Allows even distribution of medication.
g. Complete medication label with name and dose of medication, date, time, and nurse's initials. Stick it on bottle or bag (Fig. 34-1). *Optional* (check institution's policy): apply flow strip that identifies time that solution was hung and intervals indicating fluid levels.	Label can be easily read during infusion of solution. Informs nurses and physicians of contents of bag or bottle.

NURSE ALERT Do not use felt-tip markers on plastic IV bag surface. The ink can penetrate the plastic and leak into the IV solution.

h. Spike bag or bottle with IV tubing, prime IV tubing if necessary, and	Ensures that medication is given over appropriate amount of time.

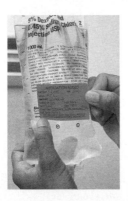

Fig. 34-1 Label affixed to IV bag.

Step	Rationale

hang. Regulate
infusion at ordered rate.

11. **To add medication to existing container:**

NURSE ALERT Because there is no way to know exactly how much IV fluid is in an existing hanging IV container, there is no way for you to determine the exact concentration of the medication in the IV solution. Therefore it is recommended that you add medications to new containers whenever possible.

Step	Rationale
a. Prepare vented IV bottle or plastic bag:	
(1) Check volume of solution remaining in bottle or bag.	Proper minimal volume (see drug insert) is needed to dilute medication adequately.
(2) Close IV infusion clamp.	Prevents medication from directly entering circulation as it is injected into bag or bottle.
(3) Wipe medication port with alcohol or antiseptic swab.	Mechanically removes microorganisms that could enter container during needle insertion.
(4) Insert syringe needle or needleless adapter through injection port, and inject medication.	Injection port is self-sealing and prevents fluid leaks.
(5) Lower bag or bottle from IV pole, and gently mix. Rehang bag.	Ensures that medication is evenly distributed.
b. Complete medication label, and stick it to bag or bottle.	Informs nurses and physicians of contents of bag or bottle.
c. Regulate infusion to desired rate.	Ensures that medication is given over appropriate amount of time.

NURSE ALERT Certain IV medications, such as potassium chloride, can cause serious adverse reactions if infused too quickly. Check institutional policy for which IV medications require administration via an infusion pump.

Step	Rationale
12. Dispose of needles and syringe in sharps container. Do not cap needle of syringe. Specially sheathed needles are discarded as unit with needle covered.	Proper disposal of needle prevents injury to nurse and client. Capping needles increases risk of needle-stick injuries (OSHA, 2001).
13. Complete postprocedure protocol.	

Recording and Reporting

- Record on appropriate form the solution and medication added to parenteral fluid.
- Report any adverse effects to client's health care provider, and document adverse effects according to institutional policy.

Unexpected Outcomes	Related Interventions
1. Client has adverse reaction to medication.	• Follow institutional policy or guidelines for appropriate response to and reporting of adverse drug reactions. • Notify client's health care provider of adverse effects immediately.
2. Client develops signs of fluid volume excess (e.g., abnormal breath sounds [crackles], blood pressure changes, jugular venous distention, edema, shortness of breath).	• Stop IV infusion. • Notify client's health care provider of fluid excess immediately.
3. IV site indicates phlebitis or infiltrate.	See Skill 53.

Intravenous Medications: Intermittent Infusion Sets and Mini-Infusion Pumps

Administering drugs by intermittent infusion is a method in which the nurse dilutes intravenous (IV) medications in small volumes of solution and administers them over a short period. Administering drugs by this method reduces the risk of rapid drug-dose infusion and provides greater comfort and independence for the client. Clients receiving drugs by intermittent infusion have an established IV line that is kept patent by intermittent flushes of normal saline. Intermittent infusion of drugs can be administered in several ways: piggyback, tandem, volume-control administration, and mini-infusion pump.

Delegation Considerations

Administering IV medications by intermittent infusion sets and mini-infusion pumps should not be delegated to assistive personnel (AP).

- Instruct AP about potential medication side effects to report.
- Have AP report to nurse any changes in client status including discomfort at infusion site and change in vital signs.

Equipment

- Antiseptic swab
- IV pole or rack
- Medication administration record (MAR) or computer printout
- Clean gloves
- Medication label, if needed (many IV medications are premixed and dispensed from the pharmacy and arrive on the nursing unit with the medication label already affixed.)

Piggyback, Tandem, or Mini-Infusion Pump

- Medication prepared in labeled infusion bag
- Short microdrip or macrodrip tubing set for piggyback with needleless device

- Needle, 21 to 23 gauge, only if needleless system is not available; use needleless system whenever possible (OSHA, 2001)
- Mini-infusion pump
- Adhesive tape (optional)

Volume-Control Administration Set

- Volutrol or Buretrol, Pediatrol
- Infusion tubing (may have needleless system attachment)
- Syringe (1 to 20 ml)
- Vial or ampule of ordered medication

Step	Rationale

NURSE ALERT Never administer IV medications through tubing that is infusing blood, blood products, or parenteral nutrition solutions.

1. Complete preprocedure protocol.	
2. ✋ Assess patency of client's existing IV infusion line or saline lock (see Skill 52).	IV line must be patent and fluids must infuse easily for medication to reach venous circulation effectively.

NURSE ALERT If IV site is saline locked, cleanse the port with alcohol and assess the patency of the IV line by flushing it with 2 to 3 ml of sterile normal saline. Attach appropriate IV tubing to the saline lock, and administer the medication via piggyback, mini-infusion, or volume-control administration set.

3. Assess IV insertion site for signs of infiltration or phlebitis: redness, pallor, swelling, and tenderness on palpation. Discard gloves and perform hand hygiene.	Confirmation of placement of IV needle or catheter and integrity of surrounding tissues ensures that medication is administered safely.
4. Assemble supplies at bedside.	Drug preparation usually is not required. Nurse may assemble infusion tubing and bag of medication in medication area or client's room.
5. Check accuracy and completeness of MAR with prescriber's written	Verifies correct medication.

Step	Rationale
medication order. Check client's name, drug name and dose, route, and time of administration.	
6. Check name of medication on infusion bag, syringe, vial/ampule label against MAR.	Ensures that client receives correct medication.
7. Check medication's expiration date.	Medications that have expired should not be used because potency of medications changes when medications become outdated.
8. Check client's identification by looking at arm bracelet and asking client's name.	Ensures that drug is administered to correct patient. At least two patient identifiers (neither to be patient's room number) are to be used when administering medications (JCAHO, 2004).
9. Explain purpose of medication and side effects. Encourage client to report symptoms of discomfort at site.	Clients who can verbalize pain at IV site can help detect IV infiltrations early, lessening damage to surrounding tissues.
10. Administer infusion:	
a. **Piggyback infusion through existing line:**	
(1) Prepare medication by checking label on small infusion bag against MAR.	Final check ensures that client receives correct medication.
(2) Connect infusion tubing to medication bag (see Skill 52). Squeeze drip chamber, and fill half full. Allow solution to fill tubing by opening	Infusion tubing should be filled with solution and free of air bubbles to prevent air embolus.

Step	Rationale
regulator flow clamp. Once tubing is full, close clamp and cap end of tubing.	
(3) Hang piggyback medication bag above level of primary fluid bag. (Hook may be used to lower main bag.)	Height of fluid bag affects rate of flow to client. Ensures that medication will infuse correctly.
(4) Connect tubing of piggyback to appropriate connector on primary infusion line:	Establishes route for IV medication to enter main IV line.
(a) *Needleless system:* Wipe off needleless port on main IV line, and insert tip of piggyback infusion tubing. Lock into place as indicated by manufacturer of needleless system (Fig. 35-1).	Needleless connections should be used whenever possible to prevent accidental needle-stick injuries (OSHA, 2001).
(b) *Tubing port:* Connect sterile 21- to 23- gauge needle to end of piggyback infusion	Prevents introduction of microorganisms during needle insertion.

Step	Rationale

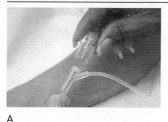 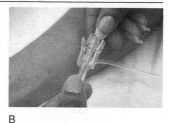

A   B

Fig. 35-1 **A,** Needleless lever lock cannula system. **B,** Blunt ended cannula inserts into ports and locks.

tubing, remove cap, cleanse injection port on main IV line, and insert needle through center of port. Consider placing piece of tape at junction where needle enters IV port to secure medication line to main IV line.	
(5) Regulate flow rate of medication solution by adjusting regulator clamp or IV pump infusion rate. Rate of flow should be determined by institutional policy. If policy does not	Provides slow, safe, intermittent infusion of medication and maintains therapeutic blood levels.

Step	Rationale
exist, consult pharmacist or drug manual. (Usually medications are recommended to infuse within 20 to 90 minutes.)	
(6) Perform hand hygiene.	Prevents spread of microorganisms.
(7) After medication has infused, check flow rate of primary infusion. Regulate main infusion line to desired rate, if necessary.	Back-check valve prevents infusion of primary line while medication is infusing. Primary infusion will automatically flow when piggyback infusion is empty. Checking and regulating flow rate ensures proper administration of IV fluids.
(8) Leave IV piggyback bag and tubing in place for future drug administration, or discard in appropriate containers. If needle used, discard in sharps container.	Establishment of IV piggyback line produces route for microorganisms to enter main line. Repeated changes in tubing increase risk of infection transmission. Check agency policy and procedure for frequency of IV tubing changes.
b. **Volume-control administration set (e.g., Volutrol):**	
(1) Prepare medication from vial or ampule (see Skill 51). Check name of drug on medication label against MAR.	Ensures that right dose of medication is prepared and ensures sterility of medication.
(2) Fill volume-control administration set	Dilution of IV medication reduces risk of infusion that is too rapid.

Step	**Rationale**
with desired amount of fluid (50 to 100 ml) by opening clamp between volume-control administration set and main IV bag.	
(3) Close clamp, and be sure clamp on air vent of volume-control administration chamber is open.	Prevents additional leakage of fluid into volume-control administration set. Air vent allows fluid in administration set to exit at regulated rate.
(4) Clean injection port on top of volume-control administration set with antiseptic swab.	Prevents introduction of microorganisms during needle insertion.
(5) Remove needle cap or sheath, and insert syringe needle through port; then inject medication (Fig. 35-2). Gently rotate volume-control administration chamber between hands.	Rotating mixes medication with solution in volume-control administration set to ensure equal distribution.
(6) Regulate IV infusion rate to allow medication to infuse in time recommended by institutional policy, pharmacist, or medication reference manual.	For optimal therapeutic effect, medication should infuse in prescribed time interval.

Step	Rationale

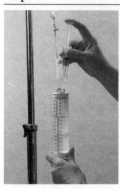

Fig. 35-2   Medication injected into volume-control set.

(7) Label volume-control administration chamber with name of medication, dosage, total volume including diluent, and time of administration.

Alerts nurses to medication being infused. Prevents other medications from being added to volume-control administration chamber.

(8) Dispose of uncapped needle or needle enclosed in safety shield and syringe in sharps container.

Prevents accidental needle sticks and prevents spread of microorganisms.

(9) After medication has infused, be sure main IV solution is infusing as ordered, or disconnect IV tubing from IV, and flush IV lock per agency policy.

Ensures accurate infusion of continuous IV fluids. Flushing IV lock maintains patent IV site.

(10) Place sterile cap on end of volume-

If tubing set is to be reused, sterility must be maintained.

Step	**Rationale**
control administration set for future use, or discard set in appropriate containers.	
c. **Administer medication using mini-infuser pump:**	
(1) Check label on prefilled syringe for drug name and dose and compare with MAR; then connect prefilled syringe to mini-infuser tubing.	Ensures that client receives correct medication. Special tubing designed to fit syringe delivers medication to main IV line.
(2) Carefully apply pressure to syringe plunger, allowing tubing to fill with medication.	Ensures that tubing is free of air bubbles to prevent air embolus.
(3) Hang infusion pump with syringe on IV pole alongside main IV bag.	
(4) Place syringe into mini-infusion pump (follow product directions). Be sure that syringe is secured (Fig. 35-3).	Syringe must be securely placed into mini-infuser to deliver medication.
(5) Connect mini-infusion tubing to main IV line:	Establishes route for IV medication to enter main IV line.
(a) *Needleless system:* Wipe off needleless port on main	Needleless connections should be used whenever possible to prevent accidental needle-stick injuries (OSHA, 2001).

Step	Rationale

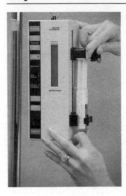

Fig. 35-3 Ensure that syringe is secure after placing it into mini-infusion pump.

IV line, and insert tip of mini-infuser tubing. Lock into place as indicated by manufacturer of needleless system.

(b) *Tubing port:* Connect sterile 21- to 23-gauge needle to mini-infuser tubing, remove cap, cleanse injection port on main IV line or saline lock, and insert needle through center of port. Consider placing tape

Cleansing reduces transmission of microorganisms. Use needles only if needleless system is not available.

Step	**Rationale**
where IV tubing enters port to keep connection secured.	
(6) Set pump to deliver medication within time recommended by institutional policy, pharmacist, or medication reference manual. Usually medications are infused over 20 to 90 minutes. Press button on pump to begin infusion. *Optional:* Set alarm.	Pump automatically delivers medication at safe, constant rate based on volume in syringe. Alarm indicates completion of infusion.
(7) After medication has infused, check flow regulator on primary infusion. Infusion should continue to flow when pump stops. Regulate main infusion line to desired rate as needed. If stopcock is used, turn off mini-infusion line.	Checking flow rate ensures proper administration of IV fluids.
(8) Leave mini-infuser pump and tubing at bedside for future drug administration, or dispose of supplies appropriately.	Mini-infuser pump tubing must remain sterile for future uses.

11. Complete postprocedure protocol.

Recording and Reporting

- Immediately record drug, dose, route, and time administered on MAR or computer printout. Correctly sign MAR according to institutional policy.
- Record volume of fluid in medication bag or Volutrol on intake and output (I&O) form to monitor total fluid intake.
- Report to client's health care provider any adverse reactions.

Unexpected Outcomes	Related Interventions
1. Client develops adverse drug reaction.	• Stop medication infusion immediately, and follow institutional policy or guidelines for appropriate response and reporting of adverse drug reactions. • Notify client's health care provider of adverse effects immediately.
2. Medication does not infuse over desired period.	• Can result from improper calculation of flow rate, malpositioning of IV needle at insertion site, or infiltration. • Determine reason, and take corrective action as indicated (e.g., correct flow rate, reposition IV, discontinue and restart IV).
3. IV site indicates philebitis or infiltrate.	See Skill 53.

Intravenous Medications: Intravenous Bolus

An intravenous (IV) bolus involves introducing a concentrated dose of a drug directly into the systemic circulation. The IV bolus allows no time to correct errors. Therefore be very careful in calculating the correct amount of the medication to give. Check your calculations with another nurse. In addition, an IV bolus may irritate the lining of blood vessels. Thus be sure that the IV catheter or needle is correctly positioned in the client's vein. Accidental injection of a medication into tissues surrounding a vein can cause pain, necrotic sloughing of tissues, and abscesses.

Administering an IV push medication too quickly can cause serious negative client outcomes, including death. The Institute for Safe Medication Practices (2003) has identified the following three strategies to reduce harm from rapid IV push medications:

- Have information regarding IV push times readily available to you.
- Use less concentrated solutions whenever possible.
- Avoid using terms in orders such as *IV push* or *IV bolus* with medications that should be administered over 1 minute or longer.

The rate of administration of IV push drugs varies from drug to drug. Therefore verify a medication's rate of administration with institutional guidelines before administering an IV bolus.

Delegation Considerations

Administering medications by IV bolus should not be delegated to assistive personnel (AP).

- Have AP report any side effects or unexpected drug reactions to the nurse.
- Have AP report discomfort at infusion site as soon as possible.
- Have AP obtain any required vital signs and report these findings to the nurse.

Equipment

- Watch with second hand
- Medication administration record (MAR) or computer printout
- Clean gloves
- Antiseptic swab

Intravenous Push (Existing Line)

- Medication in vial or ampule
- Syringe
- Needleless device or sterile needle (21 to 25 gauge)

Intravenous Push (Intravenous Lock)

- Medication in vial or ampule
- Syringe
- Vial of appropriate flush solution (saline most common, but heparin may also be used; if heparin is used, most common concentration is 10 to 100 units/ml; check agency policy)
- Needleless device or sterile needle (21 to 25 gauge)

Step	Rationale
1. Complete preprocedure protocol.	

NURSE ALERT Some IV medications can be pushed safely only when the client is being continuously monitored for dysrhythmias, blood pressure changes, or other adverse effects. Therefore some medications can be pushed only in specific areas within a health care agency. Confirm institutional guidelines regarding requirements for special monitoring, and verify that monitoring equipment is available before giving medication (Zurlinden, 2002).

Step	Rationale
2. ✋ Assess condition of IV or saline (heparin) lock insertion site for signs of infiltration or phlebitis. Discard gloves and perform hand hygiene.	Drug should not be administered if site is edematous or inflamed.
3. Assemble supplies in medication room.	Ensures sterile preparation of medications.
4. Check accuracy and completeness of MAR with prescriber's written medication order. Check client's name, drug name, and dose and route.	Verifies correct medication.
5. Check name of medication on vial/ampule label against MAR.	Ensures that client receives correct medication.

Step	Rationale
6. Check medication's expiration date.	Medications that have expired should not be used.
7. Prepare medication from vial or ampule (see Skill 51). Check dose carefully and compare MAR with drug label.	Ensures that correct medication is sterile, and correctly prepared.

NURSE ALERT Some IV medications require dilution before administration. Verify with agency policy. If a small amount of medication is given (e.g., less than 1 ml), dilute medication in 5 to 10 ml of normal saline or sterile water so that the medication does not collect in the "dead spaces" (e.g., Y site injection port, IV cap) of the IV delivery system.

Step	Rationale
8. ▧ Check client's identification by looking at arm bracelet and asking name. Compare with MAR.	Ensures that drug is administered to correct client. At least two patient identifiers (neither to be patient's room number) are to be used when administering medications (JCAHO, 2004).
9. **Intravenous push (existing line):**	
a. Select injection port of IV tubing closest to client. Whenever possible, injection port should be a needleless component.	Follows provisions of the Needle Safety and Prevention Act of 2001 (OSHA, 2001).
b. Clean injection port with antiseptic swab. Allow to dry.	Prevents introduction of microorganisms during needle insertion.
c. Connect syringe to IV line: insert needleless blunt cannula tip syringe or a small-gauge needle containing drug through center of port (Fig. 36-1).	Prevents introduction of microorganisms. Prevents damage to port diaphragm.
d. Occlude IV line by pinching tubing just above injection port (Fig. 36-2). Pull back	Final check ensures that medication is being delivered into bloodstream.

Step   Rationale

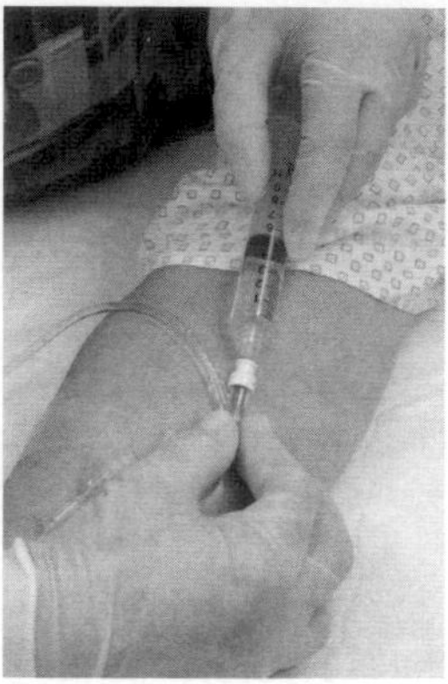

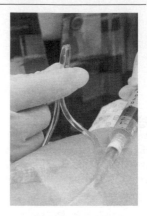

Fig. 36-1   Connecting syringe to IV line with needleless blunt cannula tip.

Fig. 36-2   Occluding IV tubing above injection port.

gently on syringe's plunger to aspirate for blood return.

NURSE ALERT   In some cases, especially with a smaller gauge IV needle, blood return may not be aspirated, even if IV is patent. If IV site does not show signs of infiltration and if IV flushes without difficulty, proceed with IV push.

e. Release tubing, and inject medication within amount of time recommended by institutional policy, pharmacist, or medication reference manual. Use watch to time administrations. IV line may be pinched while pushing medication and released when not pushing

Ensures safe drug infusion. Rapid injection of IV drug can be fatal. Allowing IV fluids to infuse while pushing IV drug will enable medication to be delivered to client at prescribed rate.

Step	**Rationale**
medication. Allow IV fluids to infuse when not pushing medication.	

NURSE ALERT If IV medication is incompatible with IV fluids, stop the IV fluids, clamp the IV line, flush with 10 ml of normal saline or sterile water, give the IV bolus over the appropriate amount of time, flush with another 10 ml of normal saline or sterile water at the same rate as the medication was administered, and then restart the IV fluids at the prescribed rate.

Step	**Rationale**
f. After injecting medication, withdraw syringe and recheck fluid infusion rate.	Injection of bolus may alter rate of fluid infusion. Rapid fluid infusion can cause circulatory fluid overload.
10. **Intravenous push (intravenous lock):**	
a. Prepare flush solutions according to hospital policy:	
(1) Saline flush method (preferred method):	
(a) Prepare two syringes filled with 2 to 3 ml of normal saline (0.9%).	Normal saline is effective in keeping IV locks patent and is compatible with wide range of medications.
(2) Heparin flush method (traditional method):	
(a) Prepare one syringe with ordered amount of heparin flush solution.	
(b) Prepare two syringes with 2 to 3 ml of normal saline (0.9%).	

Step	Rationale
b. Administer medication:	
(1) Clean lock's injection port with antiseptic swab.	Cleaning prevents introduction of microorganisms during needle insertion.
(2) Insert syringe with normal saline 0.9% through injection port of IV lock.	
(3) Pull back gently on syringe plunger, and check for blood return.	Indicates if needle or catheter is in vein.

NURSE ALERT In some cases, especially with a smaller gauge IV needle, blood return may not be aspirated, even if IV is patent. If IV site does not show signs of infiltration and if fluid is infusing without difficulty, proceed with IV push.

(4) Flush IV site with normal saline by pushing slowly on plunger.	Cleans needle and reservoir of blood. Flushing without difficulty indicates patent IV.

NURSE ALERT Closely observe area of skin above the IV catheter. Note any puffiness or swelling as you flush the IV site, which could indicate infiltration into the tissue and require removal of the catheter.

(5) Remove saline-filled syringe.	
(6) Clean lock's injection port with antiseptic swab.	Prevents transmission of infection.
(7) Insert syringe containing prepared medication through injection port of IV lock.	
(8) Inject medication within amount of	Many medication errors are associated with IV pushes being

Step	Rationale
time recommended by institutional policy, pharmacist, or medication reference manual. Use watch to time administration.	administered too quickly. Following guidelines for IV push rates promotes client safety (Karch and Karch, 2003).
(9) After administering medication, withdraw syringe.	
(10) Clean lock's injection site with antiseptic swab.	Prevents transmission of infection.
(11) Flush injection port:	
(a) Attach syringe with normal saline, and inject normal saline flush at the same rate the medication was delivered.	Irrigation with saline prevents occlusion of IV access device and ensures all medication delivered. Flushing IV site at same rate as medication ensures that any medication remaining within IV needle is delivered at correct rate.
(b) *Heparin flush option:* after instilling saline, attach syringe containing heparin flush. Inject heparin slowly, and then remove syringe.	Maintains patency of IV needle by inhibiting clot formation. *SASH method:* Saline, Administration of medication, Saline, Heparin.
11. Dispose of uncapped needles and syringes in sharps container.	Prevents accidental needle-stick injuries and follows Centers for Disease Control and Prevention (CDC) guidelines for disposal of sharps (OSHA, 2001).
12. Complete postprocedure protocol.	

Recording and Reporting

- Immediately record drug, dose, route, and time administered on MAR or computer printout. Correctly sign MAR according to institutional policy.
- Report any adverse reactions to client's health care provider.

Unexpected Outcomes	Related Interventions
1. Client develops adverse reaction to medication.	• Stop delivering medication immediately, and follow institutional policy or guidelines for appropriate response and reporting of adverse drug reactions. • Notify client's health care provider of adverse effects immediately. • Stop IV infusion immediately. • Provide extravasation care as indicated by institutional policy or prescriber.
2. IV site indicates phlebitis or infiltrate.	See Skill 53.

Isolation Precautions

As a nurse, you follow standard precautions in the care of all clients. Isolation or Barrier Precautions include the appropriate use of gowns, masks, eyewear, and other protective devices or clothing. Guidelines for Isolation Precautions are based on current epidemiological information regarding disease transmission in hospitals. Although intended primarily for care of clients in acute care, the recommendations can be applied to clients in subacute care or long-term care facilities. Standard Precautions apply to contact with (1) blood, (2) body fluids, (3) nonintact skin, and (4) mucous membranes. Box 37-1 describes standard precautions, the primary strategies for reducing risk of transmission of bloodborne and other pathogens. In 2004 the Centers for Disease Control and Prevention (CDC) added respiratory hygiene/cough etiquette to standard precautions. In cases in which clients are infected or colonized with specific microorganisms, the CDC recommends isolation precautions.

Table 37-1 lists the three types of transmission-based precautions. The precautions are designed for care of clients who are known or suspected to be infected, or colonized, with microorganisms transmitted by droplets, by airborne route, or by contact with contaminated surfaces or dry skin. The three types of Transmission-based Precautions— airborne, droplet, and contact—may be combined for diseases that have multiple routes of transmission. When used either singly or in combination, they are to be used in addition to Standard Precautions when required by the infection or colonization with a specific organism. In the case of clients with reduced immunosuppression, protective environment precautions are necessary. Box 37-2 summarizes the tiers of precautions and the types of clients requiring their use.

Delegation Considerations

This skill may be delegated to assistive personnel (AP).

- Discuss with AP the nature and type of infection a client has.
- Warn AP of high-risk factors for infection transmission that pertain to assigned client.

Equipment

- Clean gloves, mask, eyewear or goggles, and gown
- Other client care equipment (as appropriate)
- Soiled-linen and trash receptacle

BOX 37-1   Standard Precautions (Tier One)* for Use With All Clients

- Standard Precautions apply to blood, all body fluids, secretions, excretions, nonintact skin, and mucous membranes.
- Hand hygiene is performed if contaminated with blood or body fluid, immediately after gloves are removed, between client contact, and when indicated to prevent transfer of microorganisms between clients or between clients and environment.
- Gloves are worn when touching blood, body fluid, secretions, excretions, nonintact skin, mucous membranes, or contaminated items. Gloves should be removed and hand hygiene performed between client care encounters.
- Masks, eye protection, or face shields are worn if client care activities generate splashes or sprays of blood or body fluid.
- Gowns are worn if soiling of clothing is likely from blood or body fluid. Perform hand hygiene after removing gown.
- Client care equipment is properly cleaned and reprocessed, and single-use items are discarded.
- Contaminated linen is placed in leak-proof bag and is handled to prevent skin and mucous membrane exposure.
- All sharp instruments and needles are discarded in a puncture-resistant container. The CDC recommends use of needleless devices. Any needles should be disposed of uncapped or a mechanical device be used for recapping.
- A private room is unnecessary unless the client's hygiene is unacceptable. Check with infection control professional.
- Respiratory hygiene/cough etiquette. Have clients cover nose/mouth when coughing or sneezing; use tissues to contain respiratory secretions and dispose in nearest waste container; perform hand hygiene after contacting respiratory secretions and contaminated objects; contain respiratory secretrons with procedure or surgical mask; sit at least 3 feet away from others if coughing.

Modified and reprinted from Centers for Disease Control and Prevention, Hospital Infection Control Practice Advisory Committee: Guidelines for isolation precautions in hospitals, *Am J Infect Control* 24:24, 1996, with permission from the **Association for Professionals in Infection Control and Epidemiology**.

*Formerly Universal Precautions and Body Substance Isolation.

TABLE 37-1   Transmission Categories (Tier Two) (For Use With Clients Infected or Colonized With Specific Organisms)

Category	Disease	Barrier Protection
Airborne Precautions	For diseases transmitted by small droplet nuclei (smaller than 5 µm), such as measles, chickenpox, disseminated varicella zoster, pulmonary or laryngeal tuberculosis (TB).*	Private room, negative airflow of at least six air exchanges per hour; N95 particulate respirator mask or P100 respirator.
Droplet Precautions	For diseases transmitted by large droplets (larger than 5 µm), such as streptococcal pharyngitis, pneumonia, and scarlet fever in infants or small children, pertussis, mumps, meningococcal pneumonia or sepsis, pneumonic plague.	Private room or cohort client; mask when closer than 3 ft from client.
Contact Precautions	For diseases transmitted by direct client or environmental contact, such as colonization or infection with multidrug-resistant organisms, respiratory syncytial virus, major wound infections, herpes simplex, scabies, varicella zoster (disseminated).	Private room or cohort client; gloves, gowns.
Protective Environment	Allogeneic hematopoietic stem cell transplants	Private room; positive airflow with 12 or more air exchanges per hour; gloves, gowns.

Modified and reprinted from Centers for Disease Control and Prevention, Hospital Infection Control Practice Advisory Committee: Guidelines for isolation precautions in hospitals, *Am J Infect Control* 24:24, 1996, with permission from the **Association for Professionals in Infection Control and Epidemiology**.

*See CDC TB guidelines.

BOX 37-2   Synopsis of Types of Precautions for Clients Requiring the Precautions*

Standard Precautions

Use Standard Precautions for the care of all clients.

Airborne Precautions

In addition to Standard Precautions, use Airborne Precautions for clients known or suspected to have serious illnesses transmitted by airborne droplet nuclei. Examples of such illnesses include:

1. Measles
2. Varicella (including disseminated zoster)*
3. Tuberculosis†

Droplet Precautions

In addition to Standard Precautions, use Droplet Precautions for clients known or suspected to have serious illnesses transmitted by large particle droplets. Examples of such illnesses include:

1. Invasive *Haemophilus influenzae* type b disease, including meningitis, pneumonia, epiglottitis, and sepsis
2. Invasive *Neisseria meningitidis* disease, including meningitis, pneumonia, and sepsis
3. Other serious bacterial respiratory infections spread by droplet transmission, including:
   a. Diphtheria (pharyngeal)
   b. Mycoplasma pneumonia
   c. Pertussis
   d. Pneumonic plague
   e. Streptococcal pharyngitis, pneumonia, or scarlet fever in infants and young children
4. Serious viral infections spread by droplet transmission, including:
   a. Adenovirus*
   b. Influenza
   c. Mumps
   d. Parvovirus B 19
   e. Rubella

Contact Precautions

In addition to Standard Precautions, use Contact Precautions for clients known or suspected to have serious illnesses easily transmitted by direct client contact or by contact with items in the client's environment. Examples of such illnesses include:

BOX 37-2 Synopsis of Types of Precautions for
Clients Requiring the Precautions*—cont'd

---

1. Gastrointestinal, respiratory, skin, or wound infections or colonization with multidrug-resistant bacteria judged by the infection control program, based on current state, regional, or national recommendations, to be of special clinical and epidemiologic significance
2. Enteric with a low infectious dose or prolonged environmental survival, including:
   a. *Clostridium difficile*
   b. For diapered or incontinent clients: enterohemorrhagic *Escherichia coli* O157:H7, *Shigella,* hepatitis A, or rotavirus
3. Respiratory syncytial virus, parainfluenza virus, or enteroviral infections in infants and young children
4. Skin infections that are highly contagious or that may occur on dry skin, including:
   a. Diphtheria (cutaneous)
   b. Herpes simplex virus (neonatal or mucocutaneous)
   c. Impetigo
   d. Major (noncontained) abscesses, cellulitis, or decubiti
   e. Pediculosis
   f. Scabies
   g. Staphylococcal furunculosis in infants and young children
   h. Zoster (disseminated or in the immunocompromised host)*
5. Viral/hemorrhagic conjunctivitis
6. Viral hemorrhagic infections (Ebola, Lassa, or Marburg)

Modified and reprinted from Centers for Disease Control and Prevention, Hospital Infection Control Practice Advisory Committee: Guidelines for isolation precautions in hospitals, *Am J Infect Control* 24:24, 1996, with permission from the **Association for Professionals in Infection Control and Epidemiology**.

*Certain infections require more than one type of precaution.

†See CDC *Guidelines for Preventing the Transmission of Tuberculosis in Health-Care Facilities.*

Step	Rationale
1. Complete preprocedure protocol.	
2. Review laboratory test results.	Informs nurse of type of microorganism for which client is being isolated, body fluid in which it was identified, and whether client is immunosuppressed.

Step	Rationale
3. Consider types of care measures to be performed while in client's room (e.g., medication administration, dressing change).	Enables nurse to organize care items for procedures and time spent in client's room.
4. Before donning latex gloves, assess if client has known latex allergy.	Client with latex allergy can have serious allergic or sensitivity reaction even after brief exposure to gloves.
5. Prepare all equipment needed to be taken into client's room.	Prevents nurse from making more than one trip into room.
6. ![hand icon] Determine appropriate barriers to apply based on isolation category and activities to be performed for client.	Ensures adequate protection to prevent transmission of infection.
7. Prepare for entrance into isolation room. Choice of barrier protection depends on type of isolation and facility policy (Table 37-1).	Proper preparation ensures that nurse is protected from microorganism exposure.
a. Don gown, being sure it covers all outer garments. Pull sleeves down to wrist. Tie securely at neck and waist (Fig. 37-1).	Prevents transmission of infection when client has excessive drainage, discharges.
b. Apply N95 mask or a surgical mask around mouth and nose (type and fit-testing will depend on type of isolation and facility policy).	Prevents exposure to airborne microorganisms or exposure to microorganisms from splashing of fluids.
c. Apply eyewear or goggles snugly around face and eyes (when needed).	Protects nurse from exposure to microorganisms that may occur during splashing of fluids.
d. Don disposable gloves. (NOTE: latex-free	Reduces transmission of microorganisms.

Step	**Rationale**

Fig. 37-1   Nurse with protective equipment for contact and droplet infection.

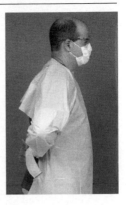

environment should be provided if client or health care worker has latex allergy.) If gloves are worn with gown, bring glove cuffs over edge of gown sleeves.	
8. Enter client's room. Arrange supplies and equipment. Place wrist watch on paper towel near client's bedside.	Prevents extra trips entering and leaving room. Prevents contamination of watch.
9. Explain purpose of isolation and precautions necessary to client and family. Offer opportunity to ask questions.	Improves client's and family's ability to participate in care and minimizes anxiety.
10. Assess vital signs:	
a. If client is infected or colonized with resistant organism (e.g., vancomycin-resistant enterococci [VRE] or methicillin-resistant *Staphylococcus aureus*	Prevents cross-contamination of other clients.

Step	Rationale
[MRSA]), equipment taken into room remains in room or is thoroughly disinfected when removed from room (see agency policy).	
b. Avoid contact of stethoscope or blood pressure cuff with infective material. Wipe with disinfectant as needed.	If used later on other clients, increases risk of infection being transmitted.
c. If stethoscope is to be reused, clean diaphragm or bell with 70% alcohol or liquid soap. Set aside on clean surface.	Systematic disinfection of stethoscopes with 70% alcohol or liquid soap will minimize chance of spreading infectious agents between clients (Bernard and others, 1999).
d. Use individual or disposable thermometers.	Prevents cross-contamination.
11. Administer medications:	
a. Give oral medication in wrapper or cup.	Supplies are handled and discarded to minimize transfer of microorganisms.
b. Dispose of wrapper or cup in plastic-lined receptacle.	
c. Administer injection, being sure gloves are worn.	Reduces risk of exposure to blood.
d. Discard disposable syringe and uncapped or sheathed needle into designated sharps container.	Reduces risk of needle-stick injury.
e. Place reusable plastic syringe (e.g., Carpuject) on clean towel for eventual removal and disinfection.	Prevents added contamination of syringe.

Step	**Rationale**
12. Administer hygiene, encouraging client to verbalize any questions or concerns regarding isolation. Informal teaching may be done at this time.	Hygiene practices further minimize transfer of microorganisms.
a. Avoid allowing isolation gown to become wet; carry wash basin outward away from gown; avoid leaning against wet tabletop.	Moisture allows organisms to travel through gown to uniform.

NURSE ALERT In case of excess soiling, a gown impervious to moisture should be worn.

b. Assist client in removing own gown; discard in impervious linen bag.	Reduces transfer of microorganisms.
c. Remove linen from bed; avoid contact with isolation gown. Place in impervious linen bag.	Linen soiled by client's body fluids is handled so as to prevent contact with clean items.
d. Provide clean bed linen and set of towels.	
e. Change gloves and perform hand hygiene if they become excessively soiled and further care is necessary.	
13. Collect specimens:	
a. Place specimen containers on clean paper towel in client's bathroom.	Container will be taken out of client's room; prevents contamination of outer surface.
b. Follow procedure for collecting specimen of body fluids.	
c. Transfer specimen to container without	Specimens of blood and body fluids are placed in well-

Step	**Rationale**
soiling outside of container. Place container in plastic bag, and label outside of bag or as per agency policy.	constructed containers with secure lids to prevent leaks during transport.
d. Check label on specimen for accuracy. Send to laboratory (warning labels may be used, depending on hospital policy).	
14. Dispose of linen, trash, and disposable items:	
a. Use single bags that are impervious to moisture and sturdy to contain soiled articles. Use double bag if outside of first bag is soiled or wet.	Linen or refuse should be totally contained to prevent exposure of personnel to infective material.
b. Tie bags securely at top in knot.	
15. Remove all reusable pieces of equipment. Clean any contaminated surfaces with hospital-approved disinfectant (see agency policy).	All items must be properly cleaned, disinfected, or sterilized for reuse.
16. Resupply room as needed. Have staff colleague hand new supplies to you.	Limiting trips of personnel into and out of room reduces nurse's and client's exposure to microorganisms. Quality time should be spent with client when in room.
17. Leave isolation room. Remember, order of removal of protective barriers depends on what is worn in room. This sequence describes steps to take if all barriers were required to be worn:	

Step	**Rationale**
a. Remove gloves. Remove one glove by grasping cuff and pulling glove inside out over hand (Fig. 37-2, *A*). Discard glove. With ungloved hand, tuck finger inside cuff of remaining glove and pull it off, inside out (Fig. 37-2, *B*).	Technique prevents nurse from contacting contaminated glove's outer surface.
b. Remove eyewear or goggles.	Hands have not been soiled.
c. Remove gown by untying neck strings and then back strings. Allow gown to fall from shoulders (Fig. 37-3). Remove hands from sleeves without touching outside of gown. Hold gown inside at shoulder seams, and fold inside out; discard in laundry bag.	Hands do not come in contact with soiled front of gown.
d. Remove mask. If mask secures over ears, remove elastic from	Ungloved hands will not be contaminated by touching only elastic or mask strings. Prevents

A 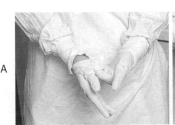 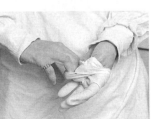 B

Fig. 37-2   Removal of gloves.

Step	Rationale

ears, pull mask away from face. For a tie-on mask, while holding strings, untie top mask string. Then hold strings while untying bottom strings. Pull mask away from face and drop into trash receptacle. (Do not touch outer surface of mask.)

top part of mask from falling down over nurse's uniform.

e. Perform hand hygiene.

Reduces transmission of microorganisms.

f. Retrieve wrist watch and stethoscope (unless it must remain in room), and record vital sign values on notepaper.

Clean hands can contact clean items.

g. Explain to client when you plan to return to room. Ask whether client requires any personal care items. Offer books, magazines, CDs, audiotapes.

Diversions help minimize boredom and feeling of social isolation.

h. Leave room and close door, if necessary. Door

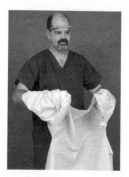

Fig. 37-3   Nurse removes gown.

Step	Rationale
should be closed if client is in negative airflow room.	
18. While in room, ask if client has had sufficient opportunity to discuss health problems, course of treatment, or other topics important to client.	Measures client's perception of adequacy of discussions with caregivers.
19. Complete postprocedure protocol.	

Recording and Reporting

- Document in nurses' progress notes the procedures performed and client's response to social isolation. Also document any client education performed and reinforced.

Unexpected Outcomes	Related Interventions
1. Client avoids social and therapeutic discussions.	• Confer with family and/or significant other, and determine best approach to reduce client's sense of loneliness and depression.
2. Client or health care worker may have allergy to latex gloves.	• Notify physician/employee health, and treat sensitivity or allergic reaction appropriately. • Use latex-free gloves for future care activities.

Mechanical Lifts

Mechanical lifts are devices to assist in transferring the dependent client or to assist the client with restricted mobility. One of the major concerns during transfer is the safety of the client and the nurse. The nurse prevents self-injury by using correct posture, minimal muscle strength, and effective body mechanics and lifting techniques. As a rule of thumb, nurses must get assistance if in doubt about their ability to transfer a client. Because of the risk of injury to nurses and their clients, the American Nurses Association (ANA) issued a position statement calling for the use of assistive equipment and devices to reposition and transfer clients to promote a safe health care environment (ANA, 2003). The use of assistive equipment, such as mechanical lifts, and continued use of proper body mechanics significantly reduce the risk of musculoskeletal injuries.

Delegation Consideration

The skills of using a mechanical lift to transfer clients may be delegated to assistive personnel (AP). Before delegating this skill, the nurse must:

- Supervise AP during the transfer of clients who are transferred for the first time after prolonged bed rest, extensive surgery, critical illness, or spinal cord trauma.
- Inform AP about the client's mobility restrictions, changes in blood pressure, or sensory alterations that may affect safe transfer.

Equipment

- *Mechanical/hydraulic lift:* Use frame, canvas strips or chains, and hammock or canvas strips

Step	Rationale
1. Complete preprocedure protocol.	
2. Assess client's physiological capacity to assist with transfer:	Determines client's ability to tolerate and assist with transfer and whether special adaptive techniques are necessary.
3. Assess presence of weakness, dizziness, or postural hypotension.	Determines risk of fainting or falling during transfer. Move from supine to vertical position redistributes about 500 ml of

Step	Rationale
	blood; immobile clients may have decreased ability for autonomic nervous system to equalize blood supply, resulting in orthostatic hypotension (Phipps and others, 2003).
4. Assess client's cognitive status:	Determines client's ability to follow directions and learn transfer techniques.
a. Ability to follow verbal instructions	May indicate clients at risk for injury.
b. Short-term memory	Clients with short-term memory deficits may have difficulty with transfer, initial learning, or consistent performance.
5. Assess client's specific risk of falling when transferred.	Certain conditions increase client's risk of falling or potential for injury. Neuromuscular deficits, motor weakness, calcium loss from long bones, cognitive and visual dysfunction, and altered balance increase risk of injury.
6. Bring lift to bedside.	Ensures safe elevation of client off bed. (Before using lift, be thoroughly familiar with its operation.) Research supports use of mechanical lifts to prevent musculoskeletal injuries (Hignett, 2003).
7. Position chair near bed, and allow adequate space to maneuver lift.	Prepares environment for safe use of lift and subsequent transfer.
8. Raise bed to high position with mattress flat. Lower side rail.	Allows nurse to use proper body mechanics.
9. Keep bed side rail up on side opposite nurse unless second nurse is assisting.	Maintains client safety.
10. Roll client on side away from nurse.	Positions client for use of lift sling.

Step	Rationale
11. Place hammock or canvas strips under client to form sling. With two canvas pieces, lower edge fits under client's knees (wide piece), and upper edge fits under client's shoulders (narrow piece).	Two types of seats are supplied with mechanical/hydraulic lift: hammock style is better for clients who are flaccid and weak and need support; canvas strips can be used for clients with normal muscle tone. Hooks should face away from client's skin. Place sling under client's center of gravity and greatest portion of body weight.
12. Raise bed rail.	Maintains client safety.
13. Go to opposite side of bed, and lower side rail.	
14. Roll client to opposite side, and pull hammock (strips) through.	Completes positioning of client on mechanical/hydraulic sling.
15. Roll client supine onto canvas seat.	Sling should extend from shoulders to knees (hammock) to support client's body weight equally.
16. Place lift's horseshoe bar under side of bed (on side with chair).	Positions lift efficiently and promotes smooth transfer.
17. Lower horizontal bar to sling level by releasing hydraulic valve. Lock valve.	Positions hydraulic lift close to client. Locking valve prevents injury to client.
18. Attach hooks on strap (chain) to holes in sling. Short chains or straps hook to top holes of sling; longer chains hook to bottom of sling (Fig. 38-1).	Secures hydraulic lift to sling.
19. Elevate head of bed.	Positions client in sitting position.
20. Fold client's arms over chest.	Prevents injury to client's arms.
21. Pump hydraulic handle using long, slow, even strokes until client is raised off bed.	Ensures safe support of client during elevation.

Step   **Rationale**

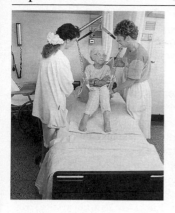

Fig. 38-1 Sling positioned under the client and attached to the lift.

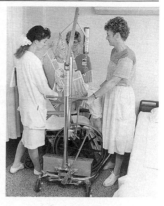

Fig. 38-2 Lowering client into the chair.

22. Use steering handle to pull lift from bed and maneuver to chair.

Moves client from bed to chair.

23. Roll base around chair.

Positions lift in front of chair in which client is to be transferred.

24. Release check valve slowly (turn to left), and lower client into chair (Fig. 38-2).

Safely guides client into chair as seat descends.

25. Close check valve as soon as client is down and straps can be released.

If valve is left open, boom may continue to lower and injure client.

26. Remove straps and mechanical/hydraulic lift.

Prevents damage to skin and underlying tissues from canvas or hooks.

27. Check client's sitting alignment, and correct if necessary.

Prevents injury from poor posture.

28. Complete postprocedure protocol.

Recording and Reporting

- Record and report procedure, including pertinent observations: weakness, ability to follow directions, weight-bearing ability, dizziness, balance, number of personnel needed to assist, and amount of assistance (muscle strength) required.

Unexpected Outcomes	Related Interventions
1. Client is unable to comprehend and follow directions for transfer.	• Cognitive impairment affects learning and retention: • Reassess continuity and simplicity of instruction. • Transfers may be difficult when client is fatigued or in pain; assess before transfer (allow for rest period before transferring, or medicate for pain if indicated).

Metered-Dose Inhalers

Inhaled medications produce local effects; for example, bronchodilators open narrowed bronchioles, and mucolytic agents liquefy thick mucous secretions. However, because these medications are absorbed rapidly through the pulmonary circulation, some have the potential for producing systemic side effects (e.g., isoproterenol [Isuprel] can cause cardiac dysrhythmias).

Clients who receive drugs by inhalation frequently suffer from chronic respiratory disease. Drugs administered by inhalation provide control of airway hyperactivity or constriction. Because clients depend on these medications for disease control, they must learn about the medications and how to administer them safely. Metered-dose inhalers (MDIs) and small-volume nebulizers are two devices that deliver medications.

Delegation Considerations

The skill of administering MDI medications should not be delegated to assistive personnel (AP).

- Instruct AP about potential side effects of medications and to report their occurrence.
- Instruct AP to report paroxysmal coughing, audible wheezing, and client's report of breathlessness or difficulty breathing.

Equipment

- MDI with medication canister
- Stethoscope
- Spacer device, such as AeroChamber or InspirEase (optional)
- Facial tissues (optional)
- Washbasin or sink with warm water
- Paper towel
- Medication administration record (MAR)

Step	Rationale
1. Complete preprocedure protocol.	
2. Assess client's ability to learn: client should not be fatigued, in pain, or in respiratory distress.	Mental or physical limitations affect client's ability to learn and methods nurse uses for instruction.

Step	Rationale
3. Assess client's ability to hold, manipulate, and depress canister and inhaler.	Any impairment of grasp or presence of hand tremors interferes with client's ability to depress canister within inhaler.
4. Assess drug schedule and number of inhalations prescribed for each dose.	Influences explanations nurse provides for use of inhaler.
5. If previously instructed in self-administration of inhaled medicine, assess client's technique in using inhaler.	Nurse's instruction may require only simple reinforcement, depending on client's level of dexterity.
6. Check accuracy and completeness of each MAR with prescriber's written medication order. Check client's name, drug name and dosage, route of administration, and time of administration.	Order sheet is most reliable source and only legal record of drugs client is to receive. Ensures that client receives correct medication.
7. Prepare medication. Check name of medication on canister against MAR.	Ensures that client receives correct medication.
8. Check client's identification bracelet, and ask name.	Ensures that correct client receives medication. At least two patient identifiers (neither to be patient's room number) are to be used whenever administering medications (JCAHO, 2004).
9. Explain procedure to client. Be specific if client wishes to self-administer drug. Explain where and how to set up in home.	Makes client participant in care and minimizes anxiety.
10. Provide adequate time for teaching session.	Prevents interruptions. Instruction should occur when client is receptive.
11. Allow client opportunity to manipulate inhaler, canister, and spacer device.	Client must be familiar with how to use equipment.

Step	Rationale

Explain and demonstrate how canister fits into inhaler.

NURSE ALERT If the client is using an MDI that is new or has not been used for several days, push a "test spray" into the air before administering the dose.

12. Explain what a metered dose is, and warn client about overuse of inhaler, including drug side effects.

    Client must not arbitrarily administer excessive inhalations because of risk of serious side effects and/or tolerance developing to medications. If drug is given in recommended doses, side effects are uncommon.

13. Explain steps for administering inhaled dose of medication (demonstrate steps when possible):

    Use of simple, step-by-step explanations allows client to ask questions at any point during procedure.

  a. Remove mouthpiece cover from inhaler.

  b. Shake inhaler well for 2 to 5 seconds (five or six shakes).

    Ensures mixing of medication in canister.

  c. Hold inhaler in dominant hand.

  d. Instruct client to position inhaler in one of two ways:

    (1) Place inhaler in mouth with opening toward back of throat, closing lips tightly around it (Fig. 39-1).

    (2) Position device 2 to 4 cm (1 to 2 inches) in front of widely

    Directs aerosol spray toward airway. Positioning mouthpiece 2 to 4 cm from mouth is

Step	Rationale

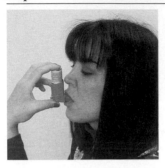

Fig. 39-1 One technique for use of an inhaler. The client opens lips and places the inhaler in the mouth with the opening toward the back of the throat.

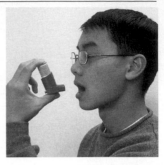

Fig. 39-2 One technique for use of an inhaler. The client positions the mouthpiece 2 to 4 cm (1 to 2 inches) from widely open mouth. This is considered the best way to deliver medication without a spacer.

Step	Rationale
opened mouth (Fig. 39-2), with opening of inhaler toward back of throat. Lips should not touch inhaler.	considered best way to deliver medication without spacer.
e. Have client take deep breath and exhale completely.	Prepares client's airway to receive medication.
f. With inhaler properly positioned, have client hold inhaler with thumb at mouthpiece and index finger and middle finger at top (Lilley and others, 2005).	Proper hand position ensures proper activation of MDI.
g. Instruct client to tilt head back slightly, inhale slowly and deeply through mouth, and depress medication canister fully.	Medication is distributed to airways during inhalation. Inhalation through mouth rather than nose draws medication into airways more effectively.

Step	**Rationale**
h. Breathe in slowly for 2 to 3 seconds; then hold breath for approximately 10 seconds.	Allows tiny drops of aerosol spray to reach deeper branches of airways.
i. Remove MDI from mouth before exhaling; then exhale slowly through nose or pursed lips.	Keeps small airways open during exhalation.
14. Explain steps to administer inhaled dose of medication using spacer device (demonstrate when possible):	
a. Remove mouthpiece cover from MDI and mouthpiece of spacer device.	Inhaler fits into end of spacer device.
b. Insert MDI into end of spacer device.	Spacer device traps medication released from MDI; client then inhales drug from device. Improves delivery of correct dose of inhaled medication (Togger and Brenner, 2001).
c. Shake inhaler well for 2 to 5 seconds (five or six shakes).	Ensures mixing of medication in canister.
d. Place spacer device mouthpiece in mouth and close lips. Do not insert beyond raised lip on mouthpiece. Do not cover small exhalation slots with lips.	Medication should not escape through mouth.
e. Breathe normally through spacer device mouthpiece.	Allows client to relax before delivering medication.
f. Depress medication canister, spraying one puff into spacer device.	Emits spray that allows finer particles to be inhaled. Large droplets are retained in spacer device.

Step	Rationale
g. Breathe in slowly and fully (for 5 seconds).	Ensures that particles of medication are distributed to deeper airways.
h. Hold full breath for 10 seconds.	Ensures full drug distribution.
15. Instruct client to wait 20 to 30 seconds between inhalations (if it is same medication), or 2 to 5 minutes between inhalations if medications are different.	Drugs must be inhaled sequentially. If bronchodilators are administered with inhaled steroids, bronchodilators should be given first to allow airway passages to be more open for second medication.
16. Instruct client against repeating inhalations before next scheduled dose.	Drugs are prescribed at intervals during day to provide constant drug levels and minimize side effects.
17. Explain that client may feel gagging sensation in throat caused by droplets of medication on pharynx or tongue.	Results when inhalant is sprayed and inhaled incorrectly.
18. For daily cleaning, instruct client to remove medication canister, rinse inhaler and cap with warm running water, and ensure that inhaler is completely dry before reuse. Twice weekly, the L-shaped mouthpiece should be washed with mild dishwashing soap and warm water, rinsed, and dried well.	Removes residual medication.
19. Complete postprocedure protocol.	

Recording and Reporting

- Immediately after administration, record on MAR the actual time each drug was administered, dosage, and concentration. Include initials or signature.

- Record client's response to medication, including pulse, respirations, breath sounds assessed, and any adverse effects.
- Document what skills were taught and client's ability to perform them.
- Report adverse effects/client response and/or withheld drugs to nurse in charge or physician.

Unexpected Outcomes	Related Interventions
1. Client experiences paroxysms of coughing.	• May need to reassess type of medication and/or delivery method. • Notify prescriber.
2. Client needs bronchodilator more than every 4 hours.	• Reassess type of medication and delivery methods. • Notify prescriber.
3. Client experiences cardiac dysrhythmias (light-headedness, syncope), especially if receiving beta-adrenergics.	• Withhold all further doses of medication. • Notify prescriber for reassessment of type of medication and delivery method.
4. Client may not be able to self-administer medication properly.	• Alternative delivery routes or devices may need to be explored.

Moist Heat (Compress and Sitz Bath)

Moist heat applications include warm compresses, commercial heat packs, warm baths and soaks, and sitz baths. A warm compress is a section of sterile or clean gauze moistened with a prescribed heated solution (e.g., normal saline, sterile water) and applied directly to an open wound or the skin's surface. A sterile compress is necessary only when there is a break in skin integrity. Commercially packaged sterile, premoistened compresses require the use of a special infrared lamp to heat. Plain sterile or clean gauze can be heated by adding the gauze to a container of warmed solution. Moist warm compresses improve circulation, relieve edema, promote consolidation of exudate in a wound, and promote comfort.

When preparing moist heat applications, remember that the client is at risk for burns to the skin. Check the water temperature of baths or soaks frequently. Keep the solution temperature constant to enhance the moist heat's therapeutic effects. Whenever you add heated solution to a soak basin or bath, first remove the client's body part and then reimmerse once the solution has mixed.

Delegation Considerations

When the client is assessed by the nurse to be stable and there are no risks or complications, the skill of applying moist heat can be delegated to assistive personnel (AP).

- Discuss with AP the need to maintain proper temperature of the application throughout the treatment and to keep the application in place for only the required length of time.
- Caution AP to inform the nurse if any discomfort develops, requiring termination of the treatment.
- Caution AP to inform the nurse if the client complains of dizziness or light-headedness.
- Instruct AP to report when treatment is complete so that the client's response can be evaluated.

Equipment

- Clean basin, tub, or sitz bath (basin may need to be sterile if body part to be soaked has an open wound)

- Prescribed solution warmed to appropriate temperature (tap water is commonly used for sitz baths)
- Absorbent gauze dressing, cloth rolls, or commercially prepared compresses
- Prescribed medication (if ordered)
- Dry bath towel
- Clean gloves
- Sterile gloves
- Waterproof pad
- Ties or tape
- Aquathermia or electric heating pad (optional)
- Bath blanket

Step	Rationale
1. Complete preprocedure protocol.	
2. Assess skin around area to be treated for sensitivity to temperature and pain by measuring light touch, pinprick, and temperature sensation.	Certain conditions alter conduction of sensory impulses that transmit temperature and pain. Clients insensitive to heat or cold sensations must be monitored closely during treatment.

NURSE ALERT Clients with diabetes, victims of stroke or spinal cord injury, and clients with peripheral neuropathy are particularly at risk for thermal injury (Stitik and Nadler, 1999).

Step	Rationale
3. Describe sensations to be felt, such as decreasing warmth and wetness. Explain precautions to prevent burning.	Minimizes client's anxiety and promotes cooperation during procedure.
4. Apply warm sterile compress/commercial heat pack:	
a. Assist client in assuming comfortable position in proper body alignment, and place waterproof pad under area to be treated.	Compress remains in place for several minutes. Limited mobility in uncomfortable position causes muscular stress. Pad prevents soiling of bed linen.

Step	Rationale
b. Expose body part to be covered with compress, and drape client with bath blanket.	Prevents unnecessary cooling and exposure of body part.
c. Prepare compress: (1) Pour solution into sterile container. (2) If using portable heating source, warm solution. Commercially prepared compresses may remain under infrared lamp until just before use.	Proper warming ensures desired therapeutic effect.

NURSE ALERT To avoid injury to client, test temperature of sterile solution by applying drop to nurse's forearm (without contaminating solution).

Step	Rationale
d. Prepare aquathermia pad (if needed) (see Skill 3)	Used to encircle compress and maintain constant warmth.
e. 🖐 Remove any existing dressing covering wound. Dispose of gloves and dressings in proper receptacle. Perform hand hygiene.	Reduces transmission of microorganisms.
f. Assess condition of wound and surrounding skin. Inflamed wound appears reddened, but surrounding skin is less red in color.	Provides baseline to determine response to moist heat.

NURSE ALERT If skin surrounding wound is reddened, application may be contraindicated.

Step	Rationale
g. Don sterile gloves.	Allows nurse to manipulate sterile dressing and touch open wound.

Step	**Rationale**
h. Pick up one layer of immersed gauze, wring out any excess solution, and apply it lightly to open wound, avoiding surrounding skin.	Excess moisture macerates skin and increases risk of burns and infection. Skin is sensitive to sudden change in temperature.
i. In few seconds, lift edge of gauze to assess for redness.	Increased redness indicates burn.
j. If client tolerates compress, pack gauze snugly against wound. Be sure all wound surfaces are covered by warm compress.	Packing of compress prevents rapid cooling from underlying air currents.
k. Cover moist compress with dry sterile dressing and bath towel. If necessary, pin or tie in place. Remove sterile gloves.	Dry sterile dressing will prevent transfer of microorganisms to wound via capillary action caused by moist compress. Towel insulates compress to prevent heat loss.
l. Apply aquathermia or waterproof heating pad over towel *(optional)* (see Skill 3). Keep it in place for desired duration of application.	Provides constant temperature to compress.

NURSE ALERT Removing warm compress after 20 minutes and then reapplying in 15 minutes, if desired, maintains vasodilation and positive therapeutic effect. Local application of heat for more than 20 minutes may cause reflex vasoconstriction (Stitik and Nadler, 1999).

m. If aquathermia pad is *not* used to maintain temperature of application, change warm compress using sterile technique every 5 to 10 minutes or as ordered during duration of therapy.	Prevents cooling and maintains therapeutic benefit of compress.

Step	Rationale
n. After prescribed time, remove pad, towel, and compress. Reassess wound and condition of skin, and replace dry sterile dressing as ordered.	Continued exposure to moisture will macerate skin. Prevents entrance of microorganisms into wound site.
5. Provide sitz bath or soak to intact, open skin:	
a. Remove any existing dressing covering wound. Dispose of gloves and dressings in proper receptacle.	Reduces transmission of microorganisms.
b. Assess condition of wound and surrounding skin. Pay particular attention to suture line.	Provides baseline to determine response to warm soak.
c. Fill basin or tub with warmed solution. Check temperature.	Checking for correct temperature reduces risk of burns.
d. Assist client to immerse body part in tub or basin.	Prevents falls.
e. Cover client with bath blanket or towel as desired.	Prevents chilling and enhances client's ability to relax.
f. Maintain constant temperature throughout 15- to 20-minute soak:	Ensures proper therapeutic effect.
(1) Keep large sheet or blanket over container or basin.	Prevents heat loss through evaporation. Therapeutic effects of soak can be obtained only from constant temperature.
(2) After 10 minutes, remove body part from soak, check to see that skin is not burned, empty	Presence of burn contraindicates completing soak. Adding warmed solution to basin with body part immersed can cause burn.

Step	Rationale
cooled solution, add newly heated solution, and reimmerse body part.	
g. ✋ After 15 to 20 minutes, remove client from soak or bath; dry body parts thoroughly. (Clean gloves are required if drainage is present.)	Avoids chilling. Enhances client's comfort.
h. Drain solution from basin or tub. Clean and place in proper storage area.	Reduces transmission of microorganisms.
6. Complete postprocedure protocol.	

Recording and Reporting

- Record in nurses' notes the procedure, noting type, location, and duration of application, as well as solution and temperature.
- Record condition of body part, wound, and skin before and after treatment and client's response to therapy.
- Record instructions given and client's ability to explain and perform procedure.
- Report any evidence of burn to skin immediately to physician.

Unexpected Outcomes	Related Interventions
1. Client's skin is reddened and sensitive to touch.	• Discontinue moist application immediately.
	• Notify physician.
2. Client complains of burning and discomfort.	• Extreme temperature for client to tolerate—reduce temperature.
	• Assess for skin breakdown.
	• Notify physician.

Mouth Care: Unconscious or Debilitated Clients

Unconscious or debilitated clients pose challenges because of their risk for having alterations of the oral cavity. The absence of saliva movement and production in the unconscious or orally intubated (artificial airway) client has serious implications. In as few as 3 days, plaque can become a host for hundreds of gram-negative bacteria.

Research has resulted in improved standards for oral care of the critically ill (Stiefel and others, 2000). Foam stick applicators, a popular substitute for the toothbrush, stimulate the mucosal tissues but are ineffective in removing debris from the teeth (Grap and others, 2003). Hydrogen peroxide, once used routinely in intensive care units (ICUs) for mouth care, removes debris and is anti-infective but if not diluted can easily cause burns of the mucosa (Grap and others, 2003).

Delegation Considerations

The skill of providing mouth care to an unconscious or debilitated client may be delegated to assistive personnel (AP). However, the nurse must first assess the client's gag reflex. The nurse provides AP with information, assistance, and direction, including:

- Informing AP of the proper way to position clients for mouth care.
- Informing AP of signs of impaired integrity of oral mucosa to report to nurse.
- Instructing AP to inform nurse if possible aspiration is suspected.

Equipment

- Small pediatric soft-bristled toothbrush
- Sponge toothette for edentulous client
- Fluoridated toothpaste
- Tongue blade
- Oral airway (optional)
- Small bulb syringe or portable suction device with catheter
- Oral airway (uncooperative client or client who shows bite reflex)
- Vaseline lip lubricant or water-based lubricant
- Cup of water
- Face towel

- Paper towels
- Emesis basin
- Disposable gloves

Step	Rationale
1. Complete preprocedure protocol.	
2. Verify presence of gag reflex by placing tongue blade on back half of tongue.	Reveals whether client is at risk for aspiration.
3. Place paper towels on over-bed table, and arrange equipment. If needed, turn on suction machine and connect tubing to suction catheter.	Prevents soiling of tabletop. Equipment prepared in advance ensures smooth, safe procedure.
4. Unless contraindicated (e.g., head injury, neck trauma) position client in side-lying position close to side of bed; keep client's head turned toward mattress. Remove dentures or partial plates if present.	Proper positioning of head prevents aspiration of secretions.
5. Place towel under client's head and emesis basin under chin.	Prevents soiling of bed linen.
6. If client is uncooperative or having difficulty keeping mouth open, insert oral airway. Insert upside down, then turn airway sideways and then over tongue to keep teeth apart. Insert when client is relaxed, if possible. Do not use force.	Prevents client from biting down on nurse's fingers and provides access to oral cavity.
7. Brush teeth with toothpaste, using up-and-down gentle motion. Clean chewing and inner tooth	Brushing action removes food particles between teeth and along chewing surfaces. Swabbing helps remove secretions and crusts

Step	Rationale
surfaces first. Clean outer tooth surfaces. Brush roof of mouth, gums, and inside cheeks. Gently brush tongue but avoid stimulating gag reflex (if present). Moisten brush with water to rinse. (Bulb syringe may also be used to rinse.) Repeat rinse several times.	from mucosa and moistens mucosa. Repeated rinsing removes all debris.

NURSE ALERT   For clients without teeth, use a toothette moistened in water or normal saline to clean oral cavity.

8. Suction secretions as they accumulate, if necessary.	Suction removes secretions and fluid that can collect in posterior pharynx. Reduces risk of aspiration.
9. Apply thin layer of moisturizing gel or water-soluble lubricant to lips.	Lubricates lips to prevent drying and cracking.
10. Complete postprocedure protocol.	

Recording and Reporting

- Record procedure on flow sheet. Record any pertinent observations (e.g., presence of gag reflex, presence of bleeding gums, dry mucosa, ulcerations, crusts on tongue).
- Report any unusual findings to nurse in charge or physician.

Unexpected Outcomes	Related Interventions
1. Localized inflammation of gums or mucosa is present.	• More frequent oral hygiene with soft-bristled toothbrush is needed. • Apply Oral Balance moisturizing gel to mucosa and massage (Fitch and others, 1999). • Chemotherapy and radiation can cause stomatitis. Clients should rinse mouth before and after meals and at bedtime, using normal saline or solution of $^1/_2$ to 1 teaspoon of salt or baking soda to 1 pint of tepid water.
2. Client aspirates secretions.	• If present, suction oral airway as secretions accumulate to maintain patent airway. • Elevate client's head of bed to facilitate breathing. • Be prepared to have chest x-ray examination performed following physician's order.

Nail and Foot Care

Feet and nails often require special care to prevent infection, odors, pain, and injury to soft tissues. Often people are unaware of foot or nail problems until discomfort or pain occurs. For proper foot and nail care, instruct your client how to protect the feet from injury, to keep the feet clean and dry, and to wear appropriate footwear.

Clients most at risk for developing serious foot problems are those with peripheral neuropathy and peripheral vascular disease. These two disorders, commonly found in clients with diabetes, cause a reduction in blood flow to the extremities and a loss of sensory, motor, and autonomic nerve function. As a result, your client may not be able to feel heat and cold, pain, pressure, and position of the foot. The reduction in blood flow impairs healing and promotes risk for infection.

Delegation Considerations

The skill of nail and foot care of the nondiabetic client and clients without circulatory compromise may be delegated to assistive personnel (AP). However, you need to provide AP with information, assistance, and direction, including:

- Informing and assisting AP in proper way to use nail clippers. (NOTE: Many agencies do not allow AP or even nurses to use nail clippers; consult agency policy.)
- Cautioning AP to use warm water.
- Instructing AP to report any changes that may indicate inflammation or injury.

Equipment

- Washbasin
- Emesis basin
- Washcloth
- Bath or face towel
- Nail clippers (check agency policy)
- Orange stick (optional)
- Emery board or nail file
- Body lotion
- Disposable gloves
- Disposable bath mat
- Paper towels

Step	Rationale
1. Complete preprocedure protocol.	
2. Inspect all surfaces of fingers, toes, feet, and nails. Pay particular attention to areas of dryness, inflammation, or cracking. Also inspect areas between toes, heels, and soles of feet. Inspect socks for stains.	Integrity of feet and nails determines frequency and level of hygiene required. Heels, soles, and sides of feet are prone to irritation from ill-fitting shoes. Socks may become stained from bleeding or draining ulcer.
3. Assess type of footwear worn by clients: Are socks worn? Are shoes tight or ill fitting? Are garters or knee-high nylons worn? Is footwear clean?	Types of shoes and footwear may predispose client to foot and nail problems (e.g., infection, areas of friction, ulcerations).
4. Identify client's risk for foot or nail problems:	Certain conditions increase likelihood of foot or nail problems.
a. Client with diabetes	Vascular changes associated with diabetes reduce blood flow to peripheral tissues. Break in skin integrity places clients with diabetes at high risk for skin infection.
b. Client with heart failure or renal disease	Both conditions can increase tissue edema, particularly in dependent areas (e.g., feet). Edema reduces blood flow to neighboring tissues.
5. Fill washbasin with warm water. Test water temperature.	Warm water softens nails and thickened epidermal cells, reduces inflammation of skin, and promotes local circulation. Proper water temperature prevents burns and injury (Armstrong and Lavery, 1998).

Step	Rationale
6. Place basin on bath mat or towel, and help client place feet in basin. Place call light within client's reach.	Clients with muscular weakness or tremors may have difficulty positioning feet. Client's safety is maintained.

NURSE ALERT The American Diabetes Association (1999) does not recommend soaking a diabetic client's feet because of risk of infection.

Step	Rationale
7. Adjust over-bed table to low position, and place it over client's lap. (Client may sit in chair or lie in bed.)	Easy access prevents accidental spills.
8. Fill emesis basin with warm water, and place basin on paper towels on over-bed table.	Warm water softens nails and thickened epidermal cells.
9. Instruct client to place fingers in emesis basin and place arms in comfortable position.	Prolonged positioning can cause discomfort unless normal anatomical alignment is maintained.
10. Clean gently under fingernails with orange stick or end of wooden applicator stick while fingers are immersed (Fig. 42-1). Remove emesis basin, and dry fingers thoroughly.	Orange stick removes debris under nails that harbors microorganisms. Thorough drying impedes fungal growth and prevents maceration of tissues.
11. With nail clippers, clip fingernails straight across and even with tops of fingers (Fig. 42-2). Shape nails with emery board or file.	Cutting straight across prevents splitting of nail margins and formation of sharp nail spikes that can irritate lateral nail margins. Filing prevents cutting nail too close to nail bed (Strauss and others, 1998).

NURSE ALERT If the client has diabetes or circulatory problems, do not cut the nail. File only.

Step	**Rationale**

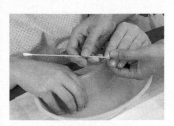

Fig. 42-1 Clean under fingernails.

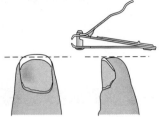

Fig. 42-2 Use nail clipper to clip fingernails straight across.

Step	**Rationale**
12. Push cuticle back gently with orange stick.	Pushing back cuticles reduces incidence of inflamed cuticles.
13. Scrub calloused areas of feet with washcloth.	Gloves prevent transmission of fungal infection. Friction removes dead skin layers.
14. Clean gently under nails with orange stick. Remove feet from basin, and dry thoroughly.	Removal of debris and excess moisture reduces chances of infection.
15. Clean and trim toenails using procedures in Steps 13 through 16. Do not file corners of toenails.	Shaping corners of toenails may damage tissues (Strauss and others, 1998).
16. Apply lotion to feet and hands, and assist client back to bed and into comfortable position.	Lotion lubricates dry skin by helping retain moisture.

NURSE ALERT The American Diabetes Association (2003) does not recommend lotion between the toes of clients with diabetes. Moisture can cause maceration and skin breakdown.

Step	**Rationale**
17. Inspect nails, areas between toes, and surrounding skin surfaces.	Inspection enables nurse to evaluate condition of skin and nails and allows nurse to note any remaining rough nail edges.
18. Complete postprocedure protocol.	

Recording and Reporting

- Record procedure and observations in nurses' notes (e.g., breaks in skin, inflammation, ulcerations).
- Report any breaks in skin or ulcerations to nurse in charge or physician.

Unexpected Outcomes	Related Interventions
1. Cuticles and surrounding tissues may be inflamed and tender to touch. Localized areas of tenderness may occur on feet with calluses or corns at point of friction.	• Repeated nail care is needed. • Change in footwear or corrective foot surgery may be needed for permanent improvement in calluses or corns. • Referral to podiatrist may be needed.
2. Ulcerations involving toes or feet may remain.	• Institute wound care policies. • Consult with wound care specialist and/or podiatrist.

Nasoenteral Tube: Placement, Irrigation, and Removal

Insertion of a nasoenteral tube involves placing a pliable, small-bore, plastic tube through the client's nasopharynx into the stomach. Small-bore tubes can be left in place for an extended period with less irritation to the nasopharyngeal, esophageal, and gastric mucosa. Because the tubes are flexible, a guidewire or stylet is used to provide rigidity to facilitate insertion and positioning; it is removed once correct placement is verified. Placing a nasoenteral tube requires a physician's order.

Small-bore feeding tubes are available in weighted (tungsten) or nonweighted designs. Weighted tubes were thought to pass more easily into the duodenum or jejunum via peristalsis; however, research has not demonstrated an advantage of the weight in promoting intestinal passage. Nonetheless, weighted tubes are used more frequently than nonweighted tubes for nasoduodenal and nasojejunal feedings because they are believed to remain in correct position longer than nonweighted tubes. Aside from the weighted tip, small-bore tubes are made of a softer material than large-bore tubes.

Delegation Considerations

This skill may not be delegated to assistive personnel (AP). However, AP may assist with client positioning during tube insertion.

Equipment

- Nasogastric (NG) or nasointestinal (NI) tube (8 to 12 Fr) with guidewire or stylet
- 60-ml or larger Luer-Lok or catheter-tip syringe
- Stethoscope
- Hypoallergenic tape and tincture of benzoin or tube fixation device
- pH indicator strip (scale 0.0 to 14.0)
- Glass of water and straw for clients able to swallow
- Emesis basin
- Towel
- Facial tissues

- Tape and rubber band
- Clean gloves
- Suction equipment in case of aspiration
- Penlight to check placement in nasopharynx
- Tongue blade

Step	Rationale
Complete preprocedure protocol.	
A. Insertion of Nasoenteral Tube	
1. Determine patency of nares. Have client close each nostril alternately and breathe. Examine each naris for patency and skin breakdown.	Nares may be obstructed or irritated, or septal defect or facial fractures may be present.
2. Assess client for gag reflex. Place tongue blade in client's mouth, touching uvula.	Assists nurse in identifying client's ability to swallow and determines if greater risk of aspiration exists.
3. Assess client's mental status.	Alert client is better able to cooperate with procedure. If vomiting should occur, alert client can usually expectorate vomitus, which can help reduce risk of aspiration.
4. Auscultate for bowel sounds.	Absence of bowel sounds may indicate decreased or absent peristalsis and increased risk of aspiration. Reassess frequently after initiation of tube feedings. Monitor residual volume.
5. Determine if physician wants prokinetic agent administered before placement of nasoenteral tube.	Prokinetic agents, such as metoclopramide, given *before* tube placement, have been shown to help advance tube into intestine (Kittinger and others, 1987).
6. Explain to client how to communicate during intubation by raising index	It is important for client to have way of communicating to alleviate stress. Nurse may pause

Step	Rationale

finger to indicate gagging or discomfort.

insertion procedure to decrease gagging.

NURSE ALERT Nasoenteral tubes may be inserted in clients with altered levels of consciousness, but the risk of inadvertent respiratory placement is increased if the gag reflex is impaired.

7. Position client sitting with head of bed elevated at least 30 degrees or high-Fowler's position. If client is comatose, place in semi-Fowler's position with head propped forward using pillow. Assistant may be necessary to help with positioning of confused or comatose clients. If client is forced to lie supine, place in reverse Trendelenburg position.

Reduces risk of pulmonary aspiration in event client should vomit. Head propped assists with closure of airway and passage of tube into esophagus. Natural response to object being inserted into nose is to tip head backward; this should be avoided because it opens airway.

8. Examine feeding tube for flaws: rough or sharp edges on distal end and closed or clogged outlet holes.

Flaws in feeding tube hamper tube intubation and can injure client. Clogged outlets do not allow passage of feeding.

9. Determine length of tube to be inserted, and mark with tape or indelible ink (Fig. 43-1).

Being aware of proper length to intubate determines approximate depth of insertion.

10. Prepare NG or NI tube for intubation:
    a. Perform hand hygiene.

    Reduces spread of microorganisms.

    b. Inject 10 ml of water from 60-ml Luer-Lok or catheter-tip syringe into tube.

    Aids in guidewire or stylet insertion.

    c. Make certain that guidewire is securely positioned against weighted tip and that

    Promotes smooth passage of tube into gastrointestinal (GI) tract. Improperly positioned stylet can induce serious trauma.

Step	Rationale

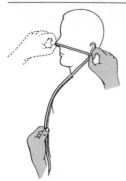

Fig. 43-1   Determine length of tube to be inserted.

both Luer-Lok connections are snugly fitted together.

11. Cut adhesive tape 10 cm (4 inches) long, or prepare tube fixation device.

12. Dip tube with surface lubricant into glass of room-temperature water, or apply water-soluble lubricant. Plastic tubes should *not* be placed in cold water or ice water.

Activates lubricant to facilitate passage of tube into nares and GI tract. Tubes will become stiff and inflexible, causing trauma to mucous membranes.

13. Hand alert client glass of water with straw or glass with crushed ice (if able to swallow).

Client will be asked to swallow water to facilitate tube passage.

14. Gently insert tube through nostril to back of throat (posterior nasopharynx). May cause client to gag. Aim back and down toward ear.

Natural contours facilitate passage of tube into GI tract.

15. Have client flex head toward chest after tube has passed through nasopharynx.

Closes off glottis and reduces risk of tube entering trachea.

Step	Rationale
16. Emphasize need to mouth breathe and swallow during procedure.	Helps facilitate passage of tube and alleviates client's fears during procedure.
17. When tube is inserted to tip of carina (approximately 25 cm [10 inches] in adult), stop and listen for air exchange from distal portion of tube.	If air can be heard, tube could be in respiratory tract; remove tube, and start over (Metheny and Titler, 2001).
18. Advance tube each time client swallows until desired length has been passed.	Reduces discomfort and trauma to client.
19. Using penlight and tongue blade, check for position of tube in back of throat.	Tube may be coiled, kinked, or entering trachea.
20. Temporarily anchor tube to nose with small piece of tape, and check placement of tube.	Movement of tube stimulates gagging. Assesses general position before anchoring tube more securely.
21. Remove gloves.	
22. Obtain x-ray of chest/ abdomen and confirm x-ray results.	Proper position is essential before initiating feedings.
23. Remove guidewire or stylet after x-ray verification of correct placement.	Must remain in place until tube verification.
24. Routinely measure and observe location of external exit site marking on tube, as well as color and pH of fluid withdrawn from NG or NI tube.	Can reveal if end of tube has changed position. However, it is possible that tube can change position inside GI tract with no external evidence of change.
25. Anchor tube to nose and avoid pressure on nares. Mark exit site with indelible ink. Use one of following options for anchoring: a. **Apply tape:** (1) Apply tincture of benzoin or other	Properly secured tube allows client more mobility and prevents trauma to nasal mucosa. Helps tape adhere better. Protects skin.

Step	**Rationale**
skin adhesive on tip of client's nose, and allow it to become tacky.	
(2) Split one end of the adhesive tape strip lengthwise 5 cm (2 inches).	
(3) Wrap each of the 5-cm strips in opposite directions around tube as it exits nose (Fig. 43-2).	
b. **Apply tube fixation device** using shaped adhesive patch:	
(1) Apply wide end of patch to bridge of nose (Fig. 43-3).	
(2) Slip connector around feeding tube as it exits nose (Fig. 43-4).	
26. Fasten end of NG tube to client's gown using piece of tape. Do not use safety pins to pin tube to client's gown.	Reduces traction on nares if tube moves. Safety pins can become unfastened and injure client.

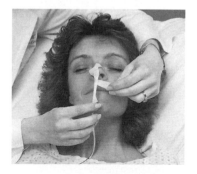

Fig. 43-2 Wrap tape to anchor nasoenteral tube.

Step   **Rationale**

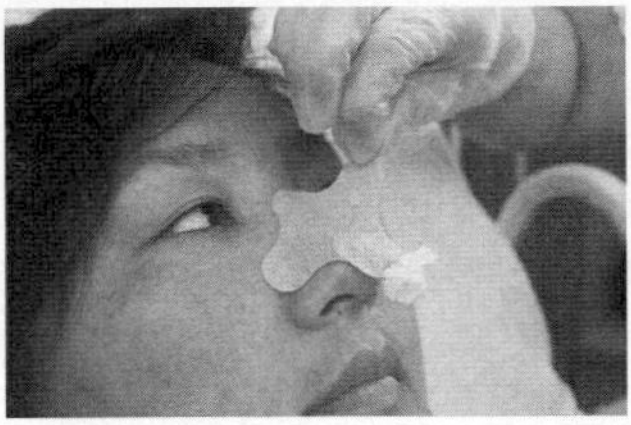

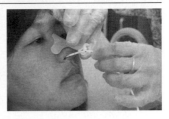

Fig. 43-3 Applying patch to bridge of nose.

Fig. 43-4 Slip connector around feeding tube.

27. Assist client to comfortable position. NOTE: Positioning client on right side does not facilitate intestinal placement.

Makes client comfortable. Researchers indicate that placing client on right side does not promote passage of tube into small intestine (Kittinger and others, 1987).

28. Administer oral hygiene. Cleanse tubing at nostril with washcloth dampened in mild soap and water.

Promotes client comfort and integrity of oral mucous membranes.

29. Remove gloves, dispose of equipment, and perform hand hygiene.

Reduces transmission of microorganisms.

B. Irrigating Feeding Tube

1. Assemble supplies:
   • 60-ml catheter-tip syringe
   • Normal saline or tap water
   • Towel
   • Disposable gloves

2. Explain procedure to client, and position in high-Fowler's position (if tolerated) or semi-Fowler's position.

Reduces risk of aspiration during irrigation.

3. Verify tube placement.

With tube correctly placed into stomach, irrigation will not increase risk of aspiration.

Step	Rationale
a. Draw up 30 ml of air into 60-ml syringe, and then attach to end of feeding tube. Flush tube with air before attempting to aspirate.	Burst of air aids in aspirating fluid more easily (Metheny and others, 1993). Smaller syringes generate unnecessary high pressures inside tube.
b. Draw back on syringe slowly, and obtain 5-10 ml of gastric aspirate (Fig. 43-5).	Quickly aspirating gastric contents increases pressure within tube and may cause tube to collapse.
c. Gently mix aspirate in syringe. Measure pH of aspirated contents by dipping pH strip into aspirated gastric contents (Fig. 43-6).	Mixing ensures equal distribution of contents for pH testing. Range of 1 to 4 is reliable indictor for stomach placement of tube (Metheny and others, 1999).
4. Draw up 30 ml of normal saline or tap water into syringe (Fig. 43-7).	This amount of fluid will flush length of tube. Irrigation fluids should be not used from multidose bottles that are used on other clients.
5. Kink feeding tube while disconnecting it from feeding-bag tubing or while removing plug at end of tube (Fig. 43-8). Place end of feeding-bag tubing on towel.	Prevents leakage of gastric secretions.

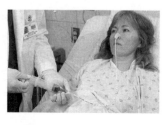

Fig. 43-5 Obtaining gastric aspirate.

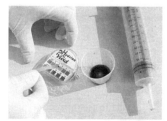

Fig. 43-6 Compare color test on pH strip with color on chart.

Step	Rationale

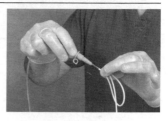

Fig. 43-8 Kink tubing while unplugging feeding tube.

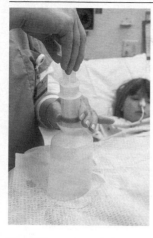

Fig. 43-7 Draw up 30 ml of solution into syringe.

6. Insert tip of catheter into end of feeding tube. Release kink, and slowly instill irrigating solution.

Infusion of fluid clears tubing.

7. If unable to instill fluid, reposition client on left side and try again

Tip of tube may be against stomach wall. Repositioning may move tip away from stomach wall.

8. When irrigation complete, remove syringe and reconnect feeding tube to tube feeding bag. Resume tube feedings as ordered.

9. Remove gloves, dispose of supplies, and perform hand hygiene

C. Removal of Feeding Tube

1. Verify order to discontinue feeding tube.

Order is needed for procedure.

2. Explain procedure to client.

Step	Rationale
3. ![icon] Disconnect tube feeding, and place feeding bag away from client's bed. Remove tape or fixation device from bridge of nose, and remove tube from gown.	Feeding tube is free of connections before removal.
4. Stand on client's right side, if right-handed; or left side, if left-handed.	Allows easy manipulation of tube.
5. Place clean towel across client's chest, and hand client tissue. Instruct client to take deep breath and hold.	Towel keeps bedding from getting soiled. Client may wish to blow nose immediately after tube is removed. Holding breath reduces risk for aspiration.
6. Clamp or kink tube securely, and then pull tube out in steady, smooth motion. Place tube on towel.	Clamping prevents residual feeding in tube from draining into client's oropharynx.
7. Measure any drainage. Dispose of tube and equipment properly.	
8. Clean nares, and provide oral hygiene.	Promotes client comfort.
9. Observe client to determine response to NG or NI tube intubation. Have client speak. Check vital signs and oxygen saturation.	Client who is comfortable, able to speak without difficulty, and has normal oxygen saturation is likely to have correctly placed tube.
10. Observe nares for irritation and redness.	Indicates pressure on nares from feeding tube.

Recording and Reporting

- Record and report type and size of tube placed, location of distal tip of tube, client's tolerance of procedure, and confirmation of tube position by x-ray examination. Documentation of nonrespiratory placement by x-ray examination is standard practice when small-bore tube is initially inserted. Record and report any type of unexpected outcome and interventions performed.

Unexpected Outcomes	Related Interventions
1. Placement of tube into respiratory tract. This may not be discovered until x-ray report. Small-bore or large-bore tube can enter airway without causing obvious respiratory symptoms, particularly in semiconscious or unconscious client.	• Remove tube, and report incident to physician; obtain order for reinsertion.
2. Aspiration of stomach contents into respiratory tract (immediate response) in alert client, evidenced by coughing, dyspnea, cyanosis, or decreases in oxygen saturation values during procedure.	• Position client on side to protect airway. • Suction client nasotracheally or orotracheally to try to remove aspirated substance. • Report event immediately to physician.
3. Clogging of feeding tube.	• Irrigate tube.
4. Nasal mucosa becomes inflamed, tender, and/or eroded.	• Retape tube in different position to relieve pressure on mucosa. • If tube has been in same site for extended period, consider reinsertion of tube in opposite naris (physician's order required).

Nasogastric Tube for Gastric Decompression: Insertion and Removal

Sometimes after major surgery or as a result of conditions affecting the gastrointestinal (GI) tract, normal peristalsis temporarily becomes altered. Because peristalsis is slowed or absent, a client cannot eat or drink fluids without causing abdominal distention. The temporary insertion of a nasogastric (NG) tube into the stomach serves to decompress the stomach, keeping it empty until normal peristalsis returns.

The Levin and Salem sump tubes are the most common for stomach decompression. The Levin tube is a single-lumen tube with holes near the tip. It may be connected to a drainage bag or an intermittent suction device to drain stomach secretions. The Salem sump tube is preferable for stomach decompression. The tube has two lumina: one for removal of gastric contents and one to provide an air vent. A blue "pigtail" is the air vent that connects with the second lumen. When the sump tube's main lumen is connected to suction, the air vent permits free, continuous drainage of secretions. *The air vent should never be clamped off, connected to suction, or used for irrigation.*

Delegation Considerations

The skill of inserting and maintaining an NG tube may not be delegated to assistive personnel (AP). You are responsible for the proper function and drainage of the NG tube, all relevant assessments, and determining the client's level of comfort. You may direct AP to:

- Measure and record the drainage from an NG tube.
- Provide oral and nasal hygiene measures.
- Perform selected comfort measures, such as positioning, offering ice chips if allowed.
- Anchor the tube to the client's gown during routine care to prevent accidental displacement.

Equipment

- 14- or 16-Fr NG tube (smaller-lumen catheters are not used for decompression in adults because they cannot remove thick secretions)
- Water-soluble lubricating jelly

- pH test strips (measure gastric aspirate acidity)
- Tongue blade
- Flashlight
- Emesis basin
- Asepto bulb or catheter-tip syringe
- 1-inch– (2.5-cm–) wide hypoallergenic tape or commercial fixation device
- Tape and rubber band
- Clamp, drainage bag, or suction machine or pressure gauge if wall suction is to be used
- Towel
- Glass of water with straw
- Facial tissues
- Normal saline
- Tincture of benzoin (optional)
- Suction equipment
- Disposable gloves

Step	Rationale
1. Complete preprocedure protocol.	
2. See Skill 43, Steps 1–11.	
3. Check medical record for physician's order, type of NG tube to be placed, and whether tube is to be attached to suction or drainage bag.	Procedure requires physician's order. Adequate decompression depends on NG suction.
4. Stand on client's right side if right-handed; left side if left-handed.	Allows easier manipulation of tubing.
5. Instruct client to relax and breathe normally while occluding one naris. Then repeat this action for other naris. Select nostril with greater airflow.	Tube passes more easily through naris that is more patent.
6. Curve 10 to 15 cm (4 to 6 inches) of end of tube tightly around index finger; then release.	Curving tube tip aids insertion and decreases stiffness of tube.

Step	**Rationale**
7. Lubricate 7.5 to 10 cm (3 to 4 inches) of end of tube with water-soluble lubricating gel.	Minimizes friction against nasal mucosa and aids insertion of tube. Water-soluble lubricant is less toxic than oil-soluble if aspirated.
8. Alert client that procedure is to begin.	Decreases client anxiety and increases client cooperation.
9. Initially instruct client to extend neck back against pillow; insert tube slowly through naris with curved end pointing downward (Fig. 44-1).	Facilitates initial passage of tube through naris.
10. Continue to pass tube along floor of nasal passage, aiming down toward ear. When resistance is felt, apply gentle downward pressure to advance tube (do not force past resistance).	Minimizes discomfort of tube rubbing against upper nasal turbinates. Resistance is caused by posterior nasopharynx. Downward pressure helps tube curl around corner of nasopharynx.
11. If resistance is met, try to rotate tube and see if it advances. If still resistant, withdraw tube, allow client to rest, relubricate tube, and insert into other naris.	Forcing against resistance can cause trauma to mucosa. Helps relieve client's anxiety.
12. Continue insertion of tube until just past nasopharynx by gently rotating tube toward opposite naris.	

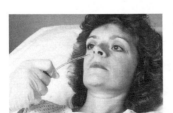

Fig. 44-1 Insertion of NG tube with curved end pointing downward.

Step	**Rationale**
a. Once past nasopharynx, stop tube advancement, allow client to relax, and provide tissues.	Relieves client's anxiety; tearing is natural response to mucosal irritation, and excessive salivation may occur because of oral stimulation.
b. Explain to client that next step requires that client swallow. Give client glass of water unless contraindicated.	Sipping of water aids passage of NG tube into esophagus.
13. With tube just above oropharynx, instruct client to flex head forward, take small sip of water, and swallow. Advance tube 2.5 to 5 cm (1 to 2 inches) with each swallow of water. If client is not allowed fluids, instruct to dry-swallow or suck air through straw. Advance tube with each swallow.	Flexed position closes off upper airway to trachea and opens esophagus. Swallowing closes epiglottis over trachea and helps move tube into esophagus. Swallowing water reduces gagging or choking. Water can be removed later from stomach by suction.
14. If client begins to cough, gag, or choke, withdraw tube slightly and stop tube advancement. Instruct client to breathe easily and take sips of water.	Tubing may accidentally enter larynx and initiate cough reflex, and withdrawal of tube reduces risk of laryngeal entry. Gagging is eased by swallowing water, which must be given cautiously to reduce risk of aspiration.

NURSE ALERT If vomiting occurs, assist client in clearing airway; oral suctioning may be needed. Do not proceed until airway is cleared.

15. If client continues to cough during insertion, pull tube back slightly.	Tube may enter larynx and obstruct airway.

Step	Rationale
16. If client continues to gag and cough or complains that tube feels as though it is coiling in back of throat, check back of oropharynx using flashlight and tongue blade. If tube is coiled, withdraw it until tip is back in oropharynx. Then reinsert with client swallowing.	Tube may coil around itself in back of throat and stimulate gag reflex.
17. After client relaxes, continue to advance tube with swallowing until tape or mark on tube is reached, which signifies tube is in desired distance. Temporarily anchor tube to client's cheek with piece of tape until tube placement is verified.	Tip of tube should be in stomach to decompress properly. Anchoring of tube prevents accidental displacement while tube placement is verified.
18. Verify tube placement. (Check agency policy for preferred methods for checking tube placement.)	
a. Ask client to talk.	Client is unable to talk if NG tube has passed through vocal cords.
b. Inspect posterior pharynx for presence of coiled tube.	Tube is pliable and can coil up in back of pharynx instead of advancing into esophagus.
c. Gently aspirate gastric contents with syringe, observing color (see Skill 43).	Gastric contents are usually cloudy and green but may be off-white, tan, bloody, or brown in color. Aspiration of contents provides means to measure fluid pH and thus determine tube tip placement in GI tract.

Step	Rationale
	Other common aspirate colors include the following: duodenal placement (yellow or bile stained), esophagus (may or may not have saliva-appearing aspirate).
d. Measure pH of aspirate with color-coded pH paper with range of whole numbers from 1 to 14 (see Skill 43).	Gastric aspirates have decidedly acidic pH values, preferably 4 or less, compared with intestinal aspirates, which are usually greater than 4, or respiratory secretions, which are usually greater than 5.5 (Metheny and others, 1993, 1994, 1998; Metheny and Titler, 2001).
e. Have ordered x-ray examination performed of chest/abdomen.	X-ray film verifies initial placement of tube (Metheny and Titler, 2001).
f. If tube is not in stomach, advance another 2.5 to 5 cm (1 to 2 inches) and repeat Steps 18, a through d, to check tube position.	Tube must be in stomach to provide decompression.

19. Anchoring tube (see Skill 43, Step 25).
20. Unless physician orders otherwise, head of bed should be elevated 30 degrees.

    Helps prevent esophageal reflux and minimizes irritation of tube against posterior pharynx.

21. Removal of NG tube:

a. Verify order to discontinue NG tube.	Physician's order required for procedure.
b. Explain procedure to client, and reassure that removal is less distressing than insertion.	Minimizes anxiety and increases cooperation. Tube passes out smoothly.

Step	Rationale
c. Turn off suction, and disconnect NG tube from drainage bag or suction. Remove tape or fixation device from bridge of nose, and untape tube from gown.	Have tube free of connections before removal.
d. Stand on client's right side if right-handed; left side if left-handed.	Allows easier manipulation of tube.
e. Hand client facial tissue; place clean towel across chest. Instruct client to take and hold deep breath.	Client may wish to blow nose after tube is removed. Towel may keep gown from getting soiled. Airway will be temporarily obstructed during tube removal.
f. Clamp or kink tubing securely, and then pull tube out steadily and smoothly into towel held in other hand while client holds breath.	Clamping prevents tube contents from draining into oropharynx. Reduces trauma to mucosa and minimizes client's discomfort. Towel covers tube, which can be an unpleasant sight. Holding breath helps prevent aspiration.
g. Measure amount of drainage, and note character of content. Dispose of tube and drainage equipment into proper container.	Provides accurate measure of fluid output. Reduces transfer of microorganisms.
h. Clean nares, and provide mouth care.	Promotes comfort.
i. Position client comfortably, and explain procedure for drinking fluids, if not contraindicated.	Depends on physician's order. Sometimes clients are allowed nothing by mouth (NPO) for up to 24 hours. When fluids are allowed, order usually begins with small amount of ice chips each hour and increases as client is able to tolerate more.

Step	Rationale
22. Observe amount and character of contents draining from NG tube. Ask if client feels nauseated.	Determines if tube is decompressing stomach of contents.
23. Palpate client's abdomen periodically, noting any distention, pain, and rigidity, and auscultate for the presence of bowel sounds. Turn off suction while auscultating.	Determines success of abdominal decompression and the return of peristalsis. Sound of suction apparatus may be transmitted to abdomen and be misinterpreted as bowel sounds.
24. Inspect condition of nares and nose.	Evaluates onset of skin and tissue irritation.
25. Complete postprocedure protocol.	

Recording and Reporting

- Record length, size, and type of gastric tube inserted and through which nostril it was inserted, client's tolerance of procedure, confirmation of tube placement, character of gastric contents, pH value, whether tube is clamped or connected to drainage or to suction, and amount of suction supplied.
- Record on intake and output (I&O) sheet the difference between amount of normal saline instilled and amount of gastric aspirate removed. Record in nurses' notes or flowsheet amount and character of contents draining from NG tube every shift.

Unexpected Outcomes	Related Interventions
1. Client's abdomen is distended and painful.	• Assess patency of tube. • Irrigate tube. • Verify that suction is on as ordered.
2. Client complains of sore throat from dry, irritated mucous membranes.	• Perform oral hygiene more frequently. • Ask physician whether client can suck on ice chips or throat lozenges.
3. Client develops irritation or erosion of skin around naris.	• Provide frequent skin care to area. • Retape tube to avoid pressure on naris. • Consider switching tube to other naris.

Oral Medications

The easiest and most desirable way to administer medications is by mouth. Clients usually are able to ingest or self-administer oral drugs with a minimum of problems. However, contraindications to clients receiving medications by mouth include presence of gastrointestinal (GI) alterations, the inability of a client to swallow food or fluids, and the use of gastric suction. Always prepare medications in an area designed for medication preparation or at the unit-dose cart.

Delegation Considerations

The skill of administering oral medications should not be delegated to assistive personnel (AP).

- Instruct AP about potential side effects of medications and to report their occurrence.

Equipment

- Medication cart or tray
- Disposable medication cups
- Glass of water, juice, or preferred liquid
- Drinking straw
- Pill-crushing or cutting device (optional)
- Paper towels
- Medication administration record (MAR)

Step	Rationale
1. Complete preprocedure protocol.	
2. Assess risk for aspiration (see Skill 4). Is client able to swallow? Assess client's swallow, cough, and gag reflexes. Determine client's ability to swallow oral medications safely.	Aspiration occurs when food, fluid, or medication intended for GI administration is inadvertently administered into respiratory tract. Clients with altered ability to swallow oral medications are at higher risk for aspiration.

NURSE ALERT Clients with neuromuscular disorders, esophageal strictures, or lesions of the mouth; those who are unresponsive or comatose and cannot swallow; and those with high risk for aspiration should not receive

Step	Rationale

medications orally. Request that the prescriber order medications by an alternate route (e.g., intravenously [IV]). When oral medications are contraindicated or if you are in doubt about the client's ability to swallow, temporarily withhold the medication and inform the prescriber.

3. Check accuracy and completeness of each MAR with prescriber's written medication order. Check client's name, drug name and dosage, route of administration, and time of administration. Compare MAR with medication label. Incomplete or unclear orders should be clarified with prescriber before implementation.	Order sheet is most reliable source and only legal record of drugs client is to receive. Ensures that client receives correct medication.
4. After confirming order, recopy or reprint any portion of MAR that is illegible.	Soiled or illegible MAR forms can be source of drug error.
5. Prepare medications:	
a. Arrange medication tray and cups in medication preparation area, as per agency policy.	Organization of equipment saves time and reduces error.
b. Check expiration date on all medications.	Medications used past expiration date may be inactive or harmful to client.
c. Prepare medications for one client at a time. Keep all pages of MAR for one client together.	Prevents preparation errors.
d. Select correct drug from stock supply or unit-dose drawer. Compare label of medication with MAR.	Reading label first time and comparing it against transcribed order reduces errors.

Step	**Rationale**
e. Calculate drug dose as necessary. Double-check calculation.	Double-checking reduces risk of error.
f. To prepare tablets or capsules from floor-stock bottle, pour required number into bottle cap and transfer medication to medication cup. Do not touch medication with fingers. Extra tablets or capsules may be returned to bottle.	Drugs are very expensive; avoid waste. Tablets that are not prescored cannot be broken into equal halves, and result will be inaccurate dose.

NURSE ALERT Medications that need to be broken to administer half the dosage can be broken, using a gloved hand, or cut with a cutting device. Tablets that are to be broken in half must be prescored. Prescored tablets are identified by a manufactured line that transects the center of the tablet.

g. To prepare unit-dose tablets or capsules, place packaged tablet or capsule directly into medicine cup. (Do not remove wrapper.)	Wrapper maintains cleanliness of medications and identifies drug name and dose.

NURSE ALERT If preparing opioids, check controlled medication record for previous drug count, compare with supply available, and maintain adherence to controlled substance laws.

h. All tablets or capsules to be given to client at same time may be placed in one medicine cup except for those requiring preadministration assessments (e.g., pulse rate, blood pressure).	Keeping medications that require preadministration assessments separate from others makes it easier for nurse to withhold drugs as necessary.

Step	Rationale
i. If client has difficulty swallowing, use pill-crushing device such as mortar and pestle to crush pills. If pill-crushing device is not available, place tablet between two medication cups and grind with a blunt instrument. Mix ground tablet in small amount of soft food (custard or applesauce).	Large tablets can be difficult to swallow. Ground tablet mixed with palatable soft food is usually easier to swallow.

NURSE ALERT Not all drugs can be crushed (e.g., capsules, enteric-coated and long-acting/slow-release drugs). The coating of these drugs is designed to protect the stomach from irritation or protect the drug from destruction from stomach acids. Consult with pharmacist when in doubt (Miller and Miller, 2000).

Step	Rationale
j. Prepare liquids:	
(1) Gently shake container. If medication is in unit-dose container with correct amount to administer, no further preparation is needed.	Prevents contamination of inside of cap.
(2) If medication is in multidose bottle, remove bottle cap it and place upside down on work surface. Hold bottle with label against palm of hand while pouring. Hold medication	Spilled liquid will not drip and soil or fade label. Ensures accuracy of measurement.

Step	Rationale
cup at eye level, and fill to desired level on scale. Scale should be even with fluid level at its surface or base of meniscus, not edges.	
(3) For small doses of liquid medications, draw liquid into calibrated oral syringe. Do not use hypodermic syringe or syringe with needle or syringe cap.	Using calibrated oral syringe allows for accurate measuring of small doses of liquid medications.

NURSE ALERT When preparing opioids, check controlled substance record for previous drug count and compare with supply available.

k. Compare MAR with all prepared drugs, and continue preparation.	Reading label second time reduces errors.
l. Return stock containers or unused unit-dose medications to shelf or drawer, and read label again.	Third check of label reduces administration errors.
m. Do not leave drugs unattended.	Nurse is responsible for safekeeping of drugs.
6. Administer medications:	
a. Take medications to client at correct time. Identify client by comparing name on MAR with name on client's identification bracelet. Ask client to state name.	Ensures that correct client receives medication. At least two patient identifiers (neither to be patient's room number) are to be used whenever administering medications (JCAHO, 2004).

Step	Rationale

b. Explain to client the purpose of each medication and its action. Allow client to ask any questions about drugs.

Client has right to be informed, and client's understanding of purpose of each medication improves compliance with drug therapy.

NURSE ALERT If client refuses medication, withhold it and notify prescriber.

c. Perform any necessary preadministration assessment (e.g., blood pressure, pulse).

d. Assist client to a seated or side-lying position if sitting is contraindicated by client's condition.

Decreases risk of aspiration during swallowing.

NURSE ALERT Withhold medication if swallow, cough, or gag reflex is impaired; notify prescriber.

e. **For tablets:** Client may wish to hold solid medications in hand or cup before placing in mouth.

Client can become familiar with medications by seeing each drug.

f. **For sublingual-administered medications:** Have client place medication under tongue and allow it to dissolve completely (Fig. 45-1). Caution client against swallowing tablet.

Drug is absorbed through blood vessels of undersurface of tongue. If swallowed, drug is destroyed by gastric juices or so rapidly detoxified by liver that therapeutic blood levels are not attained.

g. **For buccal medications:** Have client place medication in mouth against mucous membranes until it dissolves (Fig. 45-2).

Ensures proper distribution of medication.

Step	**Rationale**

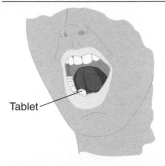

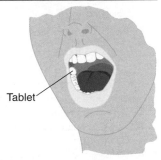

Fig. 45-1 Sublingual administration of a tablet.

Fig. 45-2 Buccal administration of a tablet.

NURSE ALERT Do not administer liquids until buccal/sublingual medications have dissolved.

h. Caution client against chewing or swallowing lozenges.	Drug acts through slow absorption through oral mucosa, not gastric mucosa.
i. **For powdered medications:** Mix with liquids at bedside, and give to client to drink.	When prepared in advance, powdered drugs may thicken and even harden, making swallowing difficult.
j. Give effervescent powders and tablets immediately after dissolving.	Effervescence improves unpleasant taste of drug and often relieves GI problems.
k. If client is unable to hold medications, place medication cup to lips and gently introduce each drug into mouth, one at a time. Do not rush.	Administering single tablet or capsule eases swallowing and decreases risk of aspiration.
l. Stay until client has completely swallowed each medication. Ask client to open mouth if uncertain whether medication has been swallowed.	Nurse is responsible for ensuring that client receives ordered dosage. If left unattended, client may not take dose or may save drugs, causing risk to health.

Step	Rationale

7. Complete postprocedure protocol.

Recording and Reporting

- Immediately after administration, record on MAR the actual time each drug was administered. Include initials or signature. Do not chart medication administration until *after* it is given to client.
- If drug is withheld, record reason in nurses' notes. Circle on MAR the time the drug normally would have been given on MAR (or follow institution's policy for noting withheld doses).
- Report adverse effects/client response and/or withheld drugs to nurse in charge or physician. Depending on medication, immediate prescriber notification may be required.

Unexpected Outcomes	Related Interventions
1. Client exhibits adverse effects such as urticaria, rash, pruritus, or wheezing.	• Withhold further doses. • Notify prescriber and pharmacy.
2. Client is unable to explain drug information.	• Further assess client's or family member's knowledge of medications and guidelines for drug safety. • Further instruction is necessary.
3. Client refuses medication.	• Assess why client is refusing medication. • Do not force client to take medications. • Notify prescriber. • Record that client refused medication and why.

Oral Medications: Nasogastric Tube Administration

Clients with nasogastric (NG) tubes usually receive nothing by mouth. Oral medications that need to be administered to these clients can be given via the tubes. Most commonly, oral medications are given through small-bore feeding tubes. Do not administer medications into nasogastric/intestinal tubes that are inserted for decompression. To administer medications by an NG or feeding tube, modify the form of a tablet to be administered by crushing and dissolving it. Medications may also be available in liquid form. *Generally, sustained-release, chewable, long-acting, or enteric-coated tablets and capsules are not administered by gastric tubes.* Consult with the hospital pharmacy when in doubt. It is essential to verify correct placement of an NG tube before administering medications (see Skill 43). If medications are ordered to be given through a percutaneous endoscopic gastrostomy (PEG) tube, follow the same steps as for giving medications through an NG tube.

Delegation Considerations

The skill of administering medications by NG tube should not be delegated to assistive personnel (AP).

- Instruct AP about potential side effects of medications and to report their occurrence.

Equipment

- 60-ml syringe: catheter tip for large-bore tubes; Luer-Lok tip for small-bore tubes
- Gastric pH test tape (scale of 0.0 to 11.0 or 14.0 preferred)
- Graduated container
- Water
- Medication to be administered
- Pill crusher if medication in tablet form
- Medication administration record (MAR)
- Clean gloves

Step	Rationale
1. Complete preprocedure protocol.	
2. ⚡ Before administration of medications, verify placement of nasogastric tube (see Skill 43). Remove gloves and perform hand hygiene.	Reduces the risk of aspiration.
3. Check accuracy and completeness of each MAR with prescriber's written medication order. Check client's name, drug name and dosage, route of administration, and time of administration.	Order sheet is most reliable source and only legal record of drugs client is to receive. Ensures that client receives correct medication.
4. Check medications' expiration dates.	Medications that have expired should not be used.
5. Prepare medications for instillation into feeding tube. Check label against MAR three times. Fill graduated container with 50 to 100 ml of tepid water.	Adequate preparation saves nursing time. Ensures that client receives correct medication.

NURSE ALERT Liquid medications are preferred to crushed tablets, but if tablets must be crushed, flush the tubing before and after the medication to prevent the drug from adhering to the inside of the tube (Lewis and others, 2004). Concentrated medications need to be thoroughly diluted. Never add crushed medications directly to tube feeding.

    a. Crush tablets using pill-crushing device to grind pills into fine powder. If pill-crushing device is not available, place tablet between two medication cups and grind with blunt instrument. Dissolve in

Step	Rationale

at least 30 ml of warm
water.

  b. *Capsules:* Open capsule
or pierce gelcap with
sterile needle, and
empty contents into
30 ml of warm water.
Gelcaps can also be
dissolved in warm water.

Ensures that contents of tablets or
capsules are fine powder or
solution so as not to occlude
NG tube.

6. Check client's identification
bracelet; ask client to state
name.

Ensures that correct client receives
medication. At least two patient
identifiers (neither to be patient's
room number) are to be used
whenever administering
medications (JCAHO, 2004).

7. Place client in high-Fowler's
position (if not
contraindicated by client's
medical condition).

Reduces risk of aspiration.

8.   Check for gastric
residual (Fig. 46-1).
Connect syringe to end of
NG tube; then pull back
evenly on plunger to
aspirate gastric contents.
Return aspirated contents
to stomach unless volume
exceeds 100 ml (or as
defined by agency policy);

Residual volume indicates if
gastric emptying is delayed.
Return of aspirate prevents fluid
and electrolyte imbalance.
Irrigation clears tubing
(Ignatavicius and Workman,
2002).

Fig. 46-1 Nurse pulls
back on syringe to aspirate
stomach contents.

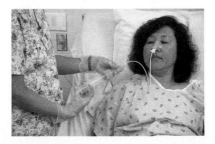

Step	Rationale

then flush tubing with at least 30 ml of water.

NURSE ALERT   If large-volume aspirate of 100 ml or more is found, return aspirate to client. Withhold medication, and notify client's health care provider. Aspirates of 100 to 150 ml indicate delayed gatric emptying, which may contribute to gastric distention, esophageal reflux, and vomiting, all of which increase the client's risk for aspiration (Mahan and Escott-Stump, 2004).

Step	Rationale
9. Pinch NG tube, and remove syringe. Draw up 30 ml of water in syringe. Reinsert tip of syringe into NG tube, release tube, and flush. Remove syringe and pinch NG tube again.	Pinching NG tube prevents leakage or spillage of stomach contents. Flushing ensures that tube is patent.
10. Remove bulb or plunger of syringe, then reinsert syringe into tube.	Removal of bulb or plunger prepares syringe for delivery of medications.
11. Administer first dose of dissolved medication by pouring into syringe.	

NURSE ALERT   If water or medication does not flow freely, a gentle push with bulb of Asepto syringe or plunger of Toomey syringe may aid flow of fluid.

Step	Rationale
a. If only one dose of medication is given, follow by pouring 30 ml of water into syringe.	Maintains patency of NG tube.
b. To administer more than one medication, give each separately and flush between medications with 10 ml of water.	Keeping medications separate allows for accurate identification of medication if dose is spilled. In addition, some medications may not be compatible with each other, which could cause clogging of tube (Phipps and others, 2003).

Step	Rationale
c. Follow last dose of medication with 30 to 60 ml of water.	Maintains patency of NG tube. Ensures passage of medication into stomach (Phipps and others, 2003).
12. Remove syringe when tube feeding is not being administered, clamp proximal end of feeding tube, and cap end of tube.	Prevents air from entering stomach between medication doses.
13. When continuous tube feeding is being administered by infusion pump:	
a. Follow medication administration Steps 1 through 11; then stop feeding for 1 hour (check agency policy).	Allows for adequate absorption of medication and avoids potential drug-food interaction between medication and enteral feeding (Ignatavicius and Workman, 2002).
14. Keep the head of the bed elevated for 1 hour after the medication is given.	Prevents aspiration (Ignatavicius and Workman, 2002).
15. Complete postprocedure protocol.	

Recording and Reporting

- Record in nurses' notes the verification of tube placement, volume of stomach aspirate, and pH of stomach aspirate.
- Immediately after administration, record on MAR the actual time each drug was administered. Include initials or signature.
- Record on proper intake and output sheet the total amount of fluid used for medication administration.
- Report adverse effects/client response and/or withheld drugs to nurse in charge or physician.

Unexpected Outcomes	Related Interventions
1. Client exhibits signs of aspiration of administered medications/fluids, which include respiratory distress, changes in vital signs, or changes in oxygen saturation.	• Stop all medications/fluids through tube. • Elevate head of bed, and stay with client. • Assess vital signs and breath sounds while another staff member notifies client's physician.
2. Client does not receive medication as prescribed because of blocked NG tube.	• Requires interventions to unclog tube to ensure drug delivery (Box 46-1).

BOX 46-1 Unclogging a Blocked Feeding Tube

- Prevent tube from becoming blocked by flushing it with at least 30 ml of tepid water before and after administering each dose of medication, before and after checking gastric residual volumes, and every 4 to 6 hours around the clock.
- If a tube becomes blocked, first try to irrigate it gently with tepid water.
- If irrigation with water is not effective, obtain an order for a pancrelipase tablet (such as Viokase) and follow manufacturer's guidelines for irrigation of the tube. In addition, a declogging stylus may be used.
- The tube may have to be removed and a new one inserted if the medication is urgent.

Modified from Lewis SM and others: *Medical-surgical nursing: assessment and management of clinical problems*, ed 6, St Louis, 2004, Mosby.

Ostomy Care (Pouching)

Immediately after surgical diversion or removal of a portion of bowel, it is necessary to place a pouch over the newly created stoma because in some incontinent ostomies, effluent may begin immediately. The pouch collects all effluent and protects the skin from irritating drainage. A pouch with its skin barrier should fit comfortably, cover the skin surface around the stoma, and create a good seal. When a new stoma is present, the postoperative pouch should allow visibility of the stoma.

The technique of pouching a newly formed stoma differs from techniques used to pouch a stoma several days or weeks old. The new stoma is edematous during the postoperative healing process for up to 6 weeks. An incision line from the bowel resection may lie close to or around the stoma.

Delegation Considerations

This skill may not be delegated to assistive personnel (AP). The one exception in some agencies is that care of an enterostomy (6-plus weeks postoperative) may be delegated to AP. When delegating this skill, the nurse must inform AP about:

- The expected amount, color, and consistency of drainage from the ostomy.
- The expected appearance of the stoma.
- Special equipment needed to complete procedure.
- When to report changes in the client's stoma and surrounding skin integrity.

Equipment

- Pouch, clear drainable colostomy/ileostomy/urostomy in correct size for two-piece system or custom cut-to-fit, one-piece type with attached skin barrier
- Pouch closure device, such as a clamp or pouch valve
- Adhesive remover (optional)
- Clean disposable gloves
- Ostomy deodorant, if needed
- Gauze pads or washcloth
- Towel or disposable waterproof barrier
- Basin with warm tap water
- Scissors

- Skin barrier such as sealant wipes or wafer
- Ostomy belt (optional)
- Stethoscope

Step	Rationale
1. Complete preprocedure protocol.	
2. Auscultate for bowel sounds.	Documents presence of peristalsis.
3. Observe existing skin barrier and pouch for leakage and length of time in place. Depending on type of pouching system used (e.g., opaque pouch), nurse may have to remove pouch to fully observe stoma. Clear pouches permit viewing of stoma without their removal.	Determines likelihood of pouch loosening from stoma and failing to collect effluent. Routine observation allows for early detection of potential problems (Thompson, 2000). Leaking may indicate need for different pouch or sealant.
4. Observe stoma for color, swelling, trauma, and healing; stoma should be moist and reddish pink. Assess type of stoma. Stomas can be almost flush with skin or be budlike protrusion on abdomen.	Stoma characteristics should be one of factors to consider when selecting appropriate pouching system (WOCN, 2005).

NURSE ALERT If the client has a new stoma, it is important to measure the stoma with each pouching system change to determine the correct size of equipment needed. New stomas change size as part of the healing process (WOCN, 2005).

5. Observe effluent from stoma, and record intake and output. Ask client about skin tenderness.	Plan on routine changing of skin barrier pouch at times of less effluent output. Generally avoid changing after meals, when gastrocolic reflex increases chance of fecal effluent output.
6. To minimize skin irritation, avoid unnecessary changing	Pouches should be emptied when one-third to one-half full

Step	**Rationale**
of entire pouching system. One-piece pouch with attached skin barriers or skin barrier of two-piece pouching system should be changed every 3 to 5 days, *not* daily.	because weight of contents may dislodge skin seal and ostomy drainage is irritating to skin. Also, pouches collect flatus (gas), which needs to be expelled because it can disrupt skin seal.
7. Assess abdomen for best type of pouching system to use. Consider:	Determines pouching system selection and need for other equipment.
a. Contour and peristomal plane	Firm/flat and round/hard abdomen usually needs flexible or soft pouching system, whereas flabby or soft abdomen usually needs firmer system (Fig. 47-1). Convexity may be needed for stomas that are retracted or in skinfolds, and different pouching systems are needed to prevent leaking.
b. Presence of scars, incisions	
c. Location and type of stoma	

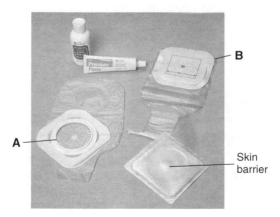

Fig. 47-1   Examples of pouching systems. A, Two-piece detachable system. (NOTE: The skin barrier would need to be custom-cut by the client according to self-stoma size obtained by measurement.) The pouch opening is already precut by the manufacturer to fit the size of the flange on the skin barrier. B, One-piece pouch with skin barrier attached.

Step	Rationale
8. Assess client's condition as to best type of pouching system to use. Assess vision, dexterity or mobility, and cognitive function (see Fig. 47-1).	Clients with poor vision may benefit by using yellow-tinted sunglasses to reduce glare and improve contrast and by using magnification mirrors (Jeffries and MacKay, 1997). Clients who also have mobility problems or spinal cord injuries may benefit by using equipment that has longer pouch, which is easier to empty independently when sitting (Erwin-Toth, 2003; Thomason, 2000).
9. Remove existing pouch, if any, by gently pushing skin from adhesive barrier; properly dispose of soiled pouch (save clamp if attached to pouch).	Prevents skin irritation and controls odor. Determines need for barrier paste to increase adherence of pouch to skin or to fill in irregularities.
10. Position client either standing or supine, and drape. If seated, position client either on or in front of toilet.	When client is supine, there are fewer skin wrinkles, which allows for ease of application of pouching system; maintains client's dignity.
11. Remove used pouch and skin barrier gently by pushing skin away from barrier. An adhesive remover may be used to facilitate removal of skin barrier.	Reduces skin trauma. Improper removal of pouch and barrier can irritate client's skin and can cause skin tears.

NURSE ALERT If portions of skin barrier remain, use an adhesive remover to gently remove remnants. Remaining skin barrier irritates the client's skin and results in poor adherence of the new pouch. When adhesive removers are used, follow up with washing the skin with water and a mild soap to remove the oily coating on the skin from the adhesive remover (WOCN, 2005).

12. Cleanse peristomal skin gently with warm tap water	Avoid use of soap because it leaves residue on skin that interferes

Step	**Rationale**
using gauze pads or clean washcloth; do not scrub skin; dry completely by patting skin with gauze or towel.	with pouch adhesion to skin (Thompson, 2000). Skin must be dry because skin barrier/pouch does not adhere to wet skin.
13. Measure stoma for correct size of pouching system needed, using manufacturer's measuring guide (Fig. 47-2).	Ensures accuracy in determining correct pouch size needed. Stoma shrinks and does not reach usual size for 6 to 8 weeks (Thompson, 2000).
14. Select appropriate pouch for client based on client assessment. With custom cut-to-fit pouch, use ostomy guide to cut opening on pouch $\frac{1}{16}$ to $\frac{1}{8}$ inch larger than stoma before removing backing. Prepare pouch by removing backing from barrier and adhesive. With ileostomy, apply thin circle of barrier paste around opening in pouch; allow to dry (Fig. 47-3).	Size of pouch opening keeps drainage off skin and lessens risk of damage to stoma during peristalsis or activity. Pouch and skin barrier are changed whenever leaking. Change when client is comfortable; before a meal is better because this avoids increased peristalsis and chance of evacuation during pouch change. Can also be changed before or after tub bath or shower. Paste facilitates seal and protects skin. Stool is alkaline and contains enzymes, and this irritates skin; fecal bacteria can colonize on skin and increase risk of infection.
15. Apply skin barrier and pouch. If creases next to	

Fig. 47-2   Measuring a stoma.

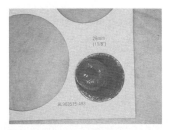

Step   Rationale

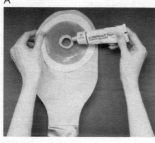

A

B

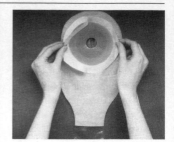

C

Fig. 47-3 A, Cut-to-fit, one-piece drainable ostomy pouch. B, Removing the backing paper for the barrier on a one-piece pouch. C, Applying barrier paste to a one-piece ostomy pouch. (Courtesy ConvaTec, Princeton, NJ.)

stoma occur, use barrier paste to fill in; let dry 1 to 2 minutes.

a. For one-piece pouching system:

　(1) Use skin sealant wipes on skin directly under adhesive skin barrier or pouch; allow to dry. Press adhesive backing of pouch and/or skin barrier smoothly against skin, starting from bottom and

Ensures smooth, wrinkle-free seal. Be aware of any irritated or open areas because skin sealant wipes often contain alcohol.

Step	**Rationale**
working up and around sides.	
(2) Hold pouch by barrier, center over stoma, and press down gently on barrier; bottom of pouch should point toward client's knees when sitting (Fig. 47-4).	Different positioning of pouch may be necessary to allow better gravity flow. For example, client confined to bed may need to have pouch positioned horizontally over side of abdomen (Thomason, 2000).
(3) Maintain gentle finger pressure around barrier for 1 to 2 minutes.	Gentle pressure and body heat assist in adhesion.
b. For two-piece pouching system:	
(1) Apply barrier-paste flange (barrier with adhesive) as in previous steps for one-piece system. Then snap on pouch, and maintain finger pressure.	Creates wrinkle-free, secure seal; decreases irritation from adhesive on skin. A snapping or clicking sound may occur with some two-piece pouching systems when attaching pouch to skin barrier.
c. For both pouching systems, gently tug on pouch in downward direction.	Determines that pouch is securely attached.

Fig. 47-4 Applying a one-piece pouch. (Courtesy ConvaTec, Princeton, NJ.)

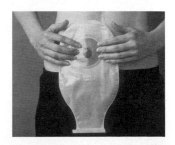

Step	Rationale
16. Gently press on pectin or karaya flange to facilitate adhesion.	Pectin, karaya, or synthetic skin barrier keeps pouch system attached securely (Erwin-Toth, 2001). Some clients may prefer belt attached to pouch for extra security.
17. Although many ostomy pouches are odor-proof, some nurses and clients like to add small amount of ostomy deodorant into pouch. Do not use "home remedies," which can harm stoma, to control ostomy odor. Do not make hole in pouch to release flatus.	Damages pouch and defeats purpose of odor-proof pouch. Hole for flatus may also allow effluent to leak.
18. Fold bottom of drainable open-ended pouches up once, and close using closure device such as clamp (or follow manufacturer's instructions for closure).	Maintains secure seal to prevent leaking.
19. Complete postprocedure protocol.	

Recording and Reporting

- Record amount and appearance of stool or drainage in pouch, size of stoma, color and texture of stool, condition of peristomal skin and sutures. Document abdominal assessment.
- Report any of the following to nurse in charge and/or physician: abnormal appearance of stoma, suture line, and peristomal skin; character of output; absence of bowel sounds; no flatus in 24 to 36 hours; and no stool by third day.

Unexpected Outcomes	Related Interventions
1. Skin around stoma is irritated, has burning sensation.	• Assess stoma as mucosal layer of stoma separates from skin. • May be caused by undermining of pouch seal by fecal contents. • May indicate allergic reaction, which can be manifested by erythema and blistering, usually confined to one area immediately under allergen (Erwin-Toth, 2000). • Remove pouch more slowly. • Obtain referral for enterostomal therapy (ET)/wound, ostomy, continence (WOC)) nurse.
2. Necrotic stoma is manifested by purple or black color, dry instead of moist texture, failure to bleed when washed gently, or presence of tissue sloughing.	• Assess circulation to stoma. • Determine presence of excessive edema or excessive tension on bowel suture line.

Oxygen Therapy: Nasal Cannula, Oxygen Mask, T Tube, or Tracheostomy Collar

Oxygen therapy is the administration of supplemental oxygen (O_2) to a client to prevent or treat hypoxia. Oxygen therapy is delivered by several methods: nasal cannula, oxygen mask, and via an artificial airway. A *nasal cannula* is a simple, comfortable device for delivering oxygen to a client. The two tips of the cannula, about 1.5 cm ($^1/_2$ inch) long, protrude from the center of a disposable tube and are inserted into the nostrils.

An *oxygen mask* is shaped to fit snugly over the client's mouth and nose and is secured in place with a strap. The two primary types of masks are those delivering a low FIO_2 and those delivering a high FIO_2. A simple face mask is used for short-term oxygen therapy. It fits loosely and delivers oxygen concentrations from 40% to 60%. A plastic face mask with a reservoir bag and a *Venturi mask* are capable of delivering higher concentrations of oxygen.

Clients with an *artificial airway* require constant humidification to the airway. An artificial airway bypasses the normal filtering and humidification process of the nose and mouth. The two devices that supply humidified gas to an artificial airway are a T tube and a tracheostomy collar. The *T tube,* also called a *Briggs adaptor,* is a T-shaped device with a 15-mm ($^3/_5$-inch) connection that connects an oxygen source to an artificial airway such as an endotracheal (ET) tube or tracheostomy. A *tracheostomy collar* is a curved device with an adjustable strap that fits around the client's neck.

Delegation Considerations

The placement of an oxygen delivery device may be delegated to assistive personnel (AP). You are responsible for assessing the client's respiratory system, response to oxygen therapy, and setup of the oxygen therapy and liter flow. Before delegating this skill:

- Discuss with AP how the system is set up and to report any differences to the nurse for further assessment.

- Instruct AP to immediately report any vital sign changes or other unexpected outcomes associated with the oxygen delivery device.

Equipment

- Oxygen delivery device as ordered by physician: Nasal cannula, oxygen mask, T tube, tracheostomy collar
- Oxygen tubing
- Humidifier, if indicated
- Sterile water for humidifier
- Oxygen source
- Oxygen flow meter
- Appropriate room signs

Step	Rationale
1. Complete preprocedure protocol.	
2. If available, note client's most recent arterial blood gas (ABG) results or pulse oximetry (SpO$_2$) value.	Objectively documents client's pH, arterial oxygen, arterial CO$_2$, or arterial oxygen saturation.
3. Attach oxygen delivery device (e.g., cannula, oxygen mask, T tube, tracheostomy collar) to oxygen tubing, and attach to humidified oxygen source adjusted to prescribed flow rate.	Humidity prevents drying of nasal and oral mucous membranes and airway secretions. Ensures correct O$_2$ delivery.
4. Adjust fit:	
a. Elastic headband on face mask or nasal cannula so that snug and comfortable fit is achieved.	Directs flow of oxygen into client's upper respiratory tract. Client is more likely to keep device in place if it fits comfortably.
b. Determine that T tube does not pull on artificial airway.	Pulling of T tube on artificial airway increases client discomfort and causes pressure from the artificial airway.
c. Observe that elastic on tracheostomy collar	

Step	Rationale
allows for direction of oxygen into the tracheostomy and does not pull on tracheostomy tube.	
5. Maintain sufficient slack on oxygen tubing, and secure to client's clothes.	Allows client to turn head without causing mask to shift position or dislodge nasal cannula.
6. Observe for proper function of oxygen delivery device:	Ensures patency of delivery device and accuracy of prescribed oxygen flow rate.
a. *Nasal cannula:* Cannula is positioned properly in nares.	Provides prescribed oxygen rate and reduces pressure on tips of nares.
b. *Nonrebreathing mask:* Apply mask over client's mouth and nose to form tight seal. Valves on mask close so exhaled air does not enter reservoir bag.	Does not allow exhaled air to be rebreathed. Valves on mask side ports permit exhalation but close during inhalation to prevent inhaling room air.
c. *Partial rebreathing mask:* Apply mask over client's mouth and nose to form tight seal. Ensure that bag remains partially inflated.	Allows exhaled air to mix with inhaled air. Ports on side of mask permit most of expired air to escape; however, bag should remain partially inflated.
d. *Venturi mask:* Apply mask over client's mouth and nose to form tight seal. Percentage of FiO$_2$ should correlate with flow rate (Fig. 48-1).	Reduces carbon dioxide buildup.
7. Assess flow meter and oxygen source for proper setup and prescribed flow rate.	Ensures delivery of prescribed oxygen therapy in conjunction with specific cannula/mask.

Step   **Rationale**

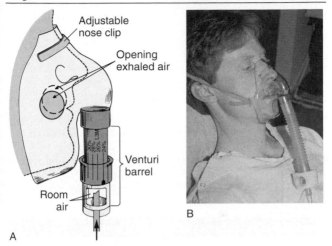

Fig. 48-1 **A,** Turning Venturi barrel of oxygen delivered to appropriate percentage, from 24% to 50%. **B,** Venturi mask in place.

8. Check oxygen delivery device every 8 hours. Keep humidification jar filled at all times.	Ensures patency of cannula and oxygen flow. Maintains inhalation of humidified oxygen.

NURSE ALERT If fluid accumulates in oxygen tubing, drain the fluid away from the client and discard in an appropriate receptacle. Excess water in the tubing is a medium for harmful bacterial growth and increases the client's risk for nosocomial infection.

9. Observe for decreased anxiety, improved level of consciousness and cognitive abilities, decreased fatigue, absence of dizziness, decreased respiratory rate, improved color, improved oxygen saturation, and return to client's baseline vital signs.	Evaluates client's response to supplemental oxygen. As client's oxygen level improves, so too should vital signs, pulse oximetry, and other physical assessment parameters associated with decreased oxygen levels.

Step	Rationale
10. Monitor ABG levels, or observe pulse oximetry for oxygen saturation.	Documents client's level of oxygenation.
11. Complete postprocedure protocol.	

Recording and Reporting

- Record respiratory assessment findings; method of oxygen delivery, flow rate, client's response; any adverse reactions or side effects; change in physician's orders.
- Report any unexpected outcome to physician or nurse in charge.

Unexpected Outcomes	Related Interventions
1. Client experiences continued hypoxia.	• Obtain physician's orders for follow-up pulse oximetry monitoring or ABG determinations. • Notify physician about continued hypoxia. • Consider measures to improve airway patency, coughing techniques, oropharyngeal or orotracheal suctioning.

Parenteral Medication Preparation: Ampules and Vials

Ampules contain single doses of injectable medication in a liquid form. An ampule is made of glass with a constricted neck that must be snapped off to allow access to the medication. A colored ring around the neck indicates where the ampule is prescored to be broken easily. Medications are easily withdrawn from the ampule by aspirating the fluid with a filter needle and syringe. The use of filter needles when preparing medications from glass ampules prevents glass particles from being drawn into the syringe with the medication (Nicoll and Hesby, 2002).

A vial is a plastic or glass container with a rubber seal at the top. A metal cap protects the sterile seal until the vial is ready to use. Vials contain liquid and/or dry forms of medication. A vial that is entered and then discarded, regardless of the amount of medication used, is called *a single-dose vial*. A vial that can be entered into several times and contains several doses of medication is called a *multidose vial*. A vial is a closed system, and air must be injected into it to permit easy withdrawal of solution.

Delegation Considerations

The skill of preparing injections from ampules and vials should not be delegated to assistive personnel (AP).

Equipment
Medication in an Ampule

- Syringe, filter needle, and needle or needleless system device
- Small gauze pad or unopened alcohol swab

Medication in a Vial

- Syringe
- Needle for drawing up medication and needle for injection (if needed)
- Blunt-tip vial access cannula (if needleless system used)
- Filter needle (if indicated)

- Small gauze pad or alcohol swab
- Diluent (e.g., normal saline or sterile water) (if indicated)

Both

- Medication administration record (MAR) or computer printout

Step	Rationale
1. Complete preprocedure protocol.	
2. Verify client's name, name of medication, dose, route of administration, and time of administration on MAR against medication order.	Ensures correct administration of medication.
3. Assess client's body build, muscle size, and weight and desired route of administration.	Determines type and size of syringe and needles to be used for injection.
4. Assemble medication and supplies at work area in medicine area.	Organization saves time and reduces risk for error.
5. Check name of medication on vial/ampule label against MAR when removing medication from supply source.	Reading label first time and comparing it against transcribed order reduces errors and ensures that client receives correct medication.
6. Check medication's expiration date printed on vial or ampule.	Medications that have expired should not be used because potency of medications changes when medications become outdated.
7. Calculate drug dose as necessary. Double-check calculation.	Reduces risk of error.
8. Ampule preparation:	
a. Tap top of ampule lightly and quickly with finger until fluid moves from neck of ampule (Fig. 49-1).	Dislodges any fluid that collects above neck of ampule. All solution moves into lower chamber.

Step   **Rationale**

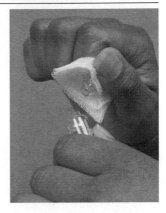

Fig. 49-1 Tapping moves fluid   **Fig. 49-2** Neck snapped away
down neck.   from hands.

b. Place small gauze pad or
   unopened alcohol swab
   around neck of ampule.

Placing pad around neck of
   ampule protects nurse's fingers
   from trauma as glass tip is
   broken off. *Do not use opened
   alcohol swab to wrap around top
   of ampule because alcohol may
   leak into ampule.*

c. Snap neck of ampule
   quickly and firmly away
   from hands (Fig. 49-2).

Protects nurse's fingers and face
   from being cut by glass.

d. Draw up medication
   quickly, using a filter
   needle long enough to
   reach bottom of ampule.

System is open to airborne
   contaminants. Needle must be
   long enough to access
   medication for preparation.
   Filter needles are used to filter
   out glass fragments (Nicoll and
   Hesby, 2002).

e. Hold ampule upside
   down, or set it on flat
   surface. Insert filter
   needle into center of

Broken rim of ampule is
   considered contaminated. When
   ampule is inverted, solution
   dribbles out of ampule if needle

Step	Rationale
ampule opening. Do not allow needle tip or shaft to touch rim of ampule.	tip or shaft touches rim of ampule.
f. Aspirate medication into syringe by gently pulling back on plunger (Fig. 49-3).	Withdrawal of plunger creates negative pressure within syringe barrel, which pulls fluid into syringe.
g. Keep needle tip under surface of liquid. Tip ampule to bring all fluid within reach of needle.	Prevents aspiration of air bubbles.
h. If air bubbles are aspirated, do not expel air into ampule.	Expelling air creates pressure that may force fluid out of ampule, and medication will be lost.
i. To expel excess air bubbles, remove needle from ampule. Hold syringe with needle pointing up. Tap side of syringe to cause bubbles	Withdrawing plunger too far will remove it from barrel. Holding syringe vertically allows air bubbles to rise to top of barrel and fluid to settle in bottom of barrel. Pulling back on plunger

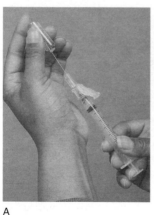
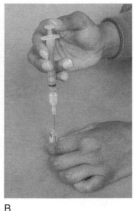

A B

Fig. 49-3 A, Medication aspirated with vial inverted. B, Medication aspirated with vial on flat surface.

Step	**Rationale**

<table>
<tr><td>

to rise toward needle. Draw back slightly on plunger, and then push plunger upward to eject air. *Do not eject fluid.*

</td><td>

allows fluid within needle to enter barrel so fluid is not expelled. Air at top of barrel and within needle is then expelled.

</td></tr>
<tr><td>

j. If syringe contains excess fluid, use sink for disposal. Hold syringe vertically with needle tip up and slanted slightly toward sink. Slowly eject excess fluid into sink. Recheck volume of medication in syringe by holding it vertically.

</td><td>

Medication is safely dispersed into sink. Position of needle allows medication to be expelled without its flowing down needle shaft and onto nurse's hand. Rechecking fluid level ensures proper dose.

</td></tr>
<tr><td>

k. Cover needle with its safety sheath or cap. Replace filter needle with needle for injection.

</td><td>

Prevents contamination of needle. Filter needles cannot be used for injection.

</td></tr>
</table>

9. **Vial containing solution:**

<table>
<tr><td>

a. Remove cap covering top of unused vial to expose rubber seal. If using multidose vial that has been opened, cap is already removed. Firmly and briskly wipe surface of rubber seal with alcohol swab, and allow it to dry.

</td><td>

Vials come packaged with cap that cannot be replaced after removal. Not all drug manufacturers guarantee that rubber seals of unused vials are sterile. Therefore rubber seals must be swabbed with alcohol before drawing up medication. Allowing alcohol to dry prevents alcohol from coating needle and mixing with medication.

</td></tr>
<tr><td>

b. Pick up syringe, and remove cap covering needleless vial access device or safety filter needle. Pull back on plunger to draw amount of air into syringe equivalent to volume of medication to be aspirated from vial.

</td><td>

Air must first be injected into vial to prevent buildup of negative pressure in vial when aspirating medication.

</td></tr>
</table>

Step	**Rationale**

NURSE ALERT Some medications and some institutions require that a filter needle be used when preparing medications from a vial. Check agency policy to determine if use of a filter needle is indicated (Nicoll and Hesby, 2002; Rodger and King, 2000).

c. With vial on flat surface, insert needleless vial access device or tip of safety filter needle with beveled tip entering first through center of rubber seal (Fig. 49-4).	Center of seal is thinner and easier to penetrate. Inserting needle with bevel up prevents coring of rubber seal, which could enter vial or needle (Nicoll and Hesby, 2002).
d. Inject air into vial's airspace, holding on to plunger with firm pressure. Hold plunger with firm pressure (plunger may be forced backward by air pressure within vial).	Air must be injected before aspirating fluid. Injecting into vial's airspace prevents formation of bubbles and inaccuracy in dose.
e. Invert vial while keeping firm hold on syringe and plunger (Fig. 49-5).	Inverting vial allows fluid to settle in lower half of container. Position of hands prevents

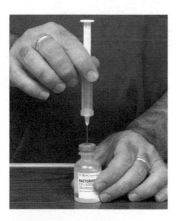

Fig. 49-4 Insert needle's adapter through center of diaphragm.

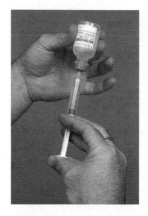

Fig. 49-5 Withdraw fluid with vial inverted.

Step	Rationale
Hold vial between thumb and middle fingers of nondominant hand. Grasp end of syringe barrel and plunger with thumb and forefinger of dominant hand to counteract pressure in vial.	forceful movement of plunger and permits easy manipulation of syringe.
f. Keep tip of needleless vial access device or filter needle below fluid level.	Prevents aspiration of air.
g. Allow air pressure from vial to fill syringe gradually with medication. If necessary, pull back slightly on plunger to obtain correct amount of medication.	Positive pressure within vial forces fluid into syringe. Pulling back too quickly or forcefully on plunger will pull unwanted air into syringe.
h. When desired volume has been obtained, position needleless vial access device or filter needle into vial's airspace; tap side of syringe barrel carefully to dislodge any air bubbles. Eject any air remaining at top of syringe into vial.	Forcefully striking barrel while needle is inserted in vial may bend needle. Accumulation of air displaces medication and causes dose errors.

NURSE ALERT Do not withdraw the last drops in a vial to reduce the likelihood of withdrawing foreign particles into the syringe (Nicoll and Hesby, 2002).

i. Remove needleless vial access device or filter needle from vial by pulling back on barrel of syringe.	Pulling plunger rather than barrel causes plunger to separate from barrel, resulting in loss of medication.

Step	Rationale
j. Hold syringe at eye level, at 90-degree angle, to ensure correct volume and absence of air bubbles. Remove any remaining air by tapping barrel to dislodge any air bubbles (Fig. 49-6). Draw back slightly on plunger; then push plunger upward to eject air. Do not eject fluid. Recheck volume of medication.	Holding syringe vertically allows air to rise to top of barrel and fluid to settle in bottom of barrel. Pulling back on plunger allows fluid within needle to enter barrel so fluid is not expelled. Air at top of barrel and within needle is then expelled.

NURSE ALERT When preparing medication from a single-dose vial, do not assume that the volume listed on the label is the total volume in the vial. Some manufacturers provide a small amount of extra liquid, expecting loss during preparation. Be sure to draw up only the desired volume.

Step	Rationale
k. If medication is to be injected into client's tissue, change needleless vial access device or filter needle for needle of appropriate gauge	A needleless vial access device must be changed for needle because it cannot pierce skin. Filter needles cannot be used for injections (Nicoll and Hesby, 2002).

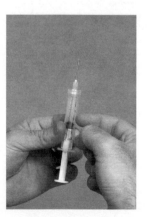

Fig. 49-6 Hold syringe upright; tap barrel to dislodge air bubbles.

Step	**Rationale**
and length according to route of medication.	
l. For multidose vial, make label that includes date of opening, mixing (if necessary), concentration of drug per milliliter, and nurse's initials.	Ensures that future doses will be prepared correctly. Some drugs must be discarded after certain number of days after opening or mixing of vial.
10. **Vial containing a powder (reconstituting medications):**	
a. Remove cap covering vial of powdered medication and cap covering vial of proper diluent. Firmly swab both rubber seals with alcohol swab, and allow alcohol to dry.	Vials come packaged with cap that cannot be replaced after removal. Not all drug manufacturers guarantee that rubber seals of unused vials are sterile. Therefore rubber seals must be swabbed with alcohol before drawing up medication. Allowing alcohol to dry prevents alcohol from coating needle and mixing with medication.
b. Draw up diluent into syringe, following Steps 9 b to j.	Prepares diluent for injection into vial containing powdered medication.
c. Insert tip of needleless vial access device or safety filter needle through center of rubber seal of vial of powdered medication. Inject diluent into vial. Remove needleless device or filter needle from vial, and cover with its cap.	Diluent begins to dissolve and reconstitute medication. Maintaining sterility of needleless vial access device and syringe allows syringe to be used to draw up medication once it is reconstituted.
d. Mix medication thoroughly. Roll in palms. Do not shake.	Ensures proper dispersal of medication throughout solution.

Step	Rationale
e. Reconstituted medication in vial is ready to be drawn into syringe. Read label carefully to determine concentration after reconstitution.	Once diluent has been added, concentration of medication (mg/ml) determines amount to be given.
f. Draw up medication into syringe without adding additional air. Follow Steps 9 b to j.	Injection of diluent creates pressure needed to withdraw medication.

NURSE ALERT Some institutions require that medications prepared for parenteral administration be verified for accuracy by another nurse. Check individual institution guidelines before administering medication.

11. Compare MAR with prepared drugs and continue.	Reading label second time reduces error.
12. Compare dose in syringe with desired dose on MAR.	Third check ensures that accurate dose has been prepared.
13. Complete postprocedure protocol.	

Unexpected Outcomes	Related Interventions
1. Air bubbles remain in syringe barrel.	• Expel air from syringe, and add medication to syringe until correct dose is prepared.
2. Excess or insufficient volume of medication is prepared.	• Be sure correct amount of medication is in syringe before administering to ensure that correct dose of medication is given.

Parenteral Medications: Mixing Medications in One Syringe

Occasionally you will mix medications from two vials or from a vial and an ampule. Mixing compatible medications avoids the need to give a client more than one injection at a time. Determine medication compatibility by referring to a compatibility chart, found in various drug reference guides, or by consulting with your pharmacist. When mixing medications, remember how to correctly aspirate fluid from each type of container. When using multidose vials, do not contaminate the vial's contents with medication from another vial or ampule.

Use caution when preparing insulin, which comes in vials. Insulin is the hormone used to treat high blood glucose levels most frequently associated with diabetes. Often clients with diabetes receive a combination of different types of insulin to control their blood glucose levels. Regular insulin is a rapid- or short-acting solution that can be given subcutaneously (Sub-Q), intravenously (IV), or intramuscularly (IM). Other types of insulin contain the addition of a protein that slows absorption. Intermediate- or long-acting insulin preparations cannot be given IV or IM. Some insulins can be mixed in the same syringe. However, when insulins are mixed, chemical changes may occur either immediately or over time. This can result in a client response to insulin that is different from the response that would occur if the insulins had been given separately. Box 50-1 lists recommendations from the American Diabetes Association for mixing insulins.

Delegation Considerations

The skill of mixing medications from two vials or from a vial and an ampule should not be delegated to assistive personnel (AP).

Equipment

- Single-dose or multidose vials and ampules containing medications
- Syringe with needleless vial access device or filter needle and syringe
- Extra needle for injection
- Alcohol swab

BOX 50-1   Recommendations for Mixing Insulins

- Clients whose blood sugar levels are well controlled on a mixed insulin dose should maintain their individual routine when preparing and administering their insulin.
- Insulin should not be mixed with any other medications or diluent unless approved by the prescribing physician or advanced practice nurse.
- Insulin glargine should not be mixed with any other forms of insulin.
- Commercially available premixed insulins may be used if the ratio of the insulins within the vial matches the client's current insulin requirements.
- Injections that mix NPH and short-acting insulins may be administered immediately or they may be stored for future use.
- Rapid-acting insulin may be mixed with NPH, Lente, and Ultralente.
- Mixtures of rapid-acting insulin with either an intermediate- or long-acting insulin should be injected within 15 minutes before a meal.
- Short-acting and Lente insulins should not be mixed unless the client's blood sugar levels are currently under control with this mixture.
- Phosphate-buffered insulins (e.g., NPH) should not be mixed with Lente insulins. If they are mixed, a precipitate may form and the time of onset and peak action of the insulins will change.
- Insulin formulations may change. Follow manufacturer's guidelines if the manufacturer's guidelines conflict with the American Diabetes Association guidelines.

- Sharps container for disposing of syringes, needles, and glass
- Medication administration record (MAR) or computer printout

Step	Rationale
1. Complete preprocedure protocol.	
2. Consider medications to be mixed, compatibility of medications, and type of injection.	Determines if medications can be mixed, order of drawing up medications, and size of syringe.
3. Assemble medication and supplies at work area in	Organization saves time and reduces risk of error.

Step	Rationale

medication preparation
area.

4. Check name of medication
   on vial/ampule label
   against MAR.

Reading label first time and
comparing it against transcribed
order reduce errors and ensure
that client receives correct
medication.

5. Check medication's
   expiration date printed on
   vial or ampule.

Medications that have expired
should not be used because
potency of medications changes
when medications become
outdated.

6. **Mixing medications from
   two vials:**
   a. Using syringe with
      needleless vial access
      device or filter needle,
      aspirate volume of air
      equivalent to first dose
      of medication (vial A).

   Air must be introduced into vial
   to create positive pressure
   needed to withdraw solution.

   b. Inject air into vial A,
      making sure needleless
      device or filter needle
      does not touch solution
      (Fig. 50-1, *A*).

   Prevents cross contamination.

   c. Holding on to plunger,
      withdraw needleless vial
      access device or filter
      needle and syringe from
      vial A. Aspirate air
      equivalent to second
      dose of medication
      (vial B).

   If plunger is not held in place,
   injected air may escape from vial
   A. Air is injected into vial B to
   create positive pressure needed
   to withdraw desired dose.

   d. Insert needleless vial
      access device or filter
      needle into vial B, inject
      air, and then withdraw
      proper volume of
      medication from vial
      (see Fig. 50-1, *B*).

   First portion of dose has been
   prepared.

Step	Rationale

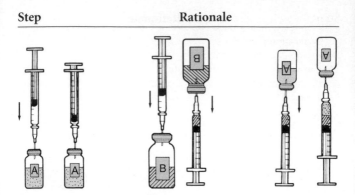

Fig. 50-1   **A,** Injecting air into vial A. **B,** Injecting air into vial B and withdrawing dose. **C,** Withdrawing medication from vial A; medications are now mixed.

e. Withdraw needleless access device or filter needle and syringe from vial B. Ensure that proper volume has been obtained.

Ensures that correct dose is prepared.

f. Determine at which point on syringe scale combined volume of medications should measure.

Prevents accidental withdrawal of too much medication from second vial.

g. Insert needleless access device or filter needle into vial A, being careful not to push plunger and expel medication into vial. Invert vial, and carefully withdraw correct amount of medication into syringe (see Fig. 50-1, *C*).

Positive pressure within vial A allows fluid to fill syringe without need to aspirate.

h. Withdraw needleless access device or filter needle, and expel any

Air bubbles should not be injected into tissues. Excess fluid causes incorrect dose.

Step	Rationale

excess air or fluid from syringe. Check fluid level in syringe. Medications are now mixed.

NURSE ALERT If too much medication is withdrawn from second vial, discard syringe and start over. Do not push medication back into vial.

   i. Change needleless access device for appropriate-size needle if medication is being injected. Replace filter needle with needleless system or with appropriate-size needle according to route of medication. Keep needleless device or needle capped until administration time.

     A needleless vial access device must be changed for needle if medication is to pierce skin. Filter needles cannot be used for injections (Nicoll and Hesby, 2002).

7. **Mixing insulin:**
   a. If mixing rapid- or short-acting insulin with intermediate- or long-acting insulin, use insulin syringe to aspirate volume of air equivalent to dose to be withdrawn from cloudy insulin first. If two modified forms of insulin are mixed, it makes no difference which vial is prepared first.

     Air must be introduced into vial to create pressure needed to withdraw solution.

NURSE ALERT If the long-acting insulin glargine (Lantus) is ordered, note that this is a clear insulin that should not be mixed with other insulin.

   b. Inject air into vial of intermediate- or long-

     Prevents cross contamination.

Step	Rationale
acting insulin. Be sure that needle does not touch solution.	
c. Withdraw needle and syringe from vial without aspirating medication. Aspirate air equivalent to dose to be withdrawn from rapid- or short-acting insulin.	Air will be injected into vial to withdraw desired dose.
d. Insert needle into vial of rapid- or short-acting insulin, inject air, and then fill syringe with correct insulin dose.	First portion of dose has been prepared. Always fill syringe with rapid- or short-acting insulin first to prevent contamination with intermediate- or long-acting insulin.
e. Withdraw needle and syringe from vial by pulling on barrel; remove any air bubbles, and check dose.	Prevents accidental pulling of plunger, which may cause loss of medication. Ensures that correct dose is prepared.

NURSE ALERT Some institutions require insulin doses to be verified by another nurse for accuracy. Check institutional policy. Have dose of clear insulin verified before mixing, and then have combined dose verified after the medications are mixed as well.

Step	Rationale
f. Determine at which point on syringe scale combined units of insulin should measure by adding number of units of both insulins together (e.g., 5 units Regular + 12 units NPH = 17 units total).	Prevents accidental withdrawal of too much insulin from second vial.
g. Insert needle into vial of intermediate- or long-acting insulin. Be careful not to push	Positive pressure within vial of intermediate- or long-acting insulin allows fluid to fill syringe without need to aspirate.

Step	Rationale

plunger and expel
medication into vial.
Invert vial, and carefully
withdraw desired
amount of insulin into
syringe.

h. Withdraw needle, and
check fluid level in
syringe. Keep needle of
prepared syringe
sheathed or capped
until administering
medication.

Ensures accurate dose. Inaccurate
doses of insulin can cause
serious hypoglycemia or
hyperglycemia. Keeping needle
capped or sheathed keeps needle
sterile for insulin administration.

8. **Mixing medications from
vial and ampule:**

a. Prepare medication
from vial first, Skill 49.

Medication administration from
vial requires insertion of air into
vial. Therefore vial medication is
prepared first.

b. Determine at which
point on syringe scale
combined volume of
medication should
measure.

Prevents accidental withdrawal of
too much medication from
ampule.

NURSE ALERT If needleless vial access device was used in preparing
medication from vial, change needleless system to filter needle.

c. Prepare medication
from ampule (Skill 49).

Ensures that appropriate amount
of medication is prepared.

d. Withdraw filter needle
from ampule, and verify
fluid level in syringe.
Change filter needle to
appropriate needleless
device or needle with
appropriate gauge.

Ensures accurate dose. Keeping
needle or needleless device
capped maintains sterility for
medication administration.

e. Perform hand hygiene.

Reduces transmission of infection.

9. Check syringe carefully for
total combined dose of
medications.

Accurate dose ensures safe
medication administration.

Step	Rationale
10. Compare MAR with prepared drugs and continue.	Reading label second time reduces error.
11. Compare dose in syringe with desired dose on MAR.	Third check ensures that accurate dose is prepared.
12. Complete postprocedure protocol.	

Unexpected Outcomes   Related Interventions

See Skill 49.

Patient-Controlled Analgesia

Patient-controlled analgesia (PCA) is an interactive method of pain management that permits client control over pain through self-administration of analgesics (Pasero, 2003). A client simply depresses the button on a PCA device, and a regulated dose of analgesic is delivered. Thus it is crucial that candidates for PCA be able to understand how, why, and when to self-administer the medication (American Pain Society, 2003). It is used extensively in clients with acute (e.g., postoperative) and chronic (e.g., cancer) pain. Family-controlled analgesia (FCA) has been used in children with cognitive or physical disabilities (Lehr and BeVier, 2003). PCA is not recommended in situations in which oral analgesics could easily manage pain (American Pain Society, 2003).

The PCA has several advantages. It allows more constant serum levels of the opioid and, as a result, avoids the peaks and troughs of a large bolus. Because the blood level is maintained within a narrow range of the minimum effective analgesic concentration for the individual, pain relief is enhanced and the incidence of side effects, such as sedation and respiratory depression, is decreased (Pasero, 2003). A second advantage is that when used postoperatively, fewer complications may arise because earlier and easier ambulation occurs as a result of effective pain relief. Increased client control and independence are other advantages of PCA.

Delegation Considerations

The administration of PCA may not be delegated to assistive personnel (AP). However, certain aspects of the client's care, such as hygiene and vital signs, might be delegated. The nurse must instruct AP:

- To report to the nurse signs of unrelieved pain and/or sedation.
- To immediately report any new symptom or change in client status to the nurse.
- To never administer a PCA dose for the client.

Equipment

- PCA system
- Identification label and time tape (may already be attached and completed by pharmacy)
- 18- or 20-gauge needle (if not using a needleless system)
- Alcohol swab
- Adhesive tape
- Disposable gloves, if applicable

Step	Rationale
1. Complete preprocedure protocol.	
2. Assess for physical, behavioral, emotional, and cognitive signs and symptoms of pain or discomfort.	Combination of signs and symptoms may reveal source and nature of pain.
3. Assess patency of existing intravenous (IV) infusion line (see Skill 53).	IV line must be patent, with fluid infusing, for medication to reach venous circulation.
4. Assess venipuncture site for infiltration or inflammation (see Skill 53).	Confirmation of placement of IV needle or catheter and integrity of surrounding tissues ensures that medication is administered safely.
5. Check client's history of drug allergies.	Avoids placing client at risk for allergic reaction.
6. Check infuser and patient-control module for accurate labeling or evidence of leaking.	Avoids medication error. Damage to system can occur in shipping and handling; inspect to avoid injury or harm to client, self, or others.
7. Program computerized PCA pump to deliver prescribed medication dose and lockout interval.	Ensures safe, therapeutic drug administration.
8. Prepare prescribed medication. Verify client identification, using two identifiers, neither of which	Minimizes risk of medication error and harm to client.

Step	Rationale
can be the patient's room number. Follow the "six rights" to be sure of correct medication. Check client's identification band, and call client by name.	
9. Attach drug reservoir to infusion device, and prime tubing.	Locks system and prevents air from infusing into IV tubing.
10. ✍ Attach 18- or 19-gauge needle to exit tubing adapter of patient-control module, or attach needleless system adapter.	Needed to connect with IV line.
11. Wipe injection port of maintenance IV line with alcohol if closed port is being used.	Alcohol is a topical antiseptic that minimizes entry of surface microorganisms during needle insertion.
12. Insert needleless adapter or needle into injection port nearest client.	Establishes route for medication to enter main IV line. Prevents delay of medication delivery to client.
13. Secure connection with tape, and immobilize PCA tubing.	Prevents dislodging of needle from port. Facilitates ambulation.
14. Administer loading dose of analgesic as prescribed.	A one-time dose may be given manually by nurse or programmed into PCA pump.
15. Complete postprocedure protocol.	

Recording and Reporting

- Record drug, dose, and time begun on appropriate medication form. Specify concentration and diluent. Note lockout time, demand and/or basal dose.
- Record regular periodic assessments of client status on PCA medication form if required, in narrative notes, pain assessment flowsheet, or other documentation tool used in institution.

Unexpected Outcomes	Related Interventions
1. Client verbalizes continued or worsening discomfort, or displays nonverbal behaviors indicative of pain.	• Perform complete pain assessment. • Assess for possible complications. • Inspect IV site for possible catheter occlusion or infiltration. • Evaluate number of attempts and deliveries initiated by client. • Check that maintenance IV fluid is continuously running. • Evaluate pump for operational problems. • Consult with physician.
2. Client is sedated and not readily aroused.	• Stop PCA. • Elevate head of bed 30 degrees, unless contraindicated. • Assess vital signs. • Notify physician. • Prepare to administer an opioid reversing agent as ordered. • Observe client frequently.

Peripheral Intravenous Care: Regulating Intravenous Flow Rate, Changing Tubing and Solution, Dressing Care, Discontinuation

After an intravenous (IV) infusion is initiated and the line is patent, the nurse is responsible for regulating the rate of infusion, changing the tubing and solutions as needed, maintaining the dressing, and discontinuing the IV line according to the physician's orders.

A client receiving IV therapy may require frequent changes of IV solutions, especially if the client's condition is unstable. It is important that proper technique is followed to ensure the sterility of the IV fluid container. In addition, the "six rights" of medication administration must be adhered to when changing solutions. Ideally, infusion tubing should be changed when hanging a new fluid container. However, that is not always possible.

IV dressings are done when the IV is inserted or when the IV site is changed. The insertion site is the most common source of colonization and infections for IV cannulas. A peripheral IV dressing must be securely applied and changed when it becomes wet, soiled, or loosened (CDC, 2002). Transparent dressings should be changed with cannula site rotation and immediately if the integrity is compromised. Gauze dressings are changed every 48 hours. The gauze used under a transparent dressing is considered a gauze dressing and should be changed every 48 hours as well (CDC, 2002; INS, 2006).

Delegation Considerations

The skill of peripheral IV catheter care may not be delegated to assistive personnel (AP). However, AP may be delegated other aspects of care, and the nurse must instruct AP to notify the nurse when:

- The electronic infusion device alarm signals, the fluid container is almost empty, and the client complains of any discomfort at the IV site.
- The IV dressing is wet, soiled, or dislodged.
- The IV tubing separates or contains air or blood.
- The client complains of pain, burning, or swelling or if the insertion site is cold or moist.

Equipment
Regulating IV Flow Rate
- Watch with second hand
- Calculator or pad and pen/pencil
- Tape
- Label
- IV regulating device (electronic infusion device [EID], volume-control device [optional])

Changing IV Solutions
- Bottle/bag of IV solution/medication as ordered by physician
- Time tape

Changing IV Tubing
If a new IV dressing must be applied, assemble additional equipment:
- Disposable, nonsterile gloves
- Label or tape
- 2 × 2 gauze (optional)

Continuous IV Infusion
- Infusion tubing

Intermittent Saline/Heparin Lock
- Syringe filled with normal saline or heparin flush solution (check agency policy)
- Loop of extension tubing, injection cap
- Antiseptic swab or stick (e.g., chlorhexidine, povidone-iodine, alcohol)

Changing IV Dressing
- Antiseptic swab
- Adhesive remover (if needed)

- Skin protectant swab
- Disposable gloves, mask, gown
- Strips of nonallergenic tape
- Hand or arm board or IV housing device if needed

For Transparent Dressing

- Sterile transparent dressing

For Gauze Dressing

- Sterile 2 × 2 gauze pad

Discontinuing Peripheral Intravenous Access

- Disposable gloves
- Sterile 2 × 2 or 4 × 4 gauze sponge
- Antiseptic swab
- Tape

Step	Rationale
1. Complete preprocedure protocol.	
2. Check client's medical record for correct solution and additives. Follow "six rights" of medication administration. Usual order includes solution, additives or medications (if included), infusion rate or volume in specified time period. Occasionally, IV order contains only 1 L to keep vein open (KVO).	IV fluids are medications. "Six rights" prevent medication administration error.
a. When changing IV fluids or replacing existing IV fluid, verify solution with current order and follow "six rights" of medication administration.	When IV fluid container runs dry or hang time exceeds CDC (2002) recommendations, IV solution must be replaced and replacement fluid must be consistent with prescribed fluid orders. If new solution is to be hung, new solution must be consistent with new fluid order.

Step	Rationale
b. Determine compatibility of all IV fluids and additives by consulting appropriate literature or pharmacist.	Incompatibilities may lead to precipitate formation and cause physical, chemical, and therapeutic changes.
3. Perform hand hygiene. Observe for patency of IV line and cannula.	For fluid to infuse at proper rate, IV line and cannula must be free of kinks and thrombi.
a. Puncture of infusion tubing requires immediate change.	Punctured tubing results in fluid leakage and bacterial contamination.
b. Contamination of tubing (e.g., separation of connections) requires immediate change.	Contamination of tubing allows entry of pathogens into client's bloodstream.
c. Occlusions in tubing, from transfusion of blood or blood products, requires immediate change.	Whole blood or blood products can occlude or partially occlude infusion tubing because viscous solutions adhere to wall of tubing and decrease size of lumen.
4. Inspect IV site, determine if there is pain or burning. Palpate site for tenderness.	Pain or burning may be early indication of phlebitis (see Tables 53-1 and 53-2, p. 371). Includes client in decision making.

5. Know calibration (drop factor) in drops per milliliter (gtt/ml) of infusion set used by agency:
Microdrip: 60 gtt/ml
Macrodrip (Metheny, 2000):
  Abbott: 15 gtt/ml
  Travenol: 10 gtt/ml
  McGaw: 15 gtt/ml
	Microdrip tubing, also called *pediatric tubing,* universally delivers 60 gtt/ml and is used when small or very precise volumes are to be infused. However, there are different commercial parenteral administration sets for macrodrip tubing. Macrodrip tubing should be used when large quantities or fast rates are necessary.

6. Select one of the following formulas to calculate flow rate after determining ml/hr:	Once hourly rate has been determined (see next page), these formulas give correct flow rate.

Step	Rationale

ml/hr/60 min = ml/min
Drop factor × ml/min = drops/min
Or
ml/hr × drop factor/ 60 min = drops/min

7. **Regulate IV infusion rate:**

a. Obtain prescribed IV solution/medication and appropriate tubing material. IV fluids may be ordered for 24-hour period, indicating how long each liter of fluid should run.

Use of correct tubing ensures more accurate infusion delivery. Determines volume of fluid that should infuse hourly.

b. Determine hourly rate by dividing volume by hours; for example:
ml/hr = total infusion (ml)/hours of infusion
1000 ml/8 hr = 125 ml/hr
or if 3 L is ordered for 24 hours
3000 ml/24 hr = 125 ml/hr

Provides even infusion of fluid over prescribed hourly rate.

c. Place marked adhesive tape or commercial fluid indicator tape on IV container next to volume markings.

Time taping IV bag gives nurse visual cue as to whether fluids are being administered over correct period of time. Time tapes should be used for all IV infusions, including those on therapies infused via EIDs.

d. After hourly rate is determined, calculate minute rate based on drop factor of infusion set (see Step 5).

Allows nurse to calculate minute flow rate for regulation of infusion.

e. Determine flow rate by counting drops in drip chamber for 1 minute

Regulate to prescribed rate.

Step	Rationale

by watch; then adjust roller clamp to increase or decrease rate of infusion.

f. Follow this procedure for infusion gravity controller or EID pump:

  (1) Consult manufacturer's directions for setup of infusion. Place electronic eye over drip chamber (Fig. 52-1). If gravity controller is used, ensure that IV container is 36 inches above IV site.

IV controller works by gravity.

  (2) Insert IV tubing into chamber of control mechanism (see manufacturer's directions).

Most electronic infusion pumps use positive pressure to infuse.

  (3) Required drops per minute or volume per hour is selected, door to control

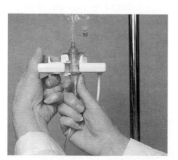

Fig. 52-1 Electronic eye placed over drip chamber.

Step	Rationale

chamber is closed, power button is turned on, and start button is pressed.

(4) Open drip regulator completely while EID is in use.

Ensures that pump freely regulates infusion rate.

(5) Monitor infusion rate and IV site for infiltration according to agency policy. Rate of infusion should be checked by comparing volume in container with calculated amount that should have been infused even when EID is used.

Infusion controllers or pumps are fallible and do not replace frequent, accurate nursing evaluation. Infusion pumps may continue to infuse IV fluids after infiltration has begun.

(6) Assess patency of system when alarm signals.

Alarm on infusion pump can be triggered by empty solution container, tubing obstruction, closed drip regulator, infiltration, thrombus formation, air in tubing, and/or low battery.

g. Follow this procedure for gravity volume-control device:

(1) Place gravity volume-control device between IV container and insertion spike of infusion set, using aseptic technique.

Delivers small volume but must be refilled as it becomes low.

(2) Place no more than 2 hours' allotment of fluid into device by opening clamp

Allows safeguard for nurse if unable to return in exactly 60 minutes. Should infusion rate accidentally increase in rate,

Step	Rationale
between IV bag and device.	allows, at most, only 2-hour allotment of fluid to infuse.
(3) Assess system at least hourly; add fluid to volume-control device. Regulate flow rate.	Maintains patency of system.
8. Hanging new IV solution:	
a. Prepare new solution for changing. If using plastic bag, remove protective cover from IV tubing port (see Skill 52). If using glass bottle, remove metal cap and metal disk over rubber stopper.	Permits quick, smooth, and organized change from old to new solution.
b. Move roller clamp to stop flow rate on existing infusion.	Prevents solution remaining in drip chamber from emptying while changing solutions.
c. Remove old IV solution from IV pole.	Brings work to nurse's eye level. Prevents fluid from pouring when spike is removed.
d. Quickly remove spike from old solution container and, without touching tip, insert spike into new container.	Reduces risk of solution in drip chamber running dry, and maintains sterility.
e. Hang new container of solution.	Position allows gravity to assist with delivery of fluid into drip chamber.
f. Observe for air in tubing, and remove appropriately. Close roller clamp, stretch tubing down, and tap tubing with finger to cause bubbles to rise in fluid to drip chamber.	Reduces risk for air embolus. Use of air-eliminating filter also reduces this risk.

Step	**Rationale**
g. Ensure that drip chamber is one-third to one-half full.	Reduces risk of air entering tubing. If chamber is too full, drip rate cannot be observed and not accurately regulated. In addition, electronic eye of EID will not be able to detect drop.
h. Regulate flow to prescribed rate, and apply time tape to side of container. Do not mark on container.	Ensures administration of prescribed rate of fluid. Ink may leach into PVC containers.
i. Apply label to IV solution. Be sure label contains date and time hung.	Provides mechanism to communicate when new solution was initiated.

9. **Changing infusion tubing:**
   a. *For continuous IV infusion:*

(1) Move roller clamp on new IV tubing to "off" position.	Prevents spillage of solution after container is spiked.
(2) Slow rate of existing infusion by regulating drip rate on old tubing. Be sure rate is at KVO rate.	Prevents complete infusion of solution remaining in tubing. Complete infusion of solution remaining in tubing increases risk of occlusion of IV cannula.
(3) Compress drip chamber of old tubing, and fill chamber.	Provides surplus of fluid in drip chamber so there is enough fluid to maintain IV patency while changing tubing.
(4) Remove existing container from IV pole.	Brings work to nurse's eye level.
(5) Invert container, and remove old tubing from container; keep spike sterile until new tubing	Allows fluid to continue to flow through IV cannula while nurse is preparing new tubing.

Step	Rationale
connected. *Option:* Tape old drip chamber to IV pole without contaminating spike.	
(6) Place insertion spike of new tubing into old solution container opening, and hang solution container on IV pole.	Permits flow of fluid from solution into new infusion tubing.
(7) Compress and release drip chamber on new tubing; slowly fill drip chamber one-third to one-half full (see Skill 52).	Allows drip chamber to fill, and promotes rapid, smooth flow of solution through new tubing.
(8) Slowly open roller clamp, remove protective cap from adapter (if necessary), and flush tubing with solution. Stop infusion. Replace cap. Place end of adapter near client's IV site.	Removes air from tubing and replaces it with fluid. Positions equipment for quick, smooth connection of new tubing.
(9) Turn roller clamp on old tubing to "off " position.	Prevents spillage of fluid as tubing is removed from cannula hub.
b. *For saline/heparin lock:*	
(1) 🔲 Swab injection cap with antiseptic swab. Insert syringe with	Removes air to prevent introduction into vein.

Step	Rationale
1 to 3 ml saline or heparin flush solution, and inject through injection cap into loop or short extension tubing.	
(2) *Option:* Place 2 × 2 gauze under cannula hub.	Prevents tubing from accidentally contacting skin and collects blood that may leak from cannula hub.
(3) Stabilize cannula hub, and apply pressure over vein just above cannula tip (at least 4 cm [1½ inches] above insertion site). Gently disconnect old tubing from cannula hub, and quickly insert adapter of new tubing into cannula hub.	Allows smooth transition from old to new tubing, minimizing time system open to infection.
c. Open roller clamp on new tubing, allowing solution to run rapidly for 30 to 60 seconds; then regulate IV drip according to physician's orders, and monitor rate hourly. *Optional:* Connect new tubing to EID and regulate.	Ensures patency of cannula and maintenance of venous access.
d. Attach piece of tape or preprinted label with date and time of tubing change onto tubing below drip chamber.	Provides reference to determine next time for tubing change.

Step	Rationale
e. Form loop of tubing, and secure it to client's arm with strip of tape.	Avoids accidental pulling against site and cannula movement.
f. Remove and discard any dressing material and old IV tubing. If necessary, apply new dressing. Dispose of gloves. Perform hand hygiene.	Reduces transmission of microorganisms.

10. **Changing IV dressing:**

a. ![icon] Remove tape, gauze, and/or transparent dressing from old dressing one layer at a time by pulling toward insertion site (Fig. 52-2), leaving tape that secures IV cannula intact. Be cautious if cannula tubing becomes tangled between two layers of dressing. When removing transparent dressing, hold cannula hub and tubing with nondominant hand.

   Prevents accidental displacement of cannula.

b. Observe insertion site for signs and/or symptoms of infection: tenderness, redness, swelling, and exudate.

   Presence of infection indicates need to discontinue IV at current site.

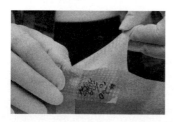

Fig. 52-2 Remove transparent dressing by pulling side laterally.

Step	Rationale
c. If complication exists or if ordered by physician, discontinue infusion.	
d. If IV is infusing properly, gently remove tape securing cannula. Stabilize cannula with one hand. Use adhesive remover to cleanse skin and remove adhesive residue, if needed.	Exposes venipuncture site. Stabilization prevents accidental displacement of cannula. Adhesive residue decreases ability of new tape to adhere securely to skin.
e. Cleanse insertion site with antiseptic swab using friction. Use first swab in horizontal plane, cleansing skin from side to side. Apply second swab on vertical plane, up and down. Apply final swab in circular pattern, moving outward from insertion site. Allow each swab to dry.	Mechanical friction in this pattern allows penetration of antiseptic solution into cracks and fissures of epidermal layer of skin (Crosby and Mares, 2001). Antiseptic solutions should be allowed to air-dry completely to effectively reduce microbial counts (INS, 2006). If antiseptic agents are used in combination, allow each to air-dry separately.
f. *Option:* Apply skin protectant solution to area where tape or dressing will be applied. Allow to dry.	Coats skin with protective solution to maintain skin integrity, prevent irritation from adhesive, and promote adhesion of dressing.
g. Tape or secure catheter: (1) Applying transparent dressing: Secure catheter with nondominant hand while preparing to apply dressing.	Prevents catheter dislodgement.
(2) Applying gauze dressing: Place narrow piece	Chevron secures cannula. Inspection of insertion site is essential.

Step	Rationale

1.25 cm [½ inch] of tape under cannula hub with adhesive side up; cross tape over hub to make chevron. Place tape only on cannula, *never over* insertion site.

h. Apply sterile dressing over site:
   (1) *Transparent dressing* (see Skill 53, Step 23a)
   (2) *Gauze dressing* (see Skill 53, Step 23b)

i. Remove and discard gloves.

Prevents transmission of microorganisms.

j. *Option:* Apply hand board or securement device if insertion site or dressing is affected by motion of joint.

Reduces risk of phlebitis and infiltration from mechanical motion.

k. Anchor IV tubing with additional pieces of tape if necessary. When using transparent dressing, avoid placing tape over dressing.

Prevents accidental displacement of IV cannula.

l. Place date and time of dressing change and size and gauge of cannula directly on dressing.

Provides information about dressing change.

11. Ensure that flow rate is accurate.

Validates that IV is patent and functioning correctly. Manipulation of cannula and tubing may affect rate of infusion.

Step	Rationale
12. Inspect condition of IV site, noting color, bleeding, erythema. Palpate for skin temperature, edema, and tenderness.	Complications such as phlebitis and infiltration require discontinuance of IV and location of another site for cannula.
13. **Discontinuing peripheral IV access:**	
a. ✋ Turn IV tubing roller clamp to "off" position or turn EID off and then turn roller clamp to "off" position.	Prevents spillage of IV fluid.
b. Remove IV site dressing, stabilizing IV device (see Step 11). Then remove tape securing cannula.	Exposes cannula with minimal discomfort.
c. Hold cannula, and clean site with antimicrobial swab.	Removes secretions around skin puncture site.
d. Place clean sterile gauze over venipuncture site, apply light pressure, and remove cannula by pulling straight away from insertion site in slow, steady motion. Keep cannula parallel to skin during withdrawal. Inspect catheter for intactness after removal.	Dry pad causes less irritation to puncture site. Prevents damage to client's vein; determines if catheter tip is intact. Tips of catheter can break off, causing embolus and emergency situation. Notify physician immediately if tip is broken.
e. Keep gauze in place, and apply continuous pressure to site for 2 to 3 minutes.	Controls bleeding and hematoma formation. Contraction is enhanced by pressure to site for at least 2 to 3 minutes (Chukhraev and Grekov, 2000).
f. Apply clean, folded gauze dressing over insertion site, and secure with tape.	Maintains pressure to prevent bleeding and reduces bacterial entry into puncture site.

Step	Rationale

14. Complete postprocedure
    protocol.

Recording and Reporting

- Record rate of infusion, gtt/min, and ml/hr in nurses' notes or on parenteral fluid form, immediately record in nurses' notes any ordered change in IV fluid rates, indicate use of any electronic infusion device or controlling device and number on that device.
- At change of shift or when leaving on break, report rate of infusion and volume left in container to nurse in charge or next nurse assigned to care for client.

Unexpected Outcomes	Related Interventions
1. Sudden infusion of large volume of solution occurs with client having symptoms of dyspnea, crackles in lung, and increased urine output, indicating fluid overload.	• Slow infusion to KVO rate, and notify physician immediately. • Place client in high-Fowler's position. • New IV orders will be required. • Client may require diuretics. • Check condition of site. • If volume infused is deficient, consult physician/IP for new order to provide necessary fluid volume.
2. IV cannula is infiltrated, or phlebitis is present (see Tables 53-1 and 53-2).	• Stop infusion, and discontinue IV; see Step 13. • Notify physician, and start new IV as ordered; see Skill 49.
3. IV insertion site is red and/or edematous, it may or may not be painful, and exudates may or may not be present. Signs indicate possible infection at venipuncture site.	• Notify physician • Discontinue IV; see Step 13. • Obtain culture of cannula, if ordered. • Administer antibiotics if prescribed.

Peripheral Intravenous Insertion

The goal of intravenous (IV) fluid administration is correction or prevention of fluid and electrolyte disturbances in clients who are or may become acutely ill. For example, a client with third-degree burns over 40% of the body is critically ill and has severe fluid and electrolyte imbalances. A client who is NPO (nothing by mouth) after surgery receives IV fluid replacement to prevent fluid and electrolyte imbalances; the infusion is usually discontinued when the client resumes oral intake. Another reason to perform a venipuncture is to provide IV access for intermittent or emergency medication administration. Peripheral IV access should be used with caution for administration of medications that are irritants; a central venous access is preferred. Vesicants should be administered only through a central venous access site (see Skill 54).

Delegation Considerations

The skill of initiating peripheral IV therapy may not be delegated to assistive personnel (AP). However, this skill may be within the scope of practice for licensed practical (vocational) nurses in some states; verify with agency policy. If other aspects of care are delegated to AP, the nurse should instruct AP to:

- Inform nurse if client complains of burning, bleeding, swelling, or coolness at catheter insertion site.
- Inform nurse if IV dressing becomes wet.
- Inform nurse if the volume of fluid in the bag is low.

Equipment

- Correct IV solution (with time tape attached)
- Proper IV safety access device for venipuncture (will vary with client's body size and reason for IV fluid administration)
- IV start kit (available in some agencies): may contain a sterile drape to place under the client's arm, cleansing and antiseptic preparations, dressings, and a small roll of sterile tape

For IV Fluid Infusion

- Administration set (choice depends on type of solution and rate of administration; infants and children require microdrip tubing, which provides 60 gtt/ml)

- 0.22-mm filter (if required by agency policy or if particulate matter is likely)
- Extension tubing
- Antiseptic swabs (i.e., chlorhexidine, alcohol, or povidone-iodine)
- Disposable gloves
- Tourniquet (can be a source of contamination; use a single-use product)
- Arm board, if needed (used to maintain wrist or elbow joint position when catheter is placed close to or over a joint; will help prevent infiltration of IV)
- Nonallergenic tape
- Towel (to place under client's hand or arm)
- IV pole, rolling or ceiling mounted
- Special gown with snaps at shoulder seams (makes removal with IV tubing easier), if available
- Needle disposal container (also called *sharps container*)

For Heparin or Normal Saline Lock

- Injection cap (also called *IV plug, PRN adapter*)
- IV loop or short piece of extension tubing, if necessary
- 1 to 3 ml of normal saline or heparin flush (10 units/ml as ordered)
- Syringes and 25-gauge needles

Transparent Dressing Only

- Transparent dressing

Gauze Dressing Only

- 2 × 2 or 4 × 4 sterile gauze sponge
- Sterile tape

Step	Rationale
1. Complete preprocedure protocol.	
2. Review physician's order for type and amount of IV fluid and rate of fluid administration. Nurse follows "six rights" of medication administration.	An order requesting initiation of peripheral IV access and administration of IV solution must be made by physician before initiation of this therapy.

Step	**Rationale**
3. Assess for clinical factors/ conditions that will respond to or be affected by IV fluid administration:	Provides baseline to determine effect IV fluids have on client's fluid and electrolyte balance.
a. Peripheral edema—can be rated for severity by assessing pitting over bony prominences.	Indicates expanded interstitial volume. This is usually most evident in dependent areas (e.g., feet and ankles). Fluid overload will worsen edema.
b. Body weight.	Daily weights document fluid retention or loss. Change in body weight of 1 kg corresponds to 1 L of fluid retention or loss.
c. Blood pressure changes.	Elevated blood pressure may indicate volume excess caused by increase in stroke volume. Decreased blood pressure may indicate fluid volume deficit caused by decrease in stroke volume.
d. Irregular pulse rhythm; increased pulse rate.	Rhythm changes may occur with potassium, calcium, and/or magnesium abnormalities; rate change may occur with fluid volume deficit.
e. Auscultation of crackles or rhonchi in lungs.	May signal fluid buildup in lungs caused by fluid volume excess.
f. Decreased urine output.	During dehydration, kidneys attempt to restore fluid balance by reducing urine production.
4. Determine if client is to undergo any planned surgeries or is to receive blood infusion later.	Allows nurse to anticipate and place large-gauge catheter for fluid infusion and avoids placement of catheter in area that will interfere with medical procedures.
5. Check client's identity using two forms of identification.	Ensures that right client receives right IV fluid.

Step	Rationale

6. Change client's gown to more easily removed gown with snaps at shoulder, if available.

Use of special IV gown facilitates safe removal of gown once IV has been inserted.

7. Using aseptic technique, Prepare IV infusion tubing and solution:

   a. Make sure prescribed additives, such as potassium and vitamins, have been added. Check solution for color, clarity, and expiration date.

IV solutions are medications and should be carefully checked to reduce risk of error. Solutions that are discolored, contain particles, or are past expiration date are not to be used. Leaky bags present opportunity for infection and must not be used.

   b. Open infusion set, maintaining sterility of both ends of tubing. Many sets allow for priming of tubing without removal of end cap.

Prevents microorganisms from entering infusion equipment and bloodstream.

   c. Place roller clamp about 2 to 5 cm (1 to 2 inches) below drip chamber, and move roller clamp to "off" position.

Proximity of roller clamp to drip chamber allows more accurate regulation of flow rate. Moving clamp to "off" position prevents accidental spillage of IV fluid on client, nurse, bed, or floor.

   d. Remove protective sheath over IV tubing port on plastic IV solution bag (Fig. 53-1).

Provides access for insertion of infusion tubing into solution.

   e. Insert infusion set into fluid bag or bottle: Remove protector cap from tubing insertion spike, not touching spike, and insert spike into opening of IV bag. Cleanse rubber stopper

Flat surface on top of bottled solution may contain contaminants, whereas opening to plastic bag is recessed. Prevents contamination of bottled solution during insertion of spike.

Step	**Rationale**

Fig. 53-1 Removing protective sheath from IV bag port.

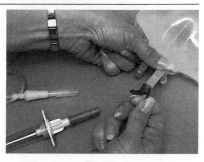

on bottled solution with antiseptic, and insert spike into black rubber stopper of IV bottle.

NURSE ALERT Do not touch the spike because it is sterile. If contamination occurs (e.g., the spike is accidentally dropped on a nonsterile surface), discard that IV tubing and obtain a new one.

Step	**Rationale**
f. Prime infusion tubing by filling with IV solution: Compress drip chamber and release, allowing it to fill one-third to one-half full.	Ensures that tubing is cleared of air before connection with IV site. Creates suction effect; fluid enters drip chamber to prevent air from entering tubing.
g. Remove protector cap on end of tubing (some tubing can be primed without removal), and slowly open roller clamp to allow fluid to travel from drip chamber through tubing to needle adapter. Return roller clamp to "off" position after tubing is primed (filled with IV fluid).	Slow fill of tubing decreases turbulence and chance of bubble formation. Removes air from tubing and permits tubing to fill with solution. Closing clamp prevents accidental loss of fluid.

Step	Rationale
h. Be certain tubing is clear of air and air bubbles. To remove small air bubbles, firmly tap IV tubing where air bubbles are located. Check entire length of tubing to ensure that all air bubbles are removed. If multiple port tubing is used, turn ports upside down and tap to fill and remove air.	Large air bubbles can act as emboli.
i. Replace cap protector on end of infusion tubing.	Maintains system sterility.
8. Prepare heparin or normal saline lock for infusion:	
a. If loop or short extension tubing is needed because of awkward IV site placement, use sterile technique to connect IV plug to loop or short extension tubing. Inject 1 to 3 ml normal saline through plug and through loop or short extension tubing before connecting to IV site.	Removes air to prevent introduction into vein. Do same with saline plug.
9. Eye protection and mask may be worn (see agency policy) if splash or spray of blood is possible.	Reduces transmission of microorganisms. Decreases exposure to HIV, hepatitis, and other blood-borne organisms (CDC, 2002) and prevents spraying of blood on nurse's mucous membranes.
10. Identify accessible vein for placement of IV cannula.	Tourniquet impedes venous return but should not occlude arterial

Step	**Rationale**
Apply flat tourniquet around arm, above antecubital fossa or 10 to 15 cm (4 to 6 inches) above proposed insertion site.	flow. If vein cannot be found in antecubital fossa, move down along arm to locate vessel in lower arm or hand.
Optional: Apply blood pressure cuff instead of tourniquet. Inflate to level just below client's normal diastolic pressure. Maintain inflation at that pressure until venipuncture is completed.	Use of blood pressure cuff creates less trauma to skin.
11. Select vein for IV insertion. Cephalic, basilic, and median cubital are preferred in adults.	Ensures adequate vein that is easier to puncture with needle and less likely to rupture.
a. Use most distal site in nondominant arm, if possible. Clip arm hair with scissors if necessary.	Venipuncture should be performed distal to proximal, which increases availability of other sites for future IV therapy. Hair impedes venipuncture and adherence of dressing.

NURSE ALERT Do not shave area. Shaving may cause microabrasions and predispose client to infection.

b. Avoid areas that are painful to palpation.	May indicate inflamed vein.
c. Select vein large enough for catheter placement.	Prevents interruption of venous flow while allowing adequate blood flow around catheter.
d. Choose site that will not interfere with client's activities of daily living or planned procedures.	Keeps client as mobile as possible.
e. With index finger, palpate vein by pressing downward and noting	Fingertip is more sensitive and is better to assess vein condition.

Step	Rationale
resilient, soft, bouncy feeling as pressure is released.	
f. If possible, place extremity in dependent position.	Permits venous dilation and visibility.
g. Select well-dilated vein.	Increases volume of blood in vein at venipuncture site.
h. Avoid sites distal to previous venipuncture site; sclerosed or hardened, cordlike veins; infiltrate site or phlebitic vessels; bruised areas; and areas of venous valves or bifurcation.	Such sites can cause infiltration of newly placed IV catheter and excessive vessel damage. Antecubital fossa area is used for blood draws; also limits mobility.
i. Avoid fragile dorsal veins in older adult clients and vessels in extremity with compromised circulation (e.g., in cases of mastectomy, dialysis graft, or paralysis).	Venous alterations can increase risk of complications (e.g., infiltration, decreased catheter dwell time).
12. Release tourniquet temporarily and carefully.	Restores blood flow while preparing for venipuncture.
13. Place connection of infusion set or IV plug nearby, maintaining sterility of system.	Permits smooth, quick connection of cannula to IV system.
14. If area of insertion appears to need cleansing, use soap and water first. Use antiseptic swab agent to cleanse insertion site using friction in horizontal plane, then vertical plane, followed with circular motion (middle to	Mechanical friction in this pattern allows penetration of antiseptic solution into cracks and fissures of epidermal layer of skin (Crosby and Mares, 2001). Antiseptic solutions should be allowed to air-dry completely to effectively reduce microbial counts (INS, 2006). If antiseptic

Step	Rationale

outward); allow agent to dry (2 to 3 minutes for povidone-iodine; 60 seconds for alcohol; 30 seconds for chlorhexidine). Refrain from touching cleansed site unless using sterile technique.

agents are used in combination, allow each to air-dry separately. Chlorhexidine 2% preparation is preferred (CDC, 2002).

Touching cleansed area introduces microorganisms from nurse's finger to site. Site would need to be prepped again.

15. Reapply tourniquet 10 to 12 cm (4 to 5 inches) above anticipated insertion site. Check presence of distal pulse.

Diminished arterial flow prevents venous filling. Pressure of tourniquet should cause vein to dilate.

16. Perform venipuncture. Anchor vein by placing thumb over vein and by gently tightening skin distal to site 4 to 5 cm (1½ to 2 inches) (Fig. 53-2). Warn client of sharp, quick stick.

Stabilizes vein for needle insertion.

   a. *Over-the-needle catheter (ONC):* Insert with bevel up at 10- to 30-degree angle slightly distal to actual site of venipuncture in direction of vein.

Places needle at 10- to 30-degree angle to vein. When vein is punctured, risk of puncturing posterior vein wall is reduced. Superficial veins require a smaller angle. Deeper veins require a greater angle.

Fig. 53-2 Stabilize vein below insertion site.

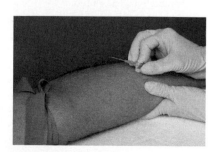

Step	**Rationale**
b. *IV catheter safety device:* Insert using same position as for ONC.	IV safety device should be available and used.
c. *Winged needle:* Hold needle at 10- to 30-degree angle with bevel up, slightly distal to actual site of venipuncture.	

NURSE ALERT   Each cannula should be used only once for each insertion.

17. Observe for blood return through flashback chamber of catheter or tubing of winged cannula, indicating that bevel of needle has entered vein. Lower needle until almost flush with skin. *(Advance catheter approximately $\frac{1}{4}$ inch into vein and then with ONC loosen stylet.)* Continue to hold skin taut, and advance catheter into vein until hub rests at venipuncture site. *Do not reinsert stylet once it is loosened.* Advance safety device by using push-off tab to thread catheter. Advance winged cannula until hub rests at venipuncture site.	Increased venous pressure from tourniquet increases backflow of blood into catheter or tubing. Allows for full penetration of vein wall, placement of catheter in vein's inner lumen, and advancement of catheter off stylet. Reduces risk of introduction of infectious microorganisms along catheter. Reinsertion of stylet can cause catheter shearing in vein and potential catheter embolization.

NURSE ALERT   No more than two attempts at initiating the IV access should be made by a single nurse.

18. Stabilize cannula with one hand, and release tourniquet with other.	Permits venous flow, reduces backflow of blood, and allows connection with administration

Step	**Rationale**
Apply gentle pressure with middle finger of nondominant hand 3 cm (1¼ inches) above insertion. Keep cannula stable with index finger. For safety device, slide catheter off stylet while gliding protective guard over stylet, or retract stylet by pushing safety tab. Click indicates device is locked over stylet. (NOTE: Techniques will vary with each IV device.) Remove stylet of ONC. Place directly into sharps container.	set with minimal blood loss. Prevents transmission of infection.
19. Quickly connect end of prepared saline lock or infusion tubing set to end of cannula. Do not touch point of entry of connection. Secure connection.	Prompt connection of infusion set maintains patency of vein and prevents risk of exposure to blood. Maintains sterility.
20. **Intermittent infusion:** Hold heparin/saline lock firmly with nondominant hand, and clean with alcohol. Insert prefilled syringe containing flush solution into injection cap (Fig. 53-3). Flush injection cap slowly with flush solution. Use positive flow adapter or withdraw syringe while still flushing.	"Positive pressure flushing" allows fluid to displace removed needle, creates positive pressure in catheter, and prevents reflux of blood during flushing (Phillips, 2001). Stabilizing cannula prevents accidental withdrawal or dislodgement.
21. **Continuous infusion:** Begin infusion by slowly opening clamp of IV tubing.	Initiates flow of fluid through IV catheter, preventing clotting of device.

Step	Rationale

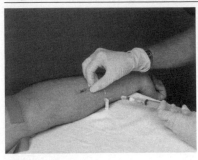

Fig. 53-3 Flush injection cap.

NURSE ALERT Be sure to calculate the rate so as not to infuse IV solution too rapidly or too slowly.

22. Secure cannula (procedures can differ; follow agency policy):

23. Apply sterile dressing over site:

   a. Transparent dressing:

     (1) Carefully remove adherent backing. Apply one edge of dressing, and then gently smooth remaining dressing over IV site, leaving connection between IV tubing and catheter hub uncovered. Remove outer covering, and smooth dressing gently over site.

     (2) Place a 2.5-cm (1-inch) piece of tape from end of hub of catheter to insertion site, over transparent dressing.

Occlusive dressing protects site from bacterial contamination. Connection between administration set and hub needs to be uncovered to facilitate changing tubing if necessary. CDC (2002) no longer recommends application of antimicrobial ointment to catheter site.

Step	**Rationale**
(3) Apply chevron, and place only over tape, not transparent dressing.	
b. Sterile gauze dressing:	
(1) Fold 2 × 2 gauze in half, and cover with 2.5 cm (1 inch–wide) tape extending about an inch from each side. Place under tubing/ catheter hub junction. Curl loop of tubing alongside arm, and place second piece of tape directly over tubing and padded 2 × 2, securing tubing in two places.	Tape on top of gauze makes it easier to access hub/tubing junction. Gauze pad elevates hub off skin to prevent pressure area. Securing loop of tubing reduces risk of dislodging catheter should IV tubing get pulled (i.e., loop would come apart before catheter dislodges).
(2) Place 2 × 2 gauze pad over insertion site and catheter hub. Secure all edges with tape. Do not cover connection between IV tubing and catheter hub.	
24. Loop tubing alongside arm, and place second piece of tape directly over tape covering transparent dressing or over padded 2 × 2.	
25. For IV fluid administration, recheck flow rate to correct drops per minute (Skill 52) and connect to electronic	Manipulation of catheter during dressing application may alter flow rate. Maintains correct rate of flow for IV solution. Flow can

Step	Rationale
infusion device (EID) as per agency policy.	fluctuate, so it must be checked at intervals for accuracy.
26. Write date and time of IV placement, cannula gauge size and length, and nurse's initials on dressing.	Provides immediate access to data as to when IV was inserted and when rotation is needed.
27. Instruct client in how to move or turn without pulling on IV catheter.	Prevents accidental dislodgement of catheter.
28. Observe client every 1 to 2 hours:	
a. Check patency of IV cannula.	Flow rate will be slowed or stopped.
b. Observe client during palpation of vessel for signs of discomfort.	Tenderness can be early sign of phlebitis.
c. Inspect insertion site, note color (e.g., redness, pallor). Inspect for presence of swelling, infiltration (Table 53-1), and phlebitis (Table 53-2). Palpate temperature of skin above dressing.	Redness or inflammation along with tenderness and warmth indicate vein inflammation or phlebitis. Swelling above insertion site and cool temperature may indicate infiltration of fluid into tissues.
23. Complete postprocedure protocol.	

Recording and Reporting

- Record in nurses' notes number of attempts at insertion, type of infusion, insertion site by vessel, flow rate, size and type of cannula, and when infusion was begun. Special parenteral therapy flowsheet may be used.
- If electronic infusion device is used, document type and rate of infusion.
- Record client's response to IV fluid, amount infused, and integrity and patency of system according to agency policy (usually hourly for vulnerable populations).
- Report to oncoming nursing staff: type of infusion, flow rate, status of venipuncture site, amount of fluid remaining in present

TABLE 53-1   Infiltration Scale

Grade	Clinical Criteria
0	No symptoms
1	Skin blanched
	Edema <1 inch in any direction
	Cool to touch
	With or without pain
2	Skin blanched
	Edema 2.5–15 cm (1–6 inches) in any direction
	Cool to touch
	With or without pain
3	Skin blanched, translucent
	Gross edema >15 cm (6 inches) in any direction
	Cool to touch
	Mild to moderate pain
	Possible numbness
4	Skin blanched, translucent
	Skin tight, leaking
	Skin discolored, bruised, swollen
	Gross edema >15 cm (6 inches) in any direction
	Deep pitting tissue edema
	Circulatory impairment
	Moderate to severe pain
	Infiltration of any amount of blood product, irritant, or vesicant

From Infusion Nurses Society: *Infusion nursing standards of practice*, Philadelphia, 2006, Lippincott, Williams and Wilkins.

TABLE 53-2   Phlebitis Scale

Grade	Clinical Criteria
0	No symptoms
1	Erythema at access site with or without pain
2	Pain at access site with erythema and/or edema
3	Pain at access site with erythema and/or edema
	Streak formation
	Palpable venous cord
4	Pain at access site with erythema and/or edema
	Streak formation
	Palpable venous cord >2.5 cm (1 inch) in length
	Purulent drainage

From Infusion Nurses Society: *Infusion nursing standards of practice*, Philadelphia, 2006, Lippincott Williams and Wilkins.

solution, expected time to hang subsequent infusion, and any side effects.

- Report to physician adverse reactions such as pulmonary congestion, shock, thrombophlebitis.

Unexpected Outcomes	Related Interventions
1. Fluid volume deficit (FVD) as manifested by decreased urine output, dry mucous membranes, decreased capillary refill, disparity in central and peripheral pulses, tachycardia, hypotension, shock.	• Notify physician. • May require readjustment of infusion rate.
2. Fluid volume excess (FVE) as manifested by crackles in lungs, shortness of breath, edema.	• Reduce IV flow rate if symptoms appear. • Notify physician.
3. Infiltration at site as indicated by swelling and possible pitting edema, pallor, coolness, pain at insertion site, possible decrease in flow rate (see Table 53-1).	• Stop infusion, and discontinue IV (see Skill 52). • Elevate affected extremity. • Restart new IV if continued therapy is necessary. • Document degree of infiltration and nursing intervention (see Table 53-1).
4. Phlebitis as indicated by pain, increased skin temperature, erythema along path of vein (see Table 53-2).	• Stop infusion, and discontinue IV (see Skill 52). • Restart new IV if continued therapy is necessary. • Place moist, warm compress over area of phlebitis. • Document degree of phlebitis and nursing interventions per agency policy and procedure (see Table 53-2).

Peripherally Inserted Central Catheter Care

Peripherally inserted central catheters (PICCs) provide alternate intravenous (IV) access when the client requires intermediate-length venous access (from longer than 7 days to 3 months). PICCs are inserted through the larger cephalic or basilic vein in the upper arm and advanced until the tip enters the central venous system (e.g., subclavian vein). When caring for clients with PICCs, it is important to understand what they are and be aware of their appropriate care and maintenance. In comparison with centrally placed venous catheters, the PICC has less risk of pneumothorax, hemothorax, or air embolism and is more cost-effective to maintain. Compared with peripheral IV catheters, PICCs have less risk of infiltration and phlebitis. This allows them to be maintained in place longer (more than 72 to 96 hours) because IV fluids and medications are diluted in the greater volume of blood flow present in the larger veins (superior vena cava) where the catheter tip resides. Complications associated with PICC use include clotting, leaking, migration, infection, and breaking of the catheter. For successful catheter placement, the client must have a usable cephalic or basilic vein located in the antecubital fossa or upper arm.

Delegation Considerations

The skill of maintaining a PICC may not be delegated to assistive personnel (AP). However, it is important to provide information and direction to AP:

- Instruct AP to immediately report any client complaint regarding the PICC.
- Instruct AP in how to position and assist clients in moving when PICC lines are in place.

Equipment
Blood Drawing

- Antimicrobial swabs (i.e., chlorhexidine, povidone-iodine, alcohol)
- Four to five syringes (preferably needleless access)
- Sterile drape
- Saline flush
- Heparin flush (100 units/ml)
- Sterile needleless access

- Blood tubes, labels, requisitions
- Gloves, masks

Dressing Change

- Antimicrobial swabs
- Gloves, mask, gown
- Sterile tape
- Transparent occlusive dressing
- Gauze dressing: 2 × 2 sterile gauze
- Steri-Strips or securement device
- Adhesive remover (if needed)

Heparinization

- Antimicrobial swabs
- Access syringe (5 ml or 10 ml—see agency policy)
- Saline flush
- Heparin flush (100 units/ml)
- Sterile needleless access

Step	Rationale
1. Complete preprocedure protocol.	
2. Review physician's order, and assess treatment schedule: times for administration of fluids, drugs, blood products, nutrition, and blood sampling.	Allows nurse to schedule use of PICC for simultaneous administration of products, to educate client about schedule of administration, and to provide for comfort and reduction of anxiety about therapy.
3. Assess type of PICC in place. Review manufacturer's directions concerning catheter and maintenance.	Care and management depend on type and size of catheter, number of lumens, purpose of therapy.

NURSE ALERT In most situations, several tests can be run from one blood tube sample. Before obtaining the blood sample, determine what laboratory tests are being ordered. Then verify with laboratory services to determine if several tests can be obtained from one sample; this reduces need to re-access PICC at later times.

Step	Rationale
4. Assess PICC placement site for skin integrity and signs of infection (i.e., redness, swelling, tenderness, exudate, bleeding).	Clients requiring long-term IV therapy often have conditions placing them at risk for alterations in skin integrity and immune function. PICC site is insult to skin integrity and provides access for pathogens through skin as well as pathogens to migrate from catheter.
5. Assess for proper function of PICC before therapy: integrity of catheter, ability to irrigate or infuse fluid, ability to aspirate blood.	Ensures proper function of PICC with minimal complications.
6. Determine frequency of irrigation and dressing change.	Provides guidelines for maintaining catheter patency and preventing infection.
7. **Administration of infusion or sampling of blood from PICC:**	
a. Don gown and goggles (check agency policy) if drawing blood sample.	Prevents transfer of body fluids.
b. Use antimicrobial preparation swabs to cleanse injection cap or catheter hub according to agency policy.	Prevents introduction of microorganisms into catheter.
c. Prepare two syringes with 10 ml normal saline each.	Used to flush catheter.
d. If injection cap will be removed, *clamp catheter*.	Catheter must be clamped if injection cap is removed to prevent entrance of air.
e. If injection cap is in place, insert needleless access syringe containing	Flushing ensures patency of catheter. Catheter must always be clamped during change of

Step	**Rationale**
10 ml normal saline and flush. If injection cap is removed, connect syringe tip to catheter hub, release clamp, flush with positive pressure, and reclamp.	syringe or tubing to prevent exposure to air.

NURSE ALERT If catheter is occluded and/or resistance is felt, do not force flushing. Vigorous flushing may cause catheter rupture or catheter emboli.

f. Connect syringe for blood sampling, and release clamp. Aspirate 5 ml fluid, reclamp, and discard aspirate. (Do not discard if drawn for blood culture.)	Discarding initial 5 ml of aspirate avoids diluting sample.
g. Attach or insert syringe of size equal to volume of blood sample to withdraw to catheter. Release clamp. Withdraw necessary blood for samples, and reclamp.	Samples should be collected at one time to minimize time with open catheter system.
h. Attach or insert syringe filled with 10 ml normal saline to catheter. If clamp is present, release, flush vigorously, and reclamp.	Catheter should be cleared of all blood or medications that may clog catheter lumen or precipitate with additives in IV fluids.
i. If no continuous infusion is indicated, flush catheter with heparin or normal saline (see agency policy). Connect syringe containing 5 ml heparin (100 units/ml) or normal saline flush	Catheter not in use must be flushed to prevent clot formation. This is commonly done with heparin; however, Groshong catheters are flushed with normal saline only.

Step	**Rationale**
solution. If clamp is present, release, flush with positive pressure, and reclamp.	
(1) Attach new cap to end of catheter, and remove clamp.	Maintains sterile seal to catheter.
j. If IV fluids will be administered, connect IV tubing to end of catheter, being sure both ends are sterile.	IV system should be closed to maintain sterility.
(1) Regulate IV infusion as ordered.	Maintains ordered fluid intake and keeps catheter patent.
(2) Secure all tubing connections.	Prevents accidental tubing disconnection and catheter displacement. Luer-Lok connections should be used.

8. **Dressing change:**
   a. Mask self and client, if indicated (check agency policy).

   Prevents exposure of catheter exit or placement site to airborne microorganisms.

   b. Carefully remove old dressing in direction catheter was inserted, noting drainage and appearance of catheter.

   Remove tape carefully because clients frequently have alterations in skin integrity. Prevents dislodgement of catheter.

   c. Inspect site for signs of redness, swelling, inflammation, tenderness, or exudate.

   This is potential site of infection.

   d. Inspect catheter and hub for intactness, and remove clean gloves.

   Catheter may become torn, cut, displaced, cracked, or split.

   e. Perform hand hygiene, and open dressing kit in sterile manner. Most agencies have dressing kits that contain all

   Reduces transmission of microorganisms.

Step	Rationale
	needed dressing change supplies.
f. Don sterile gloves.	Prevents direct transmission of microorganisms to skin exit site.
g. Clean site with antimicrobial swab, moving first in horizontal pattern. With new swab, move in vertical plane, and then use final swab in circular pattern, moving outward in concentric circles from insertion site out. Allow to dry.	It is impossible to sterilize skin. Organisms that accumulate must be eliminated by mechanical and chemical means. Mechanical friction in this pattern allows penetration of antiseptic solution into cracks and fissures of epidermal layer of skin (Crosby and Mares, 2001). Antiseptic solutions should be allowed to air-dry completely to effectively reduce microbial counts (INS, 2000). If antiseptic agents are used in combination, allow each to air-dry separately.
h. Place Steri-Strip (Fig. 54-1) or securement device over catheter.	Provides security to prevent catheter dislodgement. PICC lines may be sutured in place, preventing placement of gauze underneath.
i. Re-dress site using sterile gauze and tape or transparent dressing as indicated (see Skill 52).	Prevents entrance of bacteria into exit or placement site.

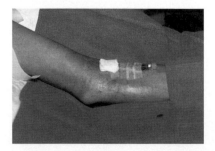

Fig. 54-1 Anchor PICC catheter hub with Steri-Strips.

Step	Rationale
j. Secure connections. Luer-Lok connections are preferred.	Prevents accidental pulling and displacement.
k. Label date, time of dressing change, and size of cannula in place.	Documents dressing change. Provides guideline for time of next change.
9. Inspect condition of catheter and connecting tubing daily for leaks, holes, tears, splits, or cracked hubs.	Break in integrity of system predisposes client to hemorrhage or air embolus.
10. Complete postprocedure protocol.	

Recording and Reporting

- Record blood samples obtained, patency of lines, and type of IV fluids administered. Note rate of fluid infusion.
- Report status of PICC, therapy being administered, and development of complications and their treatment.

Unexpected Outcomes	Related Interventions
1. There is blocked or difficult infusion of fluids through catheter, indicating occlusion that is either mechanical, nonthrombotic, or thrombotic.	• Assess tubing for kinks and inspect site to rule out external cause of obstruction. • Tight sutures may need to be removed. • Chest x-ray examination may be ordered to determine internal compression. • Know drug incompatibilities to prevent precipitation of infused solution. • Assess change in ability to aspirate or withdraw from catheter. Look for clots visible in external portion of line. Physician or independent practitioner (IP) or qualified RN may attempt aspiration of clot.

Continued

Unexpected Outcomes	Related Interventions
	• Fibrinolytic therapy may be used (see agency policy).
2. Client develops fever and elevated white blood cell count, and culture of PICC tip is positive, indicating catheter sepsis.	• Remove PICC line as ordered. • Antibiotic therapy may be ordered.
3. Client develops sudden respiratory distress, which may indicate pulmonary embolus.	• Place client in high-Fowler's position. • Notify physician or IP immediately. • Be prepared to obtain chest x-ray examination if ordered.
4. Client develops irregular pulse.	• May indicate malposition of catheter in right atrium, causing atrial irritation. Catheter may need to be withdrawn several centimeters. • Interventional radiology may be necessary to diagnose and reposition PICC.

Postoperative Exercises

Structured preoperative teaching has a positive influence on a surgical client's recovery (Shuldham, 1999). The skills of diaphragmatic breathing, controlled coughing, turning, and leg exercises are important in preventing postoperative circulatory complications (e.g., deep vein thrombosis [DVT]) and respiratory complications (e.g., pneumonia, atelectasis). In addition, the use of incentive spirometry to encourage voluntary deep breathing through an apparatus that provides visual feedback may also be included. The physician may order incentive spirometry for clients especially at risk for atelectasis or pneumonia (e.g., chronic smokers, clients on prolonged bedrest).

Delegation Considerations

The teaching of postoperative exercises may not be delegated to assistive personnel (AP). AP can reinforce and assist clients in performing postoperative exercises. The nurse should instruct AP about:

- Any precautions unique to a particular client.
- When to report if the client is unable or unwilling to perform the exercises correctly.

Equipment

- Pillow (optional; used to splint the incision to reduce discomfort when coughing)
- Incentive spirometer

Step	Rationale
1. Complete preprocedure protocol.	
2. Assess client's risk for postoperative respiratory complications (e.g., identify presence of chronic pulmonary condition, advanced pregnancy, thoracic or abdominal surgery; history of smoking; reduced hemoglobin level).	General anesthesia predisposes client to respiratory problems because lungs are not fully inflated during surgery, cough reflex is suppressed, and mucus collects within airway passages. Smoking damages ciliary clearance and increases mucus secretion. Reduced hemoglobin level can lead to reduced oxygen delivery.

Step	Rationale

NURSE ALERT If the client has a cold or signs of upper respiratory infection, notify the surgeon and/or anesthesiologist.

3. Auscultate lungs.	Establishes baseline for postoperative comparison.
4. Determine client's ability to deep breathe and cough by placing hand on client's abdomen, having client take deep breath, and observing movement of shoulders, chest wall, and abdomen. Observe chest excursion during deep breath. Ask client to cough into tissue after taking deep breath.	Diaphragmatic breathing allows for complete lung expansion and improved ventilation and increases blood oxygenation. Deep breathing also allows air to pass by partially obstructing mucous plugs, thus increasing force with which to expel mucous plug. Coughing loosens secretions and helps remove them from pulmonary alveoli and bronchi.
5. Assess client's risk for postoperative thrombus formation (older adults, immobilized clients, clients with personal or family history of clots, and women over 35 who smoke and are taking birth control pills are most at risk).	After general anesthesia, circulation is slowed, causing greater tendency for clot formation. Immobilization results in decreased muscular contraction in lower extremities, which promotes venous stasis. Physical stress of surgery creates hypercoagulable state in most individuals. Manipulation and positioning during surgery may inadvertently cause trauma to leg veins.

NURSE ALERT Homans' sign is not always present when a DVT exists (Maher and others, 2002). Checking for Homans' sign may be contraindicated in a suspected DVT because some researchers think that vigorous dorsiflexion may dislodge a thrombus. If a thrombus is suspected, notify the physician and refrain from manipulating the extremity.

6. Observe client's ability to move independently while in bed.	Clients confined to bedrest, even for limited periods, will need to turn regularly. Determines

Step	**Rationale**
	existence of any mobility restrictions.
7. Determine client's and family members' willingness and capability to learn exercises.	Capacity to learn depends on readiness, ability, and learning environment.

NURSE ALERT Highly anxious clients or those who are in severe pain have difficulty learning, and teaching of postoperative exercises may need to be repeated.

8. **Teach diaphragmatic breathing:**	
a. Assist client to comfortable semi-Fowler's or high-Fowler's position with knees flexed. If client is sitting in chair, knees should be at or higher than hips. Use stool if necessary.	Upright position facilitates diaphragmatic excursion by using gravity to keep abdominal contents away from diaphragm. Prevents tension on abdominal muscles, which allows for greater diaphragmatic excursion.
b. Face client.	Client will be able to observe breathing exercises performed by nurse.
c. Instruct client to place palms of hands across from each other along lower borders of anterior rib cage; place tips of third fingers lightly together. Demonstrate for client (Fig. 55-1).	Position of hands allows client to feel movement of chest and abdomen as diaphragm descends and lungs inside chest wall expand.
d. Have client take slow, deep breaths, inhaling through nose, and pushing abdomen against hands. Tell client to feel middle fingers separate as client inhales.	Slow, deep breath allows for more complete lung expansion and prevents panting or hyperventilation. Inhaling through nose warms, humidifies, and filters air. Explanation and demonstration focus on normal

Step	Rationale

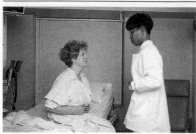

Fig. 55-1   Client and nurse practice deep breathing.

Explain that client will feel normal downward movement of diaphragm during inspiration.	ventilatory movement of chest and abdominal wall. Client learns to understand how diaphragmatic breathing feels.
e. Instruct client to avoid using chest and shoulder muscles while inhaling.	Using auxiliary chest and shoulder muscles during breathing increases unnecessary energy expenditures and does not promote full lung expansion.
f. Instruct client to take a slow, deep breath and hold for count of 3, and then slowly exhale through mouth as if blowing out candle (pursed lips).	Allows for gradual, controlled expulsion of air.
g. Repeat breathing exercise three to five times.	Allows client to observe slow, rhythmic breathing pattern.
h. Have client practice exercise. Client is instructed to take 10 slow, deep breaths every 2 hours while awake during postoperative period until mobile. Another option is to have client use incentive spirometry (Fig. 55-2).	Repetition of exercise reinforces learning. Regular deep breathing will prevent or minimize postoperative respiratory complications. Incentive spirometer gives visual incentive to breathe as deeply as possible.

Step	Rationale

Fig. 55-2 Client demonstrates incentive spirometery.

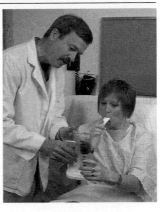

9. **Teach controlled coughing:**
   a. Explain importance of maintaining an upright position.

   Position facilitates diaphragm excursion and enhances thoracic and abdominal expansion.

   b. Instruct client to take two slow, deep breaths, inhaling through nose and exhaling through pursed lips.

   Deep breaths expand lungs fully so that air moves behind mucus and facilitates effective coughing.

   c. Instruct client to inhale deeply a third time, and hold breath to count of 3. Cough fully for two to three consecutive coughs without inhaling between coughs. (Tell client to push all air out of lungs.)

   Consecutive coughs help remove mucus more effectively and completely than one forceful cough.

NURSE ALERT Coughing may be contraindicated after brain, spinal, and eye surgeries because of elevations in intracranial pressure that occur with normal coughing.

Step	Rationale
d. Caution client against just clearing throat instead of coughing deeply.	Clearing throat does not remove mucus from deeper airways.
e. If surgical incision is thoracic or abdominal, teach client to place either hands or pillow over incisional area and place hands over pillow to splint incision (Fig. 55-3). During breathing and coughing exercises, instruct client to press gently against incisional area for splinting and support.	Surgical incision cuts through muscles, tissues, and nerve endings. Deep breathing and coughing exercises place additional stress on suture line and cause discomfort. Splinting incision with hands or pillow provides firm support and reduces incisional pulling and pain.
f. Client continues to practice coughing exercises, splinting imaginary incision. Instruct client to cough two to three times every 2 hours while awake and to examine sputum for	Value of deep coughing with splinting is stressed to effectively expectorate mucus with minimal discomfort. Sputum consistency, odor, amount, and color changes may

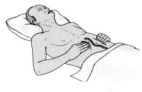
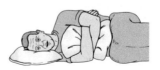
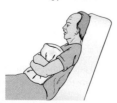

Fig. 55-3   Techniques for splinting incision when coughing or moving. (From Lewis S and others: *Medical-surgical nursing: assessment and management of clinical problems*, ed 6, St Louis, 2004, Mosby.)

Step	**Rationale**

consistency, odor, amount, and color changes. | indicate presence of pulmonary complication such as pneumonia.

NURSE ALERT For clients with preexisting pulmonary disease, know the usual characteristics of mucus (e.g., color, amount, thickness) to determine if change has occurred.

10. **Teach turning** (*Example:* turning on right side):

a. Instruct client to assume supine position and move toward left side of bed. This is easily accomplished by bending knees and pressing heels against mattress to raise buttocks. | Positioning begins in this example on left side of bed so that turning to right side will not cause client to roll off bed's edge. Buttocks lift prevents shearing force from body moving against sheets.

b. Have client place right hand or pillow over incisional area to splint it (see Fig. 55-3). | Splinting incision supports and minimizes pulling on suture line during turning.

c. Instruct client to keep right leg straight and flex left knee up. | Straight leg stabilizes client's position. Flexed left leg shifts weight for easier turning.

d. Have client grab right side rail with left hand, pull toward right, and roll onto right side. | Pulling toward side rail reduces effort needed for turning.

e. Instruct client to turn every 2 hours from side to back to other side, while awake. If client is unable to perform above maneuver, note in chart that staff or primary caregiver must turn client every 2 hours. May need to place pillows behind | Reduces risk of vascular complications by contraction of leg muscles around veins to improve venous return. Also reduces pulmonary complications by shifting mucus to prevent consolidation.

Step	Rationale
	client to help maintain side-lying position.
11. **Teach leg exercises:**	
a. Have client assume supine position in bed. Demonstrate leg exercises by performing passive range-of-motion exercises and simultaneously explaining exercise.	Provides for normal anatomical position of lower extremities and normal joint motion of each joint of lower extremities.

NURSE ALERT When a client has leg surgery, the surgeon must order specific postoperative leg exercises. The leg unaffected by surgery can be exercised safely unless the client has a preexisting thrombosis or phlebitis.

b. Rotate each ankle in complete circle. Instruct client to draw imaginary circles with big toe. Repeat five times.	Ankle circle exercises maintain joint mobility and promote venous return.
c. Alternate dorsiflexion and plantar flexion by moving both feet, pointing toes up toward head and then down toward end of mattress.	Calf pumping stretches and contracts gastrocnemius muscles, which enhances venous return.
d. Perform quadriceps setting by tightening thigh and bringing knee down toward mattress, then relaxing.	Quadriceps setting exercises contract muscles of upper legs, maintain knee mobility, and improve venous return to heart.
e. Client alternately raises each leg from bed surface; client begins by keeping leg straight and then bends leg at hip and knee.	Leg raise promotes contraction and relaxation of quadriceps muscles and promotes hip and knee movements by keeping leg straight and bending hip and knee joints.
f. Have client perform each exercise five times	Repetition of exercise sequence reinforces learning. Establishes

Step	Rationale
at least every 2 hours while awake. Instruct client to coordinate turning and leg exercises with diaphragmatic breathing, incentive spirometry, and coughing exercises.	routine for exercises that develops habit for performance. Sequence of exercises should be leg exercises, turning, deep breathing, and coughing. Exercises before coughing should enhance ability to move secretions so that they may be expectorated.
11. Observe client performing all four exercises.	Ensures that client has learned correct technique.
12. Observe client's chest excursion, and auscultate client's lungs.	Determines extent of lung expansion. Breath sounds reveal if airways are clear.
13. Observe calves for redness, warmth, and tenderness. Assess pedal pulses.	Absent signs and normal pulses usually indicate that no venous thrombosis is present.
14. Complete postprocedure protocol.	

Recording and Reporting

- Record physical assessment findings, any assessed complications and action taken, and which exercises were demonstrated to client and whether client can perform exercises independently.
- Report to nurse assigned to client on next shift any problem client has in practicing exercises.

Unexpected Outcomes	Related Interventions
1. Client is unwilling to perform exercises because of incisional pain of thorax or abdomen (deep breathing and coughing, turning) or because of surgery in lower abdomen, groin, buttocks, or legs (leg exercises).	• Instruct client to ask for pain medication 30 minutes before performing postoperative exercises or use patient-controlled analgesia immediately before exercising.
2. Client develops pulmonary complications such as atelectasis postoperatively. Breaths are shallow; cough is ineffective.	• Notify physician. • Start oxygen as ordered, and increase frequency of coughing exercises.
3. Client develops circulatory complications such as venous stasis or thrombophlebitis postoperatively. Leg exercises are inadequate.	• Notify physician. • Place client on bedrest with affected leg elevated as ordered. • Continue to have client do exercises with unaffected leg.

Pressure Ulcer Risk Assessment

The goal in preventing the development of pressure ulcers is early identification of the at-risk client and the implementation of prevention strategies. The Wound, Ostomy and Continence Nurses (WOCN) Society 2003 panel recommended that a risk assessment should be performed on entry to a health care setting and repeated on a regularly scheduled basis or when the individual's condition changes significantly. The Society suggested the use of risk assessment tools such as the Braden scale or the Norton scale. The Braden scale has the following six parameters: sensory perception (recognition of pressure), friction and shear, ability to change and control body position, skin moisture, nutritional intake, and physical activity (Ayello and Braden, 2002; Bergstrom and others, 1987, 1994, 1998). Risk cutoff scores may also vary for specific client populations. It is important to understand how to interpret the meaning of the client's total score on whatever scale you use.

Skin and bony prominences should be inspected at least daily. Devices, shoes, socks, and heel and elbow protectors should be removed for the skin inspection. All bony prominences should be inspected including the back of the head, shoulders, rib cage, elbows, hips, ischium, sacrum, knees, ankles, and heels (Fig. 56-1). Any reddened or discolored areas should be palpated with a gloved finger to determine if the erythema blanches.

Delegation Considerations

The skill of assessment of pressure ulcer risk is the responsibility of the nurse. However, certain aspects of the client's care may be delegated to assistive personnel (AP). The nurse should instruct AP to report to the nurse:

- Any redness or break in client's skin.
- Any abrasion from assistive devices.

Equipment

- Risk assessment tool
- Documentation record
- Pressure-reduction mattress, bed, and/or chair cushion
- Positioning aids
- Gloves

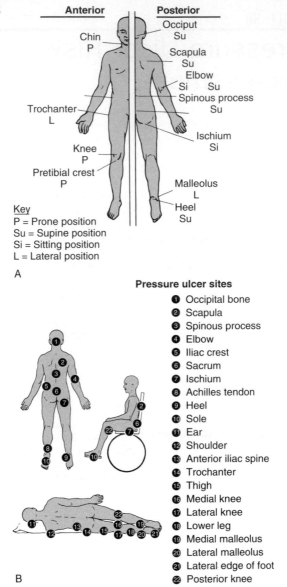

Fig. 56-1 **A,** Bony prominences most frequently underlying pressure sores. **B,** Pressure ulcer sites. (From Trelease CC: Developing standards for wound care, *Ostomy Wound Manage* 26:50, 1988. Used with permission of HMP Communications.)

Step	Rationale
1. Complete preprocedure protocol.	
2. Identify client risk factors for pressure ulcer formation, for example:	Determines need to administer preventive care and identifies specific factors placing client at risk.
a. Paralysis, or immobilization caused by restrictive devices.	Client is unable to turn or reposition independently to relieve pressure.
b. Sensory loss (e.g., hemiplegia, spinal cord injury, heavy sedation).	When sensory loss is present, client feels no discomfort from pressure and does not independently change position.
c. Circulatory disorders (e.g., diabetes mellitus).	Disorders reduce perfusion of skin's tissue layers.
d. Fever.	Increases metabolic demands of tissues. Accompanying diaphoresis leaves skin moist.
e. Anemia.	Decreased hemoglobin reduces oxygen-carrying capacity of blood and amount of oxygen available to tissues.
f. Malnutrition.	Inadequate nutrition can lead to weight loss, muscle atrophy, and reduced tissue mass. Severe protein deficiency makes tissue more susceptible to breakdown (Sager, 2002). Poor protein, vitamin, mineral, and caloric intake limits wound-healing capabilities.
g. Incontinence.	Skin becomes exposed to moist environment containing bacteria Moisture causes skin maceration.
h. Age.	There is loss of dermal thickness in older individuals, impairing ability to distribute pressure (Pieper, 2000). Neonates and very young children are at high risk, with head being most

Step	**Rationale**
	common site of pressure ulcer occurrence (WOCN Society, 2003).
i. Existing pressure ulcers.	Limits surfaces available for position changes, placing available tissues at increased risk.
3. Select a risk assessment tools. Perform risk assessment on entry to health care setting, and repeat on regularly scheduled basis or when individual's condition changes significantly (WOCN Society, 2003).	Valid and reliable risk assessment tool should be used to evaluate client's risk for developing pressure ulcer. Using risk assessment will identify risk factors that can contribute to potential for skin breakdown and pinpoint specific areas to target interventions to decrease risk of skin breakdown.
4. Assess condition of client's skin over regions of pressure (see Fig. 56-1). Body weight against bony prominences places underlying skin at risk for breakdown. Look for areas of:	Inspect skin and bony prominences at least daily. Any skin changes should be documented, including description of skin changes and any action taken (WOCN Society, 2003).
a. Skin discoloration (redness in light-tone skin; purplish or bluish in darkly pigmented skin); temperature changes (warmth or coolness); tissue consistency (firm or boggy feel) and/or sensations. See Box 56-1.	May indicate that tissue was under pressure; hyperemia is normal physiological response to hypoxemia in tissues.
b. Blanching.	If area of redness blanches (lightens in color), this indicates that tissue should not be at risk for skin breakdown. Tissue that does not blanch when palpated may indicate that there is ischemic injury.

BOX 56-1   Cultural Considerations for Skin Assessment for Pressure Ulcers: The Client With Darkly Pigmented Skin

---

Clients with darkly pigmented skin cannot be assessed for pressure ulcer risk by examining only skin color. Follow these recommended guidelines:

Assess Localized Skin Color Changes

Any of the following may appear:

- Skin color changes are different from usual skin tone.
- Color is darker than surrounding skin—purplish, bluish, eggplant. Importance of lighting for skin assessment:
- Use natural or halogen light.
- Avoid fluorescent lamps, which can give the skin a bluish tone.
- Avoid wearing tinted lenses when assessing skin color.

Tissue Consistency

- Assess for edema, swelling.
- Assess for firm or boggy feel.

Sensation

- Assess for pain or changes in skin sensation such as itching.

Skin Temperature

- Initially skin in the area of pressure ulcer may feel warmer than surrounding skin.
- Subsequently skin may feel cooler than surrounding skin.
- Feel areas of skin that are not involved in or around a pressure point to serve as a point of temperature reference.

Data from Bennett MA: Report of the task force on the implications for darkly pigmented intact skin in the prediction and prevention of pressure ulcers, *Adv Wound Care* 8(6):34, 1995; Henderson CT and others: Draft definition of stage I pressure ulcers: inclusion of persons with darkly pigmented skin, *Adv Wound Care* 10(5):16, 1997.

Step	Rationale
c. Pallor and mottling.	Persistent hypoxia in tissues that were under pressure; abnormal physiological response.
d. Absence of superficial skin layers.	Represents early pressure ulcer formation, usually partial-thickness wound.

Step	Rationale
e. Skin temperature.	Palpation of differences in temperature between area of stage I pressure ulcer and adjacent skin area may be initial indicator of ischemia (Sprigle and others, 2001).
5. Assess client for additional areas of potential pressure: a. Nares: nasogastric (NG) tube, oxygen cannula; tongue and lips: oral airway, endotracheal (ET) tube; ears: oxygen cannula, pillow.	Clients at high risk have multiple sites for pressure necrosis, in addition to bony prominences.
b. Drainage tubes; wound drainage.	Stress against tissue at exit site. Wound drainage is caustic to skin and underlying tissues, thereby increasing risk for skin breakdown.
c. Indwelling urethral (Foley) catheter.	For female clients, catheter can put pressure on labia, especially when edematous. For male clients, pressure from catheter not properly anchored can put pressure on tip of penis and urethra.
d. Orthopedic and positioning devices; pay particular attention to areas around and beneath these devices.	Improperly fitted or applied devices have potential to cause pressure on adjacent skin and underlying tissue.
6. Observe client for preferred positions when in bed or chair.	Preferred positions result in weight of body being placed on certain bony prominences.
7. Observe ability of client to initiate and assist with position changes.	Potential for friction and shear increases when client is completely dependent on others for position changes.
8. Obtain risk score, and evaluate its meaning based	Risk cutoff score will depend on instrument used. In addition,

Step	Rationale
on client's unique characteristics.	score involves identifying risk factors that contributed to score and minimizing those specific deficits.
9. Implement recommendations. (See Box 56-2.)	Reduces risk of client developing pressure ulcer.
10. If client has open, draining wounds, use disposable gloves.	Use of Standard Precautions prevents accidental exposure to body fluids.
11. Assist client with changing position. Use following positions:	Avoid positions that place client directly on an area of existing skin breakdown. It may be helpful to use schedule for position changes.
a. Supine.	Protects shoulders, trochanter, and malleolus.
b. Prone.	Used only in clients who can tolerate; breathing difficulty is normal.
c. 30-degree lateral (Fig. 56-2).	Achieved with one pillow under shoulder and one pillow under leg on same side. 30-Degree lateral position should provide pressure relief from sacrum and trochanter (WOCN Society, 2003).
12. Palpate any area of discoloration or mottling.	Early detection of pressure indicates need for more frequent

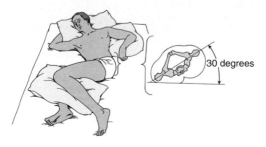

Fig. 56-2   30-Degree lateral position.

BOX 56-2 Interventions: Prevention of Pressure Ulcers

1. Assess individual risk for developing pressure ulcers:
   a. Select and use a risk assessment tool; the Braden and Norton scales have been studied most extensively.
   b. Risk assessment should be performed on entry to a health care setting and repeated on a regularly scheduled basis or when client's condition changes significantly.
2. Identify all individual risk factors (incontinence, nutritional status, immobility, friction and shear, and high-risk groups such as older adults, very young children, spinal cord injury population).
3. Assess and inspect skin at least daily. Note all pressure points; document results.
4. Institute prevention interventions as indicated by the findings of the risk assessment:
   a. Assess and treat incontinence: clean and dry skin after each incontinent episode using a pH-balanced cleanser. Use incontinence skin barriers as needed to protect and maintain skin integrity. Select underpads, diapers, or briefs that are absorbent to wick incontinence away from the skin. Consider a pouching system or collection device to contain urine or stool and to protect the skin from the effluent.
   b. Use turning or lift sheets or devices to turn or transfer clients.
   c. Maintain the head of the bed at or below 30 degrees or at the lowest level of elevation to decrease shear/friction.
   d. Schedule regular and frequent turning and repositioning for bed bound and chair bound clients. Turn at least every 2 to 4 hours.
   e. Place "at risk" individuals on pressure-reduction surface and not on an ordinary hospital mattress. Consult with trained health care professionals who have specific knowledge and expertise in this area.
   f. Relieve pressure under heels by using pillows or other devices.
   g. Maintain adequate nutrition that is compatible with the client's wishes or condition to maximize the potential for healing.
   h. Educate the client/caregiver about the causes and risk factors for pressure ulcer development and ways to minimize risk.

Modified from Wound Ostomy and Continence Nurses Society: *Guideline for prevention and management of pressure ulcers,* WOCN clinical practice guidelines series, Glenview, Ill, 2003.

Step	Rationale
Note if involved area blanches with palpation or remains discolored or red. Nonblanchable erythema or skin temperature changes may be important early indicator of stage I pressure ulcer.	position changes or use of pressure-relief device.

NURSE ALERT Do not massage any reddened or discolored pressure points because areas of nonblanchable erythema or discolored areas may indicate that deeper tissue damage is present. Massage in this area may worsen inflammation by further damaging underlying damaged blood vessels.

13. When positioning client in bed, keep head of bed at 30-degree angle or lower if client's medical condition allows.	Pressure is reduced to sacral area when head of bed is not at high elevation.
14. Observe client's skin for areas at risk for change in color or texture.	Enables nurse to evaluate success of prevention techniques.
15. Compare subsequent risk assessment scores.	Provides ongoing comparison of client's risk level to facilitate appropriateness of plan of care.
16. Complete postprocedure protocol.	

Recording and Reporting

- Record client's risk score and skin assessment, and describe positions, turning intervals, pressure-reducing devices, and other prevention measures. Note client's response to interventions.
- Report need for additional consultations for high-risk client.

Unexpected Outcomes	Related Interventions
1. Skin becomes mottled, reddened, purplish, or bluish.	• Document and communicate interval for reevaluation of risk assessment score. • Obtain physician's order (when needed) for identified consults such as wound ostomy and continence nurse, dietitian, clinical nurse specialist (CNS), and physical therapist. Reevaluate position changes.
2. Areas under pressure develop persistent discoloration, induration, or temperature changes.	• Document and communicate interval for reevaluation of risk assessment score. • Obtain physician's order (when needed) for identified consults such as wound ostomy and continence nurse, dietitian, CNS, and physical therapist.

Pressure Ulcer Treatment

The first principle of managing a client with a pressure ulcer should be to relieve or control the contributing factors. Therefore the first assessment made is to determine the etiology of the pressure ulcer.

The principle that guides the selection and use of topical dressings is to provide a wound environment that will support wound healing (Jones and others, 2004). Optimal conditions for healing are a moist environment for the wound and absence of necrotic tissue and infection in the wound. Interventions and dressings that support a clean, moist wound bed are appropriate. Before initiating wound therapy, a thorough assessment of the wound and the periwound skin is important.

Choose wound dressings to meet the characteristics of the wound bed (Baranoski and Ayello, 2004). A wound dressing will depend upon the type of wound tissue in the base of the wound, the amount of wound drainage, the presence or absence of infection, the location of the wound, the size of the wound, the ease of use, the cost-effectiveness, and comfort for the client. (See Skills 17 and 18.)

Delegation Considerations

This skill is the responsibility of the nurse. However, certain aspects of the client's care may be delegated to assistive personnel (AP). The nurse should instruct AP to report any wound drainage that might be found on linens or intact skin, which would indicate the need to change the dressing or to use an alternative dressing.

Equipment

- Disposable gloves (clean)
- Goggles and cover gown
- Plastic bag for dressing disposal
- Measuring device
- Cotton-tipped applicators
- Topical agent (as ordered)
- Cleansing agent (as ordered)
- Sterile solution container
- Washbasin, washcloths, towels
- Dressing of choice

- Hypoallergenic tape (if needed)
- Documentation records

Step	Rationale
1. Complete preprocedure protocol.	
2. Assess client's level of comfort and need for pain medication (Dallan and others, 2004).	Dressing change should not be traumatic event for client; majority of clients with pressure ulcers report pain at dressing change (Szor and Bourguignon, 1999).
3. Determine if client has allergies to topical agents.	Topical agents contain elements that may cause localized skin reactions.
4. Review order for topical agent or dressing.	Ensures that proper medication and treatment are administered.

NURSE ALERT Determine if the order for a topical agent and dressing is consistent with wound care guidelines (WOCN Society, 2003).

Step	Rationale
5. Position client to allow dressing removal, and position plastic bag for dressing disposal.	Area should be accessible for dressing change. Proper disposal of old dressing promotes proper handling of contaminated waste.
6. Assess each of client's pressure ulcer(s) and surrounding skin to determine ulcer characteristics, including the stage (see Skill 56).	Staging is way of assessing pressure ulcer, based on depth of tissue destruction. Nurse must be able to see type of tissue at base of pressure ulcer. Therefore pressure ulcer that is covered with necrotic tissue (eschar, which is black, hard, necrotic tissue) or slough (yellow, stringy, necrotic tissue) cannot be staged (National Pressure Ulcer Advisory Panel: Pressure Ulcer Stages. Revised by NPUAP, February 2007).

NURSE ALERT The base of the wound must be visible to be correctly staged. When the ulcer is covered with necrotic tissue, it cannot be staged until it is debrided (NPUAP, 2003).

Step	**Rationale**
7. Assess type of tissue in wound bed. Color type will indicate type of tissue. Black tissue is necrotic tissue, yellow tissue is slough, and red tissue is granulation tissue. Chart approximate amount of each tissue found in wound bed.	Approximate percentage of each type of tissue in wound will provide critical information on progress of wound healing and choice of dressing. Wound with high percentage of black tissue will require debridement, yellow tissue or slough tissue may indicate the presence of infection, and granulation tissue will indicate wound moving toward healing.
8. Wounds should be assessed on frequent basis. Consider using assessment tool such as Bates-Jensen Pressure Sore Status Tool (PSST) (Bates-Jensen, 1990) or the Pressure Ulcer Scale for Healing (PUSH) (Thomas and others, 1997). Reassess the wound at each dressing change to determine whether modifications are needed (WOCN Society, 2003).	Changes in appearance of wound can indicate that topical therapy should be adjusted to continue to move wound toward healing.
a. Note color, temperature, edema, moisture, and condition of skin around ulcer. Remember to modify assessment technique based on client's individual skin color (see Skill 56, Box 56-1).	Skin condition at ulcer edge may indicate progressive tissue damage. Maceration on periwound skin may show need to alter choice of wound dressing.
b. Measure wound dimensions. Measure using wound measurement guide; measure two	Consistency in how wound is measured is important for determining wound progress.

Step	Rationale
dimensions, length and width, per facility's protocol.	
c. Measure depth of pressure ulcer using sterile, cotton-tipped applicator or other device that will allow measurement of wound depth. Place applicator *gently* into pressure ulcer until it touches bottom. Mark place on applicator where it reaches top of wound, and then remove applicator from ulcer. Measure distance from tip of applicator to mark using measuring tape or ruler to determine depth of pressure ulcer.	Depth measure is important for determining amount of tissue loss.
d. Measure depth of undermining tissue (Fig. 57-1). Use cotton-	Undermining represents loss of underlying tissue. Undermining may indicate progressive tissue

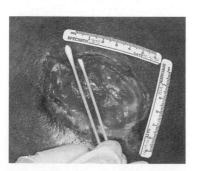

Fig. 57-1 Measuring depth of undermining of skin.

Step	**Rationale**
tipped applicator, and gently probe under skin edges.	necrosis or ongoing injury from shearing.
9. Remove gloves, discard appropriately, and perform hand hygiene.	Reduces transmission of microorganisms. Repeated hand washing is necessary as nurse assesses different pressure areas. Different wounds may be contaminated by different organisms. Failure to repeatedly perform hand hygiene can cause cross-wound contamination.
10. Prepare the following equipment and supplies:	
a. Washbasin, warm water, soap, washcloth, and bath towel.	Used to bathe surrounding skin.
b. Normal saline or other wound-cleansing agent in sterile solution container.	Ulcer surface must be cleansed before application of topical agents and new dressing.
c. Prescribed topical agent:	
(1) Enzymatic agents: Make sure manufacturer's specific directions for frequency of application are followed.	Enzymes debride dead tissue to clean ulcer surface.
OR	
(2) Topical antibiotics.	Topical antibiotics are used to decrease bioburden of wound and should be considered for use if no healing is noted after 2 to 4 weeks of optimal care (AHCPR, 1994; WOCN Society, 2003).
d. Dressing (see Skills 17 and 18).	The dressing should maintain moist environment for wound while keeping surrounding skin dry (AHCPR, 1994).
(1) Select appropriate dressing based on	

Step	Rationale
pressure ulcer characteristics, purpose for which dressing is intended, and client care setting.	
(2) Gauze.	Use as moist dressing; squeeze excessive saline from gauze, and apply over wound. Can be used to deliver solution to wound. Can be used as topper dressing when using enzymatic agent or topical antibiotics.

NURSE ALERT Determine that the selected dressing material is absorbent and adequate for the amount of wound drainage. Check that the wound does not dry out or that surrounding skin does not become macerated.

(3) Transparent dressing.	Applied over superficial ulcers and skin subjected to friction. Maintains moist environment.

NURSE ALERT Transparent membrane dressings can be used for autolytic debridement of noninfected pressure ulcers.

(4) Hydrocolloid dressing.	Maintains moist environment to facilitate wound healing while protecting wound base.
(5) Hydrogel.	Maintains moist environment to facilitate wound healing. Available in sheet or in tube.
(6) Calcium alginate.	Highly absorbent of wound exudate in heavily draining wounds.
(7) Foam.	Protective and will prevent wound dehydration; also absorbs small to moderate amounts of drainage.
e. Hypoallergenic tape or adhesive dressing sheet.	Used to secure nonadherent dressing. Prevents skin irritation and tearing.

Step	Rationale
11. Assemble needed supplies at bedside. Open sterile packages and topical solution containers. (Goggles and moisture-proof cover gown should be worn if potential for contamination from spray exists when cleansing wound.)	Maintains client privacy. Supplies should be ready for easy application so that nurse can use supplies without contaminating them; reduces transmission of microorganisms.
12. Expose ulcer and surrounding skin. Keep remaining body parts draped.	Prevents unnecessary exposure of body parts.
13. 🖐 Gently wash skin surrounding ulcer with warm water and soap. Rinse area thoroughly with water. Dry thoroughly.	Cleansing of skin surface reduces bacteria. Soap can be irritating to skin.
14. Perform hand hygiene, and change gloves.	Aseptic technique must be maintained during cleansing, measuring, and application of dressings. Refer to institutional policy regarding use of clean or sterile gloves.
15. Cleanse ulcer thoroughly with normal saline or prescribed wound-cleansing agent.	Wound should be cleansed at each dressing change, minimizing trauma to wound (WOCN Society, 2003).

NURSE ALERT Whirlpool treatments may be used to assist with wound debridement. Wound should not be positioned directly in front of water jets.

Step	Rationale
16. Apply topical agents, if prescribed:	
a. Enzymes:	Follow manufacturer's directions for frequency of application. Be aware of what solutions inactivate enzymes, and avoid their use in wound cleaning.
(1) Using wooden tongue blade, apply	Proper distribution of ointment ensures effective action. Some

Step	**Rationale**
small amount of enzyme debridement ointment directly to necrotic areas on base of pressure ulcer. Avoid getting enzyme on surrounding skin.	enzymes can cause burning, paresthesia, and dermatitis to surrounding skin.
(2) Place gauze dressing directly over ulcer, and tape it in place. Follow specific manufacturer's recommendation for type of dressing material to use to cover pressure ulcer when using enzymatic agent.	Protects wound and prevents removal of ointment during turning or repositioning.
(3) If using antibiotic solution, apply per order and cover with gauze pad. Generally applied every 12 hours.	
b. Hydrogel agents:	
(1) Cover surface of ulcer with hydrogel using applicator or gloved hand.	Provides moist environment.
(2) Apply secondary dressing, such as dry gauze, hydrocolloid, or transparent dressing, over gel to completely cover ulcer.	Holds hydrogel against wound surface because hydrogel amphorous form (in tube) or sheet form does not adhere to the wound and requires secondary dressing to hold it in place.
c. Calcium alginates:	Use in heavily draining wounds.

Step	Rationale
(1) Pack wound with alginate using applicator or gloved hand.	
(2) Apply secondary dressing, such as dry gauze, foam, or hydrocolloid, over alginate.	Holds alginate against wound surface.
17. Reposition client comfortably off pressure ulcer.	Avoids accidental removal of dressings.
18. Observe skin surrounding ulcer for inflammation, edema, and tenderness.	Clean pressure ulcer should show evidence of movement toward healing within 2 to 4 weeks.
19. Inspect dressings and exposed ulcers, observing for drainage, foul odor, and tissue necrosis. Monitor client for signs and symptoms of infection, including fever and elevated white blood cell (WBC) count.	Ulcers can become infected.
20. Use one of scales designed to measure wound healing, such as PUSH Scale (Thomas and others, 1997) or the PSST (Bates-Jensen, 1990).	Provides standard method of data collection that will demonstrate wound progress or lack thereof.
21. Complete postprocedure protocol.	

Recording and Reporting

- Record appearance of ulcer, describe type of topical agent used, dressing applied, and client's response.
- Report any deterioration in ulcer appearance to nurse in charge or physician.

Unexpected Outcomes	Related Interventions
1. Ulcer becomes deeper with increased drainage and/or development of necrotic tissue.	• Review current wound care management. • Consult with multidisciplinary team regarding changes in wound care regimen. • Obtain wound cultures.
2. Pressure ulcer extends beyond original margins.	• Monitor for systemic signs and symptoms of poor wound healing, such as abnormal laboratory results (WBC, hemoglobin/hematocrit, serum albumin, serum prealbumin, total proteins), weight loss, and fluid imbalances. • Assess and revise current turning schedule. • Consider further pressure-relieving devices.
3. See Skills 17 and 18.	

Pulse Oximetry

Pulse oximetry is the noninvasive measurement of arterial blood oxygen saturation—the percent to which hemoglobin is filled with oxygen. A pulse oximeter is a probe with a light-emitting diode (LED) connected by cable to an oximeter. The reflected light is processed by the oximeter, which calculates pulse oxygen saturation (SpO_2). SpO_2 is a reliable estimate of arterial oxygen saturation (SaO_2) (Grap, 2002). For this reason, the use of oximetry reduces the need to collect arterial blood gas (ABG) specimens for oxygen saturation analysis. In adults, the oximeter probe can be applied to the earlobe, finger, toe, or bridge of the nose, because a highly vascular area is needed to detect the degree of change in the transmitted light.

Delegation Considerations

The skill of oxygen saturation measurement can be delegated to assistive personnel (AP). Before delegating this skill, the nurse must:

- Provide AP the frequency of oxygen saturation measurements.
- Instruct AP to notify the nurse immediately of any reading lower than SpO_2 of 90%.
- Determine that AP are aware of factors that can falsely lower SpO_2.
- Caution AP to *not* use pulse oximetry as assessment of heart rate because an irregular rhythm may not be detected.

Equipment

- Oximeter
- Oximeter probe appropriate for client and recommended by oximeter manufacturer
- Acetone or nail polish remover
- Pen, pencil, vital sign flowsheet or record form

Step	Rationale
1. Complete preprocedure protocol.	
2. Assess for signs and symptoms of alterations in oxygen saturation: altered respiratory rate, depth, or rhythm;	Physical signs and symptoms may indicate abnormal oxygen saturation.

411

Step	Rationale
adventitious breath sounds; cyanotic appearance of nail beds, lips, mucous membranes, and skin; restlessness, irritability, confusion; reduced level of consciousness; labored or difficulty breathing.	
3. Assess for factors that influence measurement of SpO_2, such as oxygen therapy, respiratory therapy such as postural drainage and percussion, anemia, hypotension, temperature, and medications such as bronchodilators.	Allows nurse to accurately assess oxygen saturation variations. Peripheral vasoconstriction related to hypothermia can interfere with SpO_2 determination.
4. Determine most appropriate client-specific site (e.g., finger, earlobe, bridge of nose) for sensor probe placement by measuring capillary refill. If capillary refill less than 3 seconds, select alternative site.	Sensor requires pulsating vascular bed to identify hemoglobin molecules that absorb emitted light. Changes in SpO_2 are reflected in circulation of finger capillary bed within 30 seconds and capillary bed of earlobe within 5 to 10 seconds.
a. Site must have adequate local circulation and be free of moisture.	Moisture impedes ability of sensor to detect SpO_2 levels. Motion artifact is most common cause of inaccurate readings.
b. Artificial nails and certain nail polish colors will alter readings (Grap, 2002); place probe on finger free of polish or artificial nail.	
c. If client has tremors or is likely to move, use earlobe.	

Step	**Rationale**
d. If client is obese, clip-on probe may not fit properly; obtain a single use (tape-on) probe.	
5. If finger is to be used, remove fingernail polish with acetone or polish remover from digit to be assessed.	Opaque coatings decrease light transmission; nail polish containing blue pigment can absorb light emissions and falsely alter saturation readings.
6. Attach sensor to monitoring site. Instruct client that clip-on probe will feel like clothespin on finger but will not hurt.	Select sensor site based on peripheral circulation and extremity temperature. Peripheral vasoconstriction can alter SpO_2. Pressure of sensor's spring tension on finger or earlobe may be uncomfortable.

NURSE ALERT Do not attach the probe to the finger, ear, or bridge of nose if the area is edematous or if skin integrity is impaired. Do not attach the sensor to fingers that are hypothermic. In clients with peripheral vascular disease, attach the sensor to the ear or bridge of nose. If the client has a latex allergy, do not use disposable adhesive sensors. Do not place the sensor on the same extremity as an electronic blood pressure cuff, because when the cuff inflates, blood flow to the finger is temporarily interrupted and, as a result, an inaccurate reading occurs.

7. Once sensor is in place, turn on oximeter by activating power. Observe pulse waveform/intensity display and audible beep. Correlate oximeter pulse rate with client's radial pulse.	Pulse waveform/intensity display enables detection of valid pulse or presence of interfering signal. Pitch of audible beep is proportional to SpO_2 value. Double-checking pulse rate ensures oximeter accuracy.

NURSE ALERT If oximeter pulse rate, client's radial pulse, and apical pulse are different, reevaluate oximeter probe placement and reassess pulse rates.

8. Inform client that oximeter alarm will sound if sensor falls off or if client moves sensor.	

Step	Rationale
9. Leave sensor in place until oximeter readout reaches constant value and pulse display reaches full strength during each cardiac cycle. Read SpO$_2$ on digital display.	Reading may take 10 to 30 seconds, depending on site selected.
10. If continuous SpO$_2$ monitoring is planned, verify SpO$_2$ alarm limits, which are preset by manufacturer at low of 85% and high of 100%. Limits for SpO$_2$ and pulse rate should be determined as indicated by client's condition. Verify that alarms are on. Assess skin integrity under sensor every 2 hours. Relocate sensor at least every 4 hours and more frequently if skin integrity is altered or tissue perfusion compromised.	Alarms must be set at appropriate limits and volumes to avoid frightening clients and visitors. Spring tension of sensor or sensitivity to disposable sensor adhesive can cause skin irritation and lead to disruption of skin integrity.
11. Remove probe, and turn oximeter power off. Store sensor in appropriate location.	Batteries can be depleted if oximeter is left on. Sensors are expensive and vulnerable to damage.
12. If oxygen saturation is assessed for first time, establish SpO$_2$ as baseline if it is within acceptable range.	Used to compare future assessments of oxygen saturation.
13. Compare SpO$_2$ with client's previous baseline and acceptable SpO$_2$. Note use of oxygen therapy.	Allows nurse to assess for change in client's condition and presence of respiratory alteration.
14. During continuous monitoring, assess skin	Prevents tissue ischemia.

Step	Rationale

integrity underneath probe
at least every 2 hours,
based on client's peripheral
circulation.
15. Complete postprocedure
protocol.

Recording and Reporting

- Record SpO$_2$ on vital sign flowsheet or nurses' notes; include type
  and amount of oxygen therapy used by client during assessment.
  Assessment of O$_2$ saturation after administration of specific
  therapies should be documented in narrative form in nurses' notes;
  include any signs and symptoms of oxygen desaturation in nurses'
  notes.
- Report abnormal findings to nurse in charge or physician.

Unexpected Outcomes	Related Interventions
1. SaO$_2$ is less than 90%.	• Reposition probe and reevaluate. If SaO$_2$ is unacceptable, notify physician. An ABG level may be obtained to validate oximetry reading. • Promote oxygenation. • Position client in high-Fowler's or semi-Fowler's position. • Implement measures to reduce energy consumption. • Verify appropriate oxygen delivery system and liter flow; administer oxygen according to physician's orders.
2. Pulse waveform/intensity display is dampened or irregular.	• Locate different peripheral vascular bed, and reposition pulse oximeter probe. • Use another sensor if available. • Protect sensor from room light by covering sensor site with opaque covering or washcloth.

Rectal Suppository Insertion

Drugs administered rectally either exert a local effect on gastrointestinal mucosa, such as promoting defecation, or exert systemic effects, such as relieving nausea or providing analgesia. Rectal medications are relatively safe, because they rarely cause local irritation or side effects. Rectal medications are contraindicated in clients with rectal surgery or active rectal bleeding. Suppositories may be given through a colostomy (not ileostomy) if ordered, using a small amount of water-soluble lubricant for insertion.

Rectal suppositories have a rounded end, which prevents anal trauma during insertion. When you administer a suppository, place it past the internal anal sphincter and against the rectal mucosa. Improper placement can result in expulsion of the suppository before the medication dissolves and is absorbed into the mucosa. If a client prefers to self-administer a suppository, give specific instructions so that the medication is deposited correctly. Do not cut the suppository into sections to divide the dosage; the active drug may not be distributed evenly within the suppository, and the result may be an inaccurate dose (Lilley and others, 2005).

Delegation Considerations

The skill of rectal medication administration should not be delegated to assistive personnel (AP).

- Instruct AP about expected fecal discharge or bowel movement and to report the occurrence to the nurse.
- Instruct AP about potential side effects of medications and to report their occurrence.
- Instruct AP about informing the nurse of any rectal discharge, pain, or bleeding.

Equipment

- Rectal suppository
- Lubricating jelly (water soluble)
- Clean gloves
- Tissue
- Drape
- Medication administration record (MAR)

Step	Rationale
1. Review prescriber's order, including client's name, drug name, dosage, form, route, and time of administration.	Ensures safe and correct administration of medication.
2. Review medical record for history of rectal surgery or bleeding.	Conditions contraindicate use of suppository.

NURSE ALERT Generally, a rectal suppository is contraindicated with the presence of active rectal bleeding and diarrhea (Lilley and others, 2005). Unless the suppository is for constipation, placing a medication in a rectum filled with feces may result in poor absorption of the medication or it may be prematurely expelled with defecation.

Step	Rationale
3. Assess client's ability to hold suppository and to position self to insert medication.	Mobility restriction indicates need for nurse to assist with drug administration.
4. Review client's knowledge of purpose of drug therapy and interest in self-administering suppository.	May indicate need for health teaching. Level of motivation influences teaching approach.
5. Check accuracy and completeness of each MAR with prescriber's written medication order. Check client's name, drug name and dosage, route of administration, and time of administration. Compare MAR with medication label three times during preparation of medication.	Order sheet is most reliable source and only legal record of drugs client is to receive. Ensures that right medication is administered.
6. Check client's identification bracelet, and ask name.	Ensures that correct client receives medication. At least two identifiers (neither to be the room number) are to be used whenever administering medications (JCAHO, 2004).

Step	Rationale
7. Explain procedure to client. Be specific if client wishes to self-administer drug.	Promotes client's understanding and cooperation. Enables client to self-administer drug safely if physically able and motivated.
8. ![hand icon] Assist client in assuming a left side-lying Sims' position with upper leg flexed upward. If client has mobility limitations, assist to left lateral position. Obtain assistance from another health care provider to turn and position client. Use pillows under upper arm and leg for support.	Position exposes anus and helps client relax external anal sphincter. Left side lessens likelihood of suppository or feces being expelled.
9. Keep client draped with only anal area exposed.	Maintains privacy and facilitates relaxation.
10. Examine condition of anus externally, and palpate rectal walls as needed (e.g., if impaction is suspected). Dispose of gloves by turning them inside out and placing them in proper receptacle if they become soiled.	Determines presence of active rectal bleeding. Palpation determines whether rectum is filled with feces, which may interfere with suppository placement. Reduces transmission of infection.

NURSE ALERT Do not palpate the rectum if the client has had rectal surgery.

11. ![hand icon] Remove suppository from foil wrapper, and lubricate rounded end with water-soluble lubricant. Lubricate gloved index finger of dominant hand. If client has hemorrhoids, use liberal amount of lubricant and handle area gently.	Lubrication reduces friction as suppository enters rectal canal.

Step	Rationale
12. Ask client to take slow, deep breaths through mouth and to relax anal sphincter.	Forcing suppository through constricted sphincter causes pain.
13. Retract client's buttocks with nondominant hand. With gloved index finger of dominant hand, insert suppository gently through anus, past internal sphincter, and against rectal wall, 10 cm (4 inches) (Fig. 59-1)	Suppository must be placed against rectal mucosa for eventual absorption and therapeutic action.

NURSE ALERT Do not insert a suppository into a mass of fecal material; medication effectiveness will be reduced.

Step	Rationale
14. Withdraw finger, and wipe client's anal area.	Provides comfort.
15. Discard gloves by turning them inside out, and dispose of in appropriate receptacle.	Reduces transfer of microorganisms.
16. Ask client to remain flat or on side for 5 minutes.	Prevents expulsion of suppository.
17. If suppository contains laxative or fecal softener, place call light within	Ability to call for assistance provides client with sense of control over elimination.

Fig. 59-1 Insert rectal suppository past sphincter and against rectal wall.

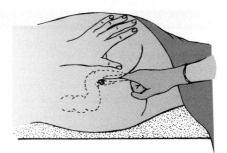

Step	Rationale
reach so client can obtain assistance to reach bedpan or toilet.	
18. If suppository was given for constipation, remind client *not* to flush commode after bowel movement.	Allows staff to evaluate results of suppository.
19. Perform postprocedure protocol.	
20. Return within 5 minutes to determine if suppository was expelled.	Determines if drug is properly distributed. Reinsertion may be necessary.
21. Evaluate client for relief of symptoms for which medication was prescribed.	Determines medication's effectiveness.

Recording and Reporting

- Immediately after administration, record on MAR actual time each drug was administered. Include initials or signature. Do not chart medication administration until *after* it is given to client.
- If drug is withheld, record reason in nurses' notes. Circle on MAR time drug normally would have been given (or follow institution's policy for noting withheld doses).
- Record client's response to medication, including any unusual reactions.
- Report adverse effects/client response and/or withheld drugs to nurse in charge or physician. Depending on medication, immediate prescriber notification may be required.

Unexpected Outcomes	Related Interventions
1. Symptoms previously reported are unrelieved.	• May require alternative therapy.
2. Client reports rectal pain during insertion.	• Suppository may need more lubrication. • Rectal route may not be suitable; assess and notify prescriber.

Respiration Assessment

Accurate assessment of respiration depends on recognizing normal thoracic and abdominal movements. Normal breathing is active and passive. On inspiration, the diaphragm contracts, causing abdominal organs to move downward and forward, thereby increasing the vertical size of the chest cavity. At the same time, the ribs lift upward and outward and the sternum lifts outward to aid the transverse expansion of the lungs. On expiration, the diaphragm relaxes upward, the ribs and sternum return to their relaxed position, and the abdominal organs return to their original position. During quiet breathing, the chest wall gently rises and falls.

Delegation Considerations

The skill of respiration measurement may be delegated to assistive personnel (AP) unless the client is considered unstable. Before delegating this skill, the nurse must:

- Inform AP if the client is at risk for increased or decreased respiratory rate or irregular respirations.
- Provide AP the frequency of measurement for the specific client.
- Inform AP of the usual values for the client.
- Instruct AP of the need to report any abnormalities that should be reconfirmed by the nurse.

Equipment

- Wristwatch with second hand or digital display
- Pen or pencil
- Vital sign flowsheet or record form

Step	Rationale
1. Complete preprocedure protocol.	
2. Assess for signs and symptoms of respiratory alterations, such as bluish or cyanotic appearance of nail beds, lips, mucous membranes, and skin; restlessness, irritability,	Physical signs and symptoms may indicate alterations in respiratory status related to ventilation.

Step	Rationale
confusion, reduced level of consciousness; pain during inspiration; labored or difficult breathing; orthopnea; use of accessory muscles; adventitious breath sounds; inability to breathe spontaneously; thick, frothy, blood-tinged, or copious sputum produced on coughing.	
3. Assess for factors that influence character of respirations:	Allows nurse to accurately assess for presence and significance of respiratory alterations.
a. Exercise.	Respirations increase in rate and depth to meet need for additional oxygen and rid body of CO_2.
b. Acute pain.	Pain alters rate and rhythm of respirations; breaths become shallow. Client may inhibit or splint chest wall movement when pain is in area of chest or abdomen.
c. Smoking.	Chronic smoking changes pulmonary airways, resulting in increased respiratory rate at rest when not smoking.
d. Medications.	Narcotic analgesics, general anesthetics, and sedative hypnotics depress rate and depth; amphetamines and cocaine may increase rate and depth; bronchodilators cause dilation of airways that ultimately can slow respiratory rate.
4. Assess pertinent laboratory values:	

Step	**Rationale**
a. Arterial blood gases (ABGs) (values may vary slightly among institutions); normal ranges are: pH: 7.35 to 7.45 PaCO$_2$: 35 to 45 mm Hg PaO$_2$: 80 to 100 mm Hg SaO$_2$: 94% to 98%	ABGs measure arterial blood pH, partial pressure of O$_2$ and CO$_2$, and arterial O$_2$ saturation, which reflects client's oxygenation status.
b. Pulse oximetry (SpO$_2$): normal SpO$_2$ 90% to 100%; 85% to 89% may be acceptable for certain chronic disease conditions; less than 85% is abnormal (Skill 58).	SpO$_2$ less than 85% is often accompanied by changes in respiratory rate, depth, and rhythm.
5. If client has been active, wait 5 to 10 minutes before assessing respirations.	Exercise increases respiratory rate and depth. Respirations should be assessed at rest to allow for objective comparison of values.
6. Assess respirations after pulse measurement in adult.	Inconspicuous assessment of respirations immediately after pulse assessment prevents client from consciously or unintentionally altering rate and depth of breathing.

NURSE ALERT Clients with difficulty breathing (e.g., dyspnea, orthopnea, which occurs in clients with congestive heart failure, abdominal ascites, pneumonia) should have their respirations assessed in the position of greatest comfort. Positioning the client supine may increase the work of breathing, which can increase respiratory rate.

7. Place client's arm in relaxed position across abdomen or lower chest, or place nurse's hand directly over client's upper abdomen (Fig. 60-1).	Similar position used during pulse assessment allows respiratory rate assessment to be inconspicuous. Client's or nurse's hand rises and falls during respiratory cycle.

Step	Rationale

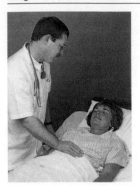

Fig. 60-1   Nurse's hand over client's abdomen to check respirations.

Step	Rationale
8. Observe complete respiratory cycle (one inspiration and one expiration).	Rate is accurately determined only after nurse has viewed respiratory cycle.
9. If rhythm is regular, count number of respirations in 30 seconds and multiply by 2. If rhythm is irregular, less than 12, or more than 20, count for 1 full minute.	Respiratory rate is equivalent to number of respirations per minute. Suspected irregularities require assessment for at least 1 minute.
10. While counting, note depth of respirations, subjectively assessed by observing degree of chest wall movement while counting rate.	Character of ventilatory movement may reveal specific disease state restricting volume of air from moving into and out of lungs.
11. If respirations are assessed for first time, establish rate, rhythm, and depth as baseline if within acceptable range.	Used to compare future respiratory assessment.
12. Compare respirations with client's previous baseline and usual rate, rhythm, and depth.	Allows nurse to assess for changes in client's condition and for presence of respiratory alterations.

Step	Rationale

13. Complete postprocedure
    protocol.

Recording and Reporting

- Record respiratory rate on vital sign flowsheet or record; record abnormal depth and rhythm in narrative form in nurses' notes. Measurement of respiratory rate after administration of specific therapies and type and amount of oxygen therapy, if used, is documented in narrative form in nurses' notes.
- Report abnormal findings to nurse in charge or physician.

Unexpected Outcomes	Related Interventions
1. Respiratory rate is less than 12 (bradypnea) or more than 20 (tachypnea). Rhythm may be irregular. Depth of respirations increased or decreased.	• Assess for conditions that restrict full expansion of chest wall. • Position client in comfortable Fowler's or high-Fowler's position. • Check for tight dressings. • Maintain patency of any existing artificial airway. • Notify physician if alteration continues, and be prepared to initiate oxygen therapy as needed. ABG test or chest x-ray examination may be ordered to evaluate nature of respiratory problem.
2. Client demonstrates Kussmaul, Cheyne-Stokes, or Biot respirations.	• Notify physician, and anticipate that immediate therapy will be ordered.

Restraint Application

Clients at risk for injury may need to be temporarily restrained. A physical restraint is any device, garment, material, or object that restricts a person's freedom of movement or access to one's body. The restraint must be clinically justified and a part of the prescribed medical treatment and plan of care, and all other less restrictive measures must be employed first (see Skill 62).

The use of restraints has been associated with several serious complications. The Food and Drug Administration (FDA), which regulates restraints as medical devices and requires manufacturers to label them "prescription only," estimates that hundreds of restraint-related injuries occur each year, with approximately 100 of them resulting in client death. Most client deaths have resulted from suffocation from a vest or jacket restraint (Lambert, 1992). Numerous institutions have stopped using vest restraints. For these reasons, the use of vest restraints is not described in this text.

When the use of restraints is the only appropriate intervention to maintain the client's safety, both the client and the family should be informed that the restraint is temporary and protective. Most institutions require a physician's order, which should specify the type of behavior or condition requiring restraint, the type of restraint, and time limitations for restraint application. A face-to-face assessment by the physician is required. Orders should be renewed according to agency policy and based on reassessment and reevaluation of the restrained client.

Delegation Considerations

Assessment of the client's behavior, level of orientation, need for restraints, and appropriate type to use and specific assessments related to oxygenation, skin integrity, and neurovascular status may not be delegated to assistive personnel (AP). However, the following aspects of the skill may be delegated to AP:

- Correctly placing the restraint.
- Observing for constriction of circulation, skin integrity, adequate breathing.
- Understanding when and how to change the client's position.
- Providing range of motion (ROM) and skin care, toileting, and opportunities for socialization.

Equipment

- Proper restraint
- Padding

Step	Rationale
1. Complete preprocedure protocol.	
2. Determine client's need for restraint if other less restrictive measures fail to prevent interruption of therapy or injury to self or others. Confer with physician or primary health care provider.	Restraints may be needed when other less restrictive measures fail to prevent interruption of therapy such as traction, intravenous (IV) infusions, or nasogastric tube feedings; to prevent confused or combative client from removing Foley catheters, surgical drains, or life support equipment; to reduce risk of injury to others by client; and at times to reduce risk of client falling out of bed or wheelchair.
3. Assess client's behavior, such as confusion, disorientation, agitation, restlessness, combativeness, or inability to follow directions.	If client's behavior continues despite attempts to eliminate cause of behavior, use of physical restraint may be needed.
4. Review agency policies regarding restraints. Check physician's order for purpose of restraint and type, location, and time or duration of restraint. Determine if signed consent for use of restraint is needed.	Physician's order is necessary to apply restraints. Least restrictive type of restraint should be ordered. Because restraints limit client's ability to move freely, nurse must make clinical judgments appropriate to client's condition and agency policy. If nurse restrains client in emergency situation because of violent or aggressive behavior that presents immediate danger, face-to-face physician assessment within 1 hour is needed (CMS, 2004).

Step	Rationale
5. Review manufacturer's instructions for restraint application before entering client's room. Determine most appropriate size restraint.	Nurse should be familiar with all devices used for client care and protection. Incorrect application of restraint device may result in client injury or death.
6. Inspect area where restraint is to be placed. Note if there is any nearby tubing or devices. Assess condition of skin, sensation, and ROM of joint (if applicable) of underlying area on which restraint is to be applied.	Restraints may compress and interfere with functioning of devices or tubes. Assessment provides baseline to monitor client's skin integrity and neuromuscular status.

NURSE ALERT Restraints should not interfere with equipment such as IV tubes. They should not be placed over vascular access devices, such as an arteriovenous (AV) dialysis shunt.

Step	Rationale
7. Approach client in calm, confident manner. Explain what you plan to do.	Reduces client anxiety and promotes cooperation.
8. Be sure client is comfortable and in correct anatomical position.	Prevents contractures and neurovascular impairment.
9. Pad skin and bony prominences (as necessary) that will be under restraint.	Reduces friction and pressure from restraint to skin and underlying tissue.
10. Apply appropriate-size restraint: *Always refer to manufacturer's directions.*	
a. **Belt restraint:** Have client in sitting position. Apply over clothes, gown, or pajamas. Remove wrinkles or creases from front and back of restraint while	Restrains center of gravity and prevents client from rolling off stretcher or sitting up while on stretcher or from falling out of bed. Tight application may interfere with ventilation.

Step	**Rationale**
placing it around client's waist. Bring ties through slots in belt. Help client lie down if in bed. Avoid placing belt too tightly across client's chest or abdomen (Fig. 61-1).	
b. **Extremity (ankle or wrist) restraint:** Restraint designed to immobilize an extremity. Commercially available limb restraints are composed of sheepskin or foam padding	Maintains immobilization of extremity to protect client from injury from fall or accidental removal of therapeutic device (e.g., IV tube, Foley catheter). Tight application may interfere with circulation.

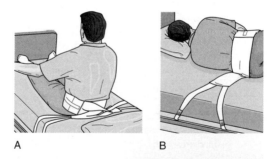

A   B

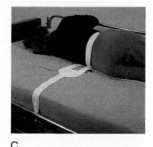

Fig. 61-1 Roll belt restraint tied to the bed frame and to an area that does not cause the restraint to tighten when the bed frame is raised or lowered. (From Sorrentino SA: *Mosby's textbook for nursing assistants,* ed 6, St Louis, 2000, Mosby.)

C

Step	Rationale

(Fig. 61-2). Limb restraint is wrapped around wrist or ankle with soft part toward skin and secured snugly in place by Velcro straps.

NURSE ALERT Clients with wrist and ankle restraints are at risk for aspiration if they are placed in the supine position; place in lateral position rather than supine.

c. **Mitten restraint:** Thumbless mitten device is used to restrain client's hands. Place hand in mitten, being sure Velcro strap(s) is around wrist and not forearm.

Prevents clients from dislodging invasive equipment, removing dressings, or scratching.

d. **Elbow restraint (freedom splint):** Restraint consists of piece of fabric with slots in which tongue blades are placed. Insert client's arm so that elbow joint rests against padded area with

Commonly used with infants and children to prevent elbow flexion (e.g., when IV placed in antecubital fossa).

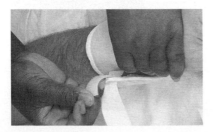

Fig. 61-2 Securing an extremity restraint. (Courtesy J.T. Posey Co., Arcadia, Calif.)

Step	**Rationale**
tongue blades, keeping joint rigid.	
11. Attach restraint straps to bed frame when head of bed is raised or lowered. *Do not attach to side rails.* Restraint may also be attached to chair frame when client is in chair or wheelchair.	Client may be injured if restraint is secured to side rail and if side rail is lowered.
12. Secure restraints with a quick-release tie (Fig. 61-3).	Allows for quick release in an emergency.
13. Insert two fingers under secured restraint.	Checking for constriction prevents neurovascular injury. Tight restraint may cause constriction and impede circulation.
14. Restraints should be removed at least every	Provides opportunity to change client's position and perform full

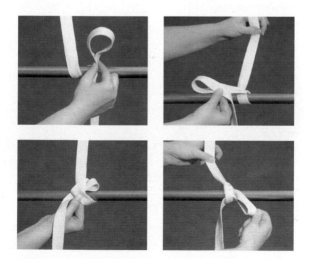

Fig. 61-3   The Posey quick-release tie. (Courtesy J.T. Posey Co., Arcadia, Calif.)

Step	Rationale
2 hours (JCAHO, 2004). If client is violent or noncompliant, remove one restraint at a time and/or have staff assistance while removing restraints.	ROM, to facilitate toileting and exercise, and to assist client's meals.
15. Secure call light or intercom system within reach.	Allows client, family, or caregiver to obtain assistance quickly.
16. Leave bed or chair with wheels locked. Bed should be in lowest position.	Locked wheels prevent bed or chair from moving if client attempts to get out. If client falls when bed is in lowest position, chances of injury are reduced.
17. Evaluate proper placement of restraint, skin integrity, pulses, temperature, color, and sensation of restrained body part *at least every 2 hours or sooner* according to client need and according to agency policy (JCAHO, 2004).	Frequent assessments prevent complications, such as suffocation, skin breakdown, and impaired circulation.
18. Inspect client for any injury, including all hazards of immobility, while restraints are in use. Also, inspect during routine removal of restraint.	Client should be free of injury and not exhibit any signs of complications from immobility.
19. Observe IV catheters, urinary catheters, and drainage tubes to determine that they are positioned correctly and that therapy remains uninterrupted.	Reinsertion can be uncomfortable and can increase risk of infection or interrupt therapy.
20. Complete postprocedure protocol.	

Step	Rationale
21. Reassess client's need for continued use of restraint at least every 24 hours or more often depending on purpose of restraint (e.g., behavioral use requires review every 2 to 4 hours). Face-to-face reassessment by physician is required and new order obtained if restraint is to be continued (see agency specific policy).	Intent is to discontinue restraint at earliest possible time (JCAHO, 2004).

Recording and Reporting

- Record nursing interventions employed to ensure client's safety before use of restraints; the type and location of restraint applied, time restraint was applied, and specific assessments related to oxygenation, skin integrity, musculoskeletal system, and peripheral vascular integrity.
- Record and report client's behavior before restraints were applied, level of orientation, and client's or family member's understanding of purpose of restraint and consent for application.
- Record and report client's behavior after restraints were applied, times client was assessed while restraints were on and findings, attempts to use alternatives to restraint and client's response, times restraints are released (temporarily and permanently), and client's response when restraints were removed.

Unexpected Outcomes	Related Interventions
1. Client experiences impaired circulation or skin integrity related to improper or prolonged use of restraint.	• Reassess need for continued use of restraint and if alternative measures can be employed. If restraint is needed to protect client or others from injury, ensure that restraint is applied correctly and provide adequate padding. • Check skin under restraint for abrasions, and remove restraints more frequently. • Institute appropriate skin/wound care. • Change wet or soiled restraints to prevent skin maceration.
2. Client exhibits increased confusion and disorientation.	• Evaluate cause for altered behavior, and attempt to eliminate cause. • Provide appropriate sensory stimulation, reorient as needed, and attempt restraint alternatives.
3. Client releases restraint and suffers fall or other traumatic injury.	• Attend to client's immediate physical needs, inform physician of fall or injury, and reassess type of restraint and its correct application.

Restraint-Free Environment

A restraint-free environment should be the goal for all clients, whether in a health care facility or nursing home. Measures can be taken to ensure safety for those clients who are at risk for self-injury by interrupting therapy and those who may inflict injury on others. The use of restraints is one safety strategy that can protect clients from injury, but they must be used with extreme caution. Physical restraints should be the last resort and used only when reasonable alternatives have failed (see Skill 61).

Recently the public, the media, and the government have grown increasingly concerned about the need to ensure basic protections for client health and safety in health care facilities, especially with regard to the use of restraints and seclusion. Regulatory agencies such as the Joint Commission on Accreditation of Healthcare Organizations (JCAHO) (2004) and the Centers for Medicaid and Medicare Services (CMS) (2004) outline standards regarding the safe use of restraints. The agencies define clients' rights and choices regarding restraints and clearly state the reasons for using physical restraints. The use of mechanical or physical restraints must be part of the prescribed medical treatment, all less restrictive interventions must be tried first, other disciplines must be used, and supporting documentation must be provided. For example, a nurse caring for a client who is attempting to dislodge a tube must try less restrictive measures first, such as camouflage or diversional activity. If the alternatives fail, the nurse may consider use of a restraint to prevent injury.

Delegation Considerations

The skills necessary to assess client behaviors and make decisions about less restrictive interventions should not be delegated to assistive personnel (AP). Promoting a safe environment (e.g., client positioning) and monitoring client behavior for risk of injury may be delegated to AP. The nurse must instruct AP to report to the nurse specific behaviors and actions, such as client confusion, getting out of bed unassisted, pulling at tubes, and combativeness.

Equipment

- Visual or auditory stimuli (e.g., calendar, clock, radio, television, pictures)
- Diversional activities (e.g., puzzle, game, music, stuffed animal, TV)

Step	Rationale
1. Complete preprocedure protocol.	
2. Assess client's physical and mental status, such as orientation; level of consciousness; ability to understand, remember, and follow directions; balance; gait; vision; hearing; bowel/bladder routine; level of pain; laboratory values; and presence of orthostatic hypotension.	Accurate assessment helps identify safety risks and physiological causes for behavior and ensures proper interventions.
3. Review prescribed medications (e.g., sedatives, hypnotics, analgesics, diuretics).	Medication interactions or side effects often contribute to falling or altered mental status.
4. Orient client and family to surroundings, introduce to staff, and explain all treatments and procedures.	Promotes client's understanding and cooperation.
5. Encourage family and friends to stay with client. Sitters or companions may be used. In some institutions, volunteers can be effective companions.	Reduces client's anxiety and increases safety when one person provides care and supervision is constant.
6. Place client in room that is easily accessible to caregivers.	Allows for frequent observation.
7. Provide appropriate visual and auditory stimuli. Choose stimulus meaningful to specific	Orients client to day, time, and physical surroundings. Strategy must be individualized to be effective.

Step	**Rationale**
client (e.g., clock, calendar, radio [with client's choice of music], television, and family pictures may be indicated).	
8. Meet client's basic needs (e.g., toileting, relief of pain, relief of hunger) as quickly as possible.	Basic needs provided in timely fashion decrease client's discomfort and anxiety.
9. Approach client and caregiver in calm, nonthreatening, professional manner.	Reduces tension in environment.
10. Provide scheduled ambulation, chair activity, and toileting. Organize treatments so client has long, uninterrupted periods throughout day.	Provides for sleep and rest periods. Constant activity may irritate client.
11. Position IV catheters, urinary catheters, tubes/drains out of client's view, or use camouflage by wrapping intravenous (IV) site with bandage or stockinet, placing undergarments on client with urinary catheter, or covering abdominal feeding tubes/drains with loose abdominal binder.	Facilitates medical treatment and reduces client's access to tubes/lines.
12. Stress-reduction techniques, such as back rub, massage, and imagery, may be employed.	Reduced stress allows client's energy to be channeled more appropriately.
13. Use diversional activities such as puzzles, games, books, folding towels, drawing/coloring, or object to hold. Be sure	Meaningful diversional activities provide distraction, help reduce boredom, and provide tactile stimulation. Minimize occurrences of wandering.

Step	Rationale
it is activity client consents to.	
14. Review medications frequently, and confer with physician if changes are needed.	Idiosyncratic reactions and drug interactions may cause changes in client behavior.
15. Determine need for continuation of invasive treatments such as IV catheters, urinary catheters, and feeding tubes and whether less invasive treatment can be substituted.	
16. Complete postprocedure protocol.	

Recording and Reporting

- Record restraint alternatives attempted, client's behaviors, and interventions to mediate these behaviors.

Unexpected Outcomes	Related Interventions
1. Client may continue to be at risk for injury, disrupt therapy, or commit violent acts toward others.	• Intensify supervision of client, and notify physician. Restraints or medication may be indicated.

Seizure Precautions

Seizure precautions include all nursing interventions to protect the client from traumatic injury: side-lying position for adequate ventilation and drainage of secretions, providing privacy, and providing support after the seizure. Traditionally, oral airways have been used with the purpose of maintaining the client's airway during a seizure. However, forcing something in the client's mouth could result in injury to the jaw, tongue, or teeth and cause stimulation of the gag reflex, causing vomiting, aspiration, and respiratory distress (National Institute of Neurological Disorders and Stroke, 2001). Forcing an airway into a client's mouth is no longer recommended. An airway is inserted only when there is clear access for insertion. Padded tongue blades do not belong at the bedside and should never be inserted into the client's mouth after a seizure begins (Ignatavicius and Workman, 2002).

Observation during a seizure is critical because it may assist in determining the type of seizure. It is important that the nurse observe the client carefully before, during, and after the seizure so that the episode can be documented accurately.

Delegation Considerations

Assessment of a client's need to be placed on seizure precautions cannot be delegated to assistive personnel (AP). Setting up seizure precautions and protecting clients at risk for seizures may be delegated to AP. Measures to emphasize if a client is at risk for a seizure include the following:

- Protecting the client from a fall.
- Avoiding attempts to restrain the client.
- Not placing anything in the client's mouth.

Equipment

- Padding for side rails and headboard
- Suction machine
- Oral airway
- Oral suction equipment
- Oxygen via nasal cannula or face mask
- Equipment for intravenous (IV) access
- Clean, disposable gloves

Step	Rationale
1. Complete preprocedure protocol.	
2. Assess client's seizure history and knowledge of precipitating factors, noting frequency of seizures, presence of aura, and sequence of events, if known. Use family as resource if necessary.	Knowledge about seizure history enables nurse to anticipate onset of seizure activity.
3. Assess for medical and surgical conditions that may lead to seizures or exacerbate existing seizure condition (e.g., electrolyte disturbances such as hypoglycemia, hyperkalemia; heart disease; excess fatigue; alcohol or caffeine consumption).	Common conditions that may precipitate seizures.
4. Assess medication history and client's adherence. Also, assess therapeutic drug levels of anticonvulsants if test results available.	Seizure medications must be taken as prescribed and not stopped suddenly. This may precipitate seizure activity.
5. Inspect client's environment for potential safety hazards if seizure occurs. Prepare bed with padded side rails and headboard, bed in low position, and client in side-lying position when possible.	Prevents client from injury sustained by striking head or body on furniture or equipment.
6. For clients with history of seizures, oxygen setup, suction apparatus, clean gloves, and pillows should be visible for immediate use in hospital setting.	This ensures prompt, organized intervention.

tep	**Rationale**
7. When seizure begins, position client safely. If client is standing or sitting, guide client to floor and protect head by cradling in nurse's lap or placing pillow under head. Clear surrounding area of furniture. If client is in bed, raise side rails, pad, and put bed in low position.	Position protects client from traumatic injury, especially head injury.
8. If possible, provide privacy. Have staff control flow of visitors in area.	Embarrassment is common after seizure, especially if others witnessed seizure.
9. If possible, turn client on side, with head flexed slightly forward.	Position prevents tongue from blocking airway and promotes drainage of secretions, thus reducing risk of aspiration.
10. Do not restrain client. Loosen clothing.	Prevents musculoskeletal injury and airway obstruction.
11. Do not force any objects into client's mouth such as fingers, medicine, tongue depressor, or airway when teeth are clenched.	Prevents injury to mouth and possible aspiration.

NURSE ALERT Injury may result from forcible insertion of hard objects. Soft objects may break or come apart and be aspirated.

12. Maintain client's airway, and suction as needed. Provide oxygen by nasal cannula or mask if ordered. *Use oral airway only if easy access to oral cavity is possible.*	Prevents episode of hypoxia during seizure activity.
13. Stay with client, observing sequence and timing of seizure activity.	Continued observation ensures adequate ventilation during and after seizure and will assist in

Step	Rationale
	documentation, diagnosis, and treatment of seizure disorder.
14. After seizure is over, explain what happened and answer client's questions.	Informing clients of type of seizure activity experienced will assist them in participating knowledgeably in their care.
15. For clients experiencing status epilepticus:	
a. 🔧 Insert oral airway when jaw is relaxed between seizure activity. Hold airway with curved side up, insert downward until airway reaches back of throat, then rotate and follow natural curve of tongue.	Airway occlusion and aspiration are potential complications.
b. Access oxygen and suction equipment, and prepare for IV insertion.	Intensive monitoring and treatment are required for this medical emergency.

NURSE ALERT Do not place fingers near or in the client's mouth. The client may inadvertently bite the nurse's fingers during a seizure. Do not forcibly insert an airway if the client's teeth are still clenched.

---

16. Pad side rails and headboard (Fig. 63-1).	Traumatic injury may be reduced. Avoid use of pillows to pad side rails because suffocation could occur.
17. After seizure, assist client to position of comfort in bed with padded side rails up and bed in lowest position. Place call light or intercom system within reach, and provide quiet, nonstimulating environment.	Provides for continued safety. Clients are often confused and sleepy after seizure.

Step	**Rationale**

Fig. 63-1   Padded side rails and headboard.

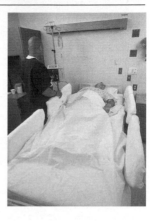

18. Offer psychosocial support; stay with client to explain what has occurred. Foster atmosphere of acceptance and respect, and provide time for client to express feelings and concerns.

Clients who accept reality of disease and integrate this reality into their own self-concept experience higher levels of self-esteem.

19. Record progression of seizure, noting type of body movement, duration.

Data assist in identification of type of seizure and source.

20. Conduct head-to-toe assessment to determine presence of any traumatic injuries resulting from seizure activity.

Injury may occur during seizure activity.

NURSE ALERT Inspect the client's oral cavity for broken teeth and breaks in mucous membrane caused by bites.

21. Assess client's mental status after seizure (level of consciousness, confusion, hallucinations).

Temporary mental status changes are common after seizure.

22. Assess for bowel or bladder incontinence.

Loss of bowel or bladder control can increase client anxiety and risk of skin breakdown.

Step	Rationale
23. Observe client's color and respiratory rate and pattern during and after seizure.	Client may experience shallow, irregular breathing during seizure, but normal color and respirations should be apparent after episode.
24. Complete postprocedure protocol.	

Recording and Reporting

- Record timing of seizure activity and sequence of events, presence of aura (if any), level of consciousness, posture, color, movements of extremities, incontinence, and client's status immediately after seizure.
- Report to physician immediately as seizure begins. Status epilepticus is emergency situation requiring immediate medical therapy.

Unexpected Outcomes	Related Interventions
1. Client suffers traumatic injury.	• Attend to client's immediate physical needs, inform physician of injury, reassess client's environment to ensure that environment is free of safety hazards, complete incident report, and communicate to other care providers measures taken to reduce risk for further injury.
2. Client's airway becomes occluded, and materials are aspirated.	• Turn onto side, insert oral airway (if possible), and apply suction to remove materials and maintain patent airway.
	• Maintain nasal oxygen.

Sequential Compression Device and Elastic Stockings

Prevention is the best method to reduce the risk of deep vein thrombosis (DVT) secondary to immobility. Early ambulation remains the most effective preventive measure (Phipps and others, 2003). However, at times, early ambulation is not an option, particularly in the critically ill client. Early application of sequential compression devices (SCDs) or elastic stockings, along with low-molecular-weight or low-dose heparin therapy, has been reported as successful in preventing the development of DVT (Boccalon and others, 2000; Merli, 2000; Phipps and others, 2003).

SCDs consist of an air pump, connecting tubing, and extremity sleeves that sequentially inflate and deflate chambers within the sleeve. The intermittent pumping action drives superficial blood into deep veins, where it is evacuated proximally by the venous valves, thus removing pooled blood and preventing both venous stasis and the accumulation of clotting factors. SCDs are believed to be more effective than elastic stockings in preventing DVT.

Delegation Considerations

The skill of applying elastic stockings and an SCD may be delegated to assistive personnel (AP). The nurse initially determines the size of elastic stockings and assesses the client's lower extremities for any signs and symptoms of impaired circulation.

- Remind AP to remove the SCD sleeves from the legs before allowing the client to get out of bed. This ensures the client's safety and avoids the client becoming tangled in the SCD.
- Instruct AP to observe for signs and symptoms of allergic reactions to elastic (e.g., redness, itching, irritation) and to report these findings immediately.
- Instruct AP to inform the nurse if one calf appears larger than the other, if a calf is red and/or warm to the touch, or if the calf is painful.

Equipment

- Tape measure
- Powder or corn starch (optional)

- Elastic support stockings
- Disposable SCD sleeve(s)
- Tubing assembly
- SCD (motor)

Step	Rationale
1. Complete preprocedure protocol.	
2. Use tape measure to measure client's legs to determine proper elastic stockings and SCD sleeve size.	Stockings must be measured according to manufacturer's directions. Elastic stockings and SCD sleeves come in two lengths: knee length and thigh length. The choice of length depends on physician's order. If too large, stockings will not adequately support extremities. If too small, stockings may impede circulation.

NURSE ALERT Compare the client's measurements with the manufacturer's sizing chart. The optimum elastic stocking pressure is 20 to 30 mm Hg at the ankle, decreasing to 8 mm Hg at the middle to upper thigh. This change in pressure produces the greatest increase in venous flow velocity that is both safe and practical (Collier, 1999; Phipps and others, 2003).

Step	Rationale
3. Position client in supine position. Elevate head of bed to comfortable level.	Promotes good body mechanics for nurse. Client position eases application. Also, elastic stockings should be applied before client stands, to prevent stagnation of blood in lower extremities.
4. Apply elastic stockings:	
a. Turn elastic stocking inside out by placing one hand into sock, holding toe of sock with other hand, and pulling (Fig. 64-1).	Allows easier application of stocking.

Step	**Rationale**

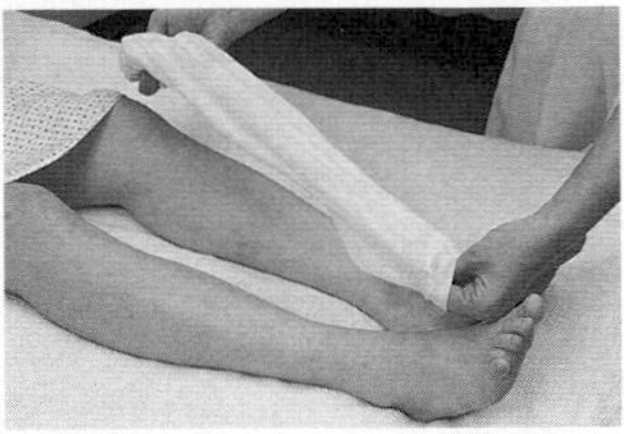

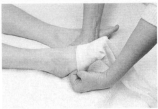

Fig. 64-1 Turn stocking inside out; hold toe and pull through.

Fig. 64-2 Place toes into foot of stocking.

b. Place client's toes into foot of elastic stocking, making sure that sock is smooth (Fig. 64-2).

Wrinkles in elastic stocking can cause constrictions and impede circulation.

c. Slide remaining portion of sock over client's foot, being sure that toes are covered. Make sure foot fits into toe and heel position of sock. Sock will now be right side out (Fig. 64-3).

If toes remain uncovered, they will become constricted by elastic and their circulation can be reduced.

d. Slide sock up over client's calf until sock is completely extended. Be sure sock is smooth and no ridges or wrinkles are present (Fig. 64-4).

e. Instruct client not to roll socks partially down.

Rolling sock partially down has constricting effect and can impede venous return.

5. Apply SCD sleeves.

a. Remove SCD sleeves from plastic, unfold, and flatten.

b. Arrange SCD sleeve under client's leg

Ensures straight and even application.

Step	**Rationale**

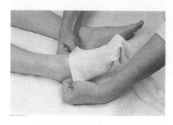

Fig. 64-3   Slide remaining portion of sock over foot.

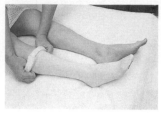

Fig. 64-4   Slide sock up leg until completely extended.

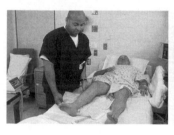

Fig. 64-5   Correct leg position on inner lining.

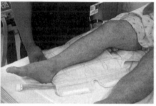

Fig. 64-6   Position back of client's knee with popliteal opening.

according to leg position indicated on inner lining of sleeve (Fig. 64-5).	
c. Place client's leg on SCD sleeve.	
d. Align back of ankle with ankle marking on inner lining of sleeve.	Correct application of SCD sleeve is important for proper functioning.
e. Position back of knee with popliteal opening (Fig. 64-6).	Prevents pressure on popliteal artery.
f. Wrap SCD sleeves securely around client's leg.	Secure fit needed for adequate compression.

Step	**Rationale**

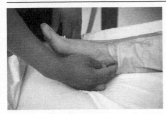

Fig. 64-7 Check fit of SCD sleeve.

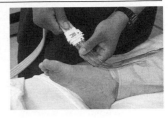

Fig. 64-8 Align arrows when connecting to mechanical unit.

g. Check fit of SCD sleeves by placing two fingers between client's leg and sleeve (Fig. 64-7).	Ensures proper fit and prevents constriction, which could impede circulation.
h. Attach SCD sleeve's connector to plug on mechanical unit. Arrows on connector line up with arrows on plug from mechanical unit (Fig. 64-8).	

NURSE ALERT Make sure the tubing and connection site are visible. Check for kinks or twisting of tubing to avoid a potential pressure ulcer.

i. Turn mechanical unit on. Green light indicates unit is functioning.	Power source initiates sequential compression cycle.
j. Monitor functioning of SCD through one full cycle of inflation and deflation.	Ensures proper functioning of unit and determines if SCD sleeves are too loose or constricting.

NURSE ALERT Remove SCD sleeves when transferring the client in and out of bed to prevent injury.

6. Complete postprocedure protocol.

Step	Rationale
7. Remove SCD sleeves or stockings at least once per shift.	

Recording and Reporting

- Record in nurses' notes the date and time of application of elastic stockings and/or SCD sleeves, condition of skin and circulatory status of lower extremities before application, length and size of elastic stockings and SCD sleeves, time elastic stockings and SCD sleeves are removed (at least once per shift), condition of skin and circulatory status after removal.
- Immediately report signs of thrombophlebitis or impeded circulation in lower extremities to charge nurse or physician.

Unexpected Outcomes	Related Interventions
1. Circulation in lower extremities decreases.	• Assess for coolness in lower extremities, cyanosis, decrease in pedal pulses, decrease in blanching, and numbness or tingling sensation. • Check that elastic stockings are not too small or have wrinkles or folds that impede circulation (Breen, 2000). • Notify physician immediately; signs and symptoms may indicate obstruction of arterial blood flow.
2. Client complains of pain in calf, tender on gentle palpation; DVT is suspected.	• Because clinical signs may be vague, obtain physician's order for more sensitive radiology tests. Doppler compression ultrasonogram (also known as *Doppler duplex*) or impedance plethysmography can rule out presence of thrombosis (Breen, 2000; Phipps and others, 2003). • Lower extremities should not be massaged because of potential for dislodging thrombus.

Unexpected Outcomes	Related Interventions
3. Client develops pulmonary embolism: tachypnea, shortness of breath, anxiety, pleuritic chest pain, cough, hemoptysis, tachycardia, and signs of right ventricular failure (i.e., distended neck veins) (Phipps and others, 2003).	• Notify physician immediately. • Monitor vital signs. • Administer supplemental oxygen as ordered. • Troubleshoot: check for kinks in tubing, air leaks, and that all connections are secure. • Get new mechanical unit.

Specialty Beds: Air-Fluidized, Air-Suspension, and Rotokinetic

Once the decision for a specialty bed is reached, it is important to determine which bed is appropriate for the client. An *air-fluidized bed* is a dynamic device designed to distribute a client's weight evenly over its support surface. The bed minimizes pressure and reduces shearing force and friction through the principle of fluidization. Fluidization is created by forcing a gentle flow of temperature-controlled air upward through a mass of microspheres that take on the properties of fluid.

Air-suspension beds are indicated for clients who are immobile or otherwise confined to the bed. The air-suspension bed supports a client's weight on air-filled cushions. The bed minimizes pressure and reduces shear in a low-air-loss system. If a client has large stage III or stage IV pressure ulcers on multiple turning surfaces, a low-air-loss bed or air-fluidized bed may be indicated (AHCPR, 1994).

The *Rotokinetic bed* is used to maintain skeletal alignment while providing constant rotation. It is used in the care of spinal cord–injured and multitrauma clients. The support structure of the bed outlines the body parts and maintains proper alignment when secured properly. This bed improves skeletal alignment with constant side-to-side rotation up to 90 degrees (Tomaselli and others, 2001). The bed rotates from side to side at a 60- to 90-degree angle every 7 minutes.

Delegation Considerations

After the nurse completes the assessment and determines the need for a specialty bed, the skill of placing the client on a specialty bed can be delegated to assistive personnel (AP). Some types of specialty beds require that the manufacturer's representative set up and maintain the system. When delegating aspects of care for a client on a support surface, the nurse must:

- Instruct AP to notify the nurse of any changes in the client's skin. The nurse then completes the skin assessment.
- Instruct AP about the normal functioning of the bed, such as inflation and deflation cycles (air-fluidized bed, air-suspension

bed), rotation of bed cycle (Rotokinetic bed), and to report to the nurse any changes in inflation, deflation, or rotation cycles or leakage of air, water, or gel (air-fluidized bed).

- Instruct AP to notify the nurse if the client becomes disoriented, becomes restless, or complains of nausea.

Equipment

- Risk assessment tool
- Specialty bed
- Gloves if drainage is present

Air-Fluidized Bed

- Foam positioning wedges, as indicated
- Filter sheet (manufacturer supplied)

Air-Suspension Bed

- Gore-Tex sheet (supplied by manufacturer)
- Disposable bed pads, if indicated

Rotokinetic Bed

- Support packs, bolsters, and safety straps as needed
- Top sheet
- Pillowcases for bolsters
- Disposable gloves (optional)

Step	Rationale
1. Complete preprocedure protocol.	
2. Determine client's risk for pressure ulcer formation using validated assessment tool. Risk factors for pressure ulcers include nutritional deficits, shear friction, alterations in mobility and perception, moisture, and abnormal serum albumin and hemoglobin levels (see Skill 56).	Risk assessment tools as suggested by Agency for Health Care Policy and Research (AHCPR) and Wound Ostomy and Continence Nurses (WOCN) (e.g., Braden scale) provide objective measure of risk consistent between nurse assessors over time (WOCN Society, 2003)
3. ![icon] Perform skin assessment. Inspect	Provides baseline to determine change in skin integrity or

Step	Rationale
condition of skin, especially over dependent sites and bony prominences.	change in existing pressure ulcer over time.
4. Assess client's level of consciousness.	Baseline used to detect change while client is on bed. Clients may become confused or disoriented from flotation sensation of bed (WOCN Society, 2003).
5. Assess client's risk for complications related to specialty beds:	Anticipates need for frequent monitoring once client is placed on support surface.
a. Air-fluidized bed:	
(1) Older adults risk dehydration from air flow.	Airflow causes insensible water loss.
(2) Risk for aspiration.	Because of inability to elevate head of bed, risk of aspiration is great, especially when feeding tube is present.
b. Air-suspension bed:	
(1) Review client's serum electrolyte levels.	Movement of air through mattress can increase client's risk for dehydration (WOCN Society, 2003).
c. Rotokinetic bed:	
(1) Determine baseline orientation level.	Rotation of bed may lead to sensory distress, especially in older adult client. This sensory distress may also present as anxiety or restlessness as well as disorientation.
6. Review instructions supplied by bed manufacturer.	Promotes safe and correct use of bed.
7. For clients with severe to moderate pain, premedicate approximately 30 minutes before transfer.	Promotes client's comfort and ability to cooperate during transfer to bed. Decreases client's energy expenditure.
8. Using safe transfer techniques, transfer client	Appropriate transfer techniques maintain alignment and reduce

Step	Rationale
to bed. Bed surface may be slippery, and transfers should not be attempted without assistance.	risk of injury during procedure. Company representative will adjust bed to client's height and weight.

a. **Air-fluidized bed** (Fig. 65-1):

Step	Rationale
(1) Turn on fluidization cycle by depressing switch; regulate temperature.	Fluidization minimizes pressure against skin's surface and reduces friction and shear force when client moves.
(2) Position client for comfort, and perform range-of-motion (ROM) exercises as appropriate.	Promotes comfort and reduces contracture formation. Bed reduces pressure on skin, but client must still be turned and exercised to avoid joint deformity or contracture (Pieper, 2000).

NURSE ALERT Never attempt to place a client face-down (prone) on an air-fluidized bed. Suffocation may occur.

Use foam wedges as needed for proper positioning. Areas supported by the foam wedges do not benefit from the bed's pressure relief surface.

Step	Rationale
(3) To turn clients, position bedpans, or perform other therapies, stop fluidization. Resume fluidization once procedure is completed.	Stopping fluidization provides firm, molded support that facilitates turning and moving client.

Fig. 65-1 Combination air-fluidized therapy and low-air-loss bed. (© 2002 Hill-Rom Services, Inc. Reprinted with permission. All rights reserved.)

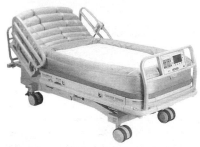

Step	Rationale

NURSE ALERT In emergencies when resuscitation is required, press cardiopulmonary resuscitation (CPR) switch and unplug unit to defluidize the bed immediately (Fig. 65-2).

b. **Air-suspension bed**
   (Fig. 65-3):
   (1) Once client is transferred, release InstaFlate™ or turn bed on by depressing switch; regulate temperature.

Pressure cushions will automatically adjust to preset levels to minimize pressure, friction, and shear (Pieper, 2000).

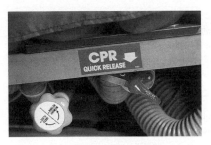

Fig. 65-2 Cardiopulmonary resuscitation switch deflates low-air-loss bed to provide hard surface.

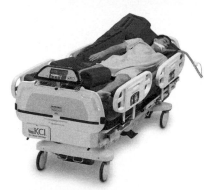

Fig. 65-3 Lateral rotation bed. (TriaDyne® Proventa™ Courtesy KCI USA, Inc. San Antonio, Tex.)

Step	Rationale
(2) Position client, and perform ROM exercises as appropriate.	Promotes comfort and reduces contracture formation. Bed reduces pressure on skin, but clients must still be turned and exercised to avoid joint deformity or contractures (AHCPR, 1994).
(3) To turn clients, position bedpans, or perform other therapies, turn on InstaFlate™ setting. Once procedure is completed, release InstaFlate™.	InstaFlate™ firms bed surface to facilitate turning and handling client. Client will not receive pressure relief while bed is in this mode.
(4) Know bed's special features, and use as needed:	
(a) Scales.	Facilitates ease of routine weights.
(b) Portable transport units to maintain inflation when primary power is interrupted.	Provides for continuous pressure relief.
(c) Availability of specialty cushions for positioning.	Reduces pressure, friction, and shearing forces.
(d) Lateral rotation (see Fig. 65-3), which allows approximately 30 degrees of turning.	Helps reduce risk and prevent pulmonary and urinary complications of reduced mobility (Cullum and others, 2003; WOCN Society, 2003).

  c. **Rotokinetic bed**
  (Fig. 65-4):
     (1) Place Rotokinetic bed in horizontal position, and

Step	Rationale

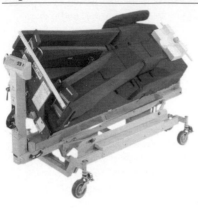

Fig. 65-4 Rotokinetic bed. (RotoRest® Delta courtesy KCI USA, Inc, San Antonio, Tex.)

remove all bolsters, straps, and supports. Close posterior hatches.	
(2) Unplug electrical cord. Lock gatch.	Prevents accidental rotation during transfer.
(3) Maintaining proper alignment of client and using appropriate transfer techniques, transfer client to Rotokinetic bed.	Reduces risk of further tissue injury during transfer. May need physician available to assist in transfer.
(4) Secure thoracic panels, bolsters, head and knee packs, and safety straps.	Maintains proper alignment and prevents sliding during rotation.
(5) Cover client with top sheet.	Prevents unnecessary exposure.
(6) Plug bed in.	
(7) Have company representative set	Rotational angle is determined by physician based on client's

Step	Rationale
optional angle as ordered by physician. May gradually increase rotation.	overall condition and tolerance to constant motion.
(8) Increase degree of rotation gradually according to client's tolerance.	Gradually increasing rotation may reduce or prevent nausea, dizziness, and orthostatic hypotension (Tomaselli and others, 2001).
(9) It is difficult to maintain eye contact when talking with clients during rotation. Provide adequate space for caregivers and family to move around bed to facilitate communication.	Allows opportunity to meet client's psychological needs.
(10) Bed may be stopped for assessment and procedures. To stop bed, permit bed to rotate to desired position, turn motor off, and push knob into lock position. If necessary, bed can be manually repositioned.	Allows nurse to assess client.
(11) Inform client that client may experience sensation of light-headedness or falling. However,	Informing client of what to expect will decrease client's anxiety.

Step	Rationale
reassure client that he or she will not fall because pads are positioned to prevent this and are checked by two people to ensure proper placement.	
9. Inspect condition of client's skin periodically while client is on bed.	Determines if any new pressure areas are forming.
10. Assess client's level of orientation.	Determines onset of perceptual changes.
11. Complete postprocedure protocol.	

Recording and Reporting

- Record in nurses' notes or skin assessment flowsheet the transfer of client to bed, tolerance of procedure, level of orientation, comfort, restlessness, and condition of skin.
- Report changes in condition of skin, level of orientation, and electrolyte levels to physician.

Unexpected Outcomes	Related Interventions
1. Existing areas of skin breakdown or pressure areas fail to heal or increase in size or depth.	• Modify skin care regimen. • Revise turning schedule. • Consult with skin care expert. • Notify physician.
2. Client is restless, confused, or agitated.	• Notify physician. • Determine need for antianxiety medication. • Evaluate alternative pressure-relief devices.
3. Client becomes nauseated.	• Provide short-term antiemetics. • If lateral rotation is used, decrease cycle frequency.

Sterile Gloving

Gloves help prevent the transmission of pathogens by direct and indirect contact. Nurses don sterile gloves before performing sterile procedures such as inserting urinary catheters, or applying sterile dressings. It is important to select the proper size glove. The gloves should not stretch so tightly over the fingers that they can easily tear, yet they should be tight enough that objects can be picked up easily. Sterile gloves are available in "one size fits all" as well as specific sizes such as 6, 6½, and 7.

Many clients and health care workers have known allergies to latex, the natural rubber used in most gloves and other medical products (DeCastro, 2002). Box 66-1 lists individuals who are at risk for latex allergy. Latex proteins enter the body through skin or mucous membranes, intravascularly, or via inhalation. The cornstarch powder used to make latex gloves slip on easily over the hands is a carrier of the latex proteins (Burt, 1998). When gloves are applied or removed, the cornstarch particles become airborne and can remain so for hours. The latex can then be inhaled or settle on clothing, skin, or mucous membranes. Reactions to latex can be mild to severe (Box 66-2). For individuals at high risk or with suspected sensitivity to latex, it is important to choose latex-free or synthetic gloves.

Delegation Considerations

The skill of donning and removing sterile gloves can be delegated to assistive personnel (AP). However, many procedures that require the use of sterile gloves cannot be delegated to AP. (Refer to specific skill recommendations.)

Equipment

- Package of proper size sterile gloves: latex or synthetic nonlatex.

Step	Rationale
1. Consider type of procedure to be performed.	Ensures proper use of sterile gloves when needed.
2. Consider client's risk for infection, for example, preexisting condition and size or extent of area being treated.	Directs nurse to follow added precautions (e.g., use of additional protective barriers) if necessary.

BOX 66-1   Individuals at Risk for Latex Allergy

- Spina bifida
- Congenital or urogenital defects
- History of indwelling catheters or repeated catheterizations
- History of using condom catheters
- High latex exposure (e.g., health care workers, housekeepers, food handlers, tire manufacturers, workers in industries that use gloves routinely)
- History of multiple childhood surgeries
- History of food allergies

Modified from Gritter M: The latex threat, *Am J Nurs* 98(9):26, 1998; and Kim KT and others: Implementation recommendations for making health care facilities latex safe, *AORN J* 67(3):615, 1998.

BOX 66-2   Levels of Latex Reactions

The following are three types of common latex reactions, listed in order of severity:
1. **Irritant dermatitis**—a nonallergic response characterized by skin redness and itching.
2. **Type IV hypersensitivity**—cell-mediated allergic reaction to chemicals used in latex processing. Reaction can be delayed up to 48 hours, including redness, itching, and hives. Localized swelling, red and itchy or runny eyes and nose, and coughing may develop.
3. **Type I allergic reaction**—a true latex allergy that can be life-threatening. Reactions vary based on type of latex protein and degree of individual sensitivity, including local and systemic. Symptoms include hives, generalized edema, itching, rash, wheezing, bronchospasm, difficulty breathing, laryngeal edema, diarrhea, nausea, hypotension, tachycardia, and respiratory or cardiac arrest.

Modified from Gritter M: The latex threat, *Am J Nurs* 98(9):26, 1998.

Step	Rationale
3. Examine glove package to determine if it is dry and intact.	Torn or wet package is considered contaminated.
4. Inspect condition of hands for cuts, open lesions, or	When strict surgical asepsis is used, presence of such lesions

Step	**Rationale**
abrasions. Lesions harbor microorganisms and should be covered with impervious dressing.	may prevent nurse from participating in procedure.
5. Assess client for following risk factors before donning latex gloves:	Determines level of client's risk for latex allergy and need to use nonlatex gloves.
a. Previous reaction to following items within hours of exposure: adhesive tape, dental or face mask, golf club grip, ostomy bag, rubber band, balloon, bandage, elastic underwear, intravenous (IV) tubing, rubber gloves, condom.	
b. Personal history of asthma, contact dermatitis, eczema, urticaria, rhinitis.	
c. History of food allergies, especially avocado, banana, peach, chestnut, raw potato, kiwi, tomato, papaya.	
d. Previous adverse reactions during surgery, dental procedure.	
e. Previous reaction to latex product.	
6. Select correct size and type of gloves.	Chance of contamination is less if correct size of gloves is worn.

NURSE ALERT Synthetic nonlatex gloves are necessary for clients at risk and for nurses who have sensitivity or allergy to latex.

7. Place glove package near work area.	Ensures availability before procedure.

Step	**Rationale**
8. Donning gloves:	
a. Perform thorough hand hygiene.	Reduces number of bacteria on skin surfaces and reduces transmission of infection.
b. Remove outer glove package wrapper by carefully separating and peeling apart sides (Fig. 66-1).	Prevents inner glove package from accidentally opening and touching contaminated objects.
c. Grasp inner package, and lay it on clean, dry, flat surface at waist level. Open package, keeping gloves on wrapper's inside surface (Fig. 66-2).	Sterile object held below waist is contaminated. Inner surface of glove package is sterile.
d. Identify right and left glove. Each glove has cuff approximately 5 cm (2 inches) wide. Glove dominant hand first.	Proper identification of gloves prevents contamination by improper fit. Gloving of dominant hand first improves dexterity.
e. With thumb and first two fingers of nondominant hand, grasp edge of cuff of glove for dominant hand. Touch only glove's inside surface (Fig. 66-3).	Inner edge of cuff will lie against skin and thus is not sterile.

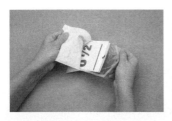

Fig. 66-1 Open outer glove package wrapper.

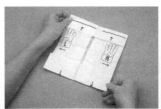

Fig. 66-2 Open inner glove package on work surface.

Step	Rationale

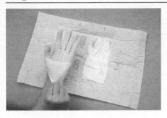

Fig. 66-3   Pick up glove for dominant hand, insert fingers, and pull glove completely over dominant hand (example is for left-handed person).

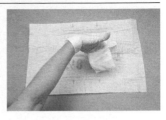

Fig. 66-4   Pick up glove for nondominant hand.

f. Carefully pull glove over dominant hand, leaving cuff and being sure cuff does not roll up wrist. Be sure thumb and fingers are in proper spaces.

If glove's outer surface touches hand or wrist, it is contaminated.

g. With gloved dominant hand, slip fingers underneath second glove's cuff (Fig. 66-4).

Cuff protects gloved fingers. Sterile touching sterile prevents glove contamination.

h. Carefully pull second glove over nondominant hand, keeping gloved dominant thumb abducted (Fig. 66-5).

Contact of gloved hand with exposed hand results in contamination.

i After second glove is on, interlock hands together, above waist level. The cuffs usually fall down after application. Be sure to touch only sterile sides.

Ensures smooth fit over fingers.

9. Glove removal:
  a. Grasp outside of one cuff with other gloved

Minimizes contamination of underlying skin.

Step	**Rationale**

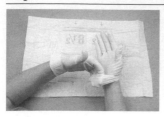 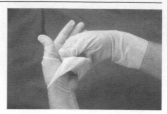

Fig. 66-5   Pull second glove over nondominant hand.

Fig. 66-6   Carefully remove first glove by turning it inside out.

hand; avoid touching wrist.

b. Pull glove off, turning it inside out (Fig. 66-6). Discard in receptacle.

Outside of glove does not touch skin surface.

c. Tuck fingers of bare hand inside remaining glove cuff. Peel glove off inside out. Discard in receptacle.

Fingers do not touch contaminated glove surface.

10. Perform hand hygiene.

Recording and Reporting

- It is not necessary to record donning of gloves. Record specific procedure performed and client's response and status.

Unexpected Outcomes	Related Interventions
1. Client develops localized or systemic signs of infection.	• Contact physician, and implement appropriate treatments as ordered.
2. Client develops allergic reaction to latex (see Box 66-2).	• Immediately remove source of latex.
	• Bring emergency equipment to bedside. Have epinephrine injection ready for administration, and be prepared to initiate IV fluids and oxygen.

Sterile Technique: Donning and Removing Cap, Mask, and Protective Eyewear

Masks, caps, and protective eyewear are worn in surgical procedure areas. However, certain surgical aseptic procedures, such as central line dressing changes performed at a client's bedside, also might require these barriers. When exposure to splattering of blood or body fluid is a risk, a mask and protective eyewear are needed. As in all situations that require protection from blood or body fluid splatters, you should follow Standard Precautions (see Skill 37).

Delegation Considerations

The skill of donning and removing cap, mask, and protective eyewear can be delegated to assistive personnel (AP). However, the procedures performed at a client's bedside that require protective barriers generally cannot be delegated (refer to specific skill recommendations).

Equipment

- Mask
- Surgical cap (NOTE: Use only if hospital policy requires, or use to secure hair if contamination of a sterile field is possible.)
- Hairpins, rubber bands, or both
- Protective eyewear (e.g., goggles or glasses with appropriate side shields)

Step	Rationale
1. Consider type of sterile procedure to be performed (consult agency policy).	Not all sterile procedures require mask, cap, or eyewear.
2. If you have symptoms of cold or respiratory infection, either avoid participating in procedure or don mask.	Greater number of pathogenic microorganisms reside within respiratory tract when infection is present.

Step	Rationale
3. Assess client's actual or potential risk for infection when choosing barriers for surgical asepsis.	Some clients are at greater risk for acquiring infection, so nurse uses additional barriers.
4. Prepare equipment, and inspect packaging for integrity and exposure to sterilization.	Ensures availability of equipment and sterility of supplies before procedure begins.
5. Don cap:	
a. If hair is long, comb back behind ears and secure.	Cap must cover all hair entirely.
b. Secure hair in place with pins.	Long hair should not fall down or cause cap to slip and expose hair.
c. Place cap over head as you would place hairnet. Be sure all hair fits under cap's edges (Fig. 67-1).	Loose hair hanging over sterile field or falling dander may result in contamination of objects on sterile field.
6. Don mask:	
a. Find top edge of mask, which usually has thin metal strip along edge.	Pliable metal fits snugly against bridge of nose.
b. Hold mask by top two strings or loops, keeping top edge above bridge of nose.	Prevents contact of hands with clean facial portion of mask. Mask will cover all of nose.
c. Tie two top strings at top of back of head, over cap (if worn), with	Position of ties at top of head provides tight fit. Strings over ears may cause irritation.

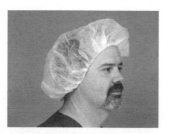

Fig. 67-1 Nurse places cap over head, covering all hair.

Step	**Rationale**

strings above ears
(Fig. 67-2).

d. Tie two lower ties
snugly around neck
with mask well under
chin (Fig. 67-3).

Prevents escape of
microorganisms through sides of
mask as nurse talks and breathes.

e. Gently pinch upper
metal band around
bridge of nose.

Prevents microorganisms from
escaping around nose.

7. Don protective
eyewear:

a. Place glasses, goggles,
or face shield
comfortably over eyes,
and check that vision is
clear (Fig. 67-4).

Positioning can affect clarity of
vision.

b. Be sure eyewear fits
snugly around forehead
and face.

Ensures that eyes are fully
protected.

Fig. 67-2 Tie top strings of mask.

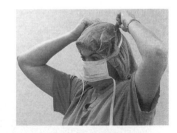

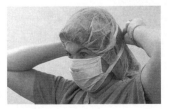

Fig. 67-3 Tie bottom strings of
mask.

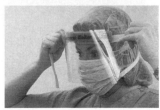

Fig. 67-4 Place face shield over cap.

Step	Rationale
8. Disposing of protective equipment and removing eyewear:	
a. Remove gloves first, if worn (see Skill 66).	Prevents contamination of hair, neck, and facial area.
b. While holding onto strings, untie top strings of mask first (Fig. 67-5).	Prevents top part of mask from falling down over nurse's uniform. Contaminated surface of mask could then contaminate uniform.
c. Hold strings while untying bottom strings of mask, and remove mask from face, holding ties securely. Discard mask in proper receptacle.	Avoids contact of nurse's hands with contaminated mask.
d. Remove eyewear, avoiding placing hands over soiled lens.	Prevents transmission of microorganisms.

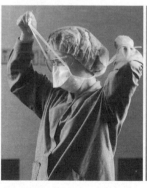 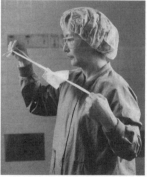

A   B

Fig. 67-5 A, Untying top mask strings. B, Removing mask from face. (From Phipps W and others: *Medical-surgical nursing: concepts and clinical practice,* ed 6, St Louis, 1999, Mosby.)

Step	Rationale
e. Grasp outer surface of cap, and lift from hair.	Minimizes contact of hands with hair.
f. Discard cap in proper receptacle, and perform hand hygiene.	Reduces transmission of infection.

Recording and Reporting

■ No recording or reporting is required for this set of skills. Record specific procedure performed in nurses' progress notes.

Subcutaneous Injections

A subcutaneous (Sub-Q) injection deposits medication into the loose connective tissue underlying the dermis. Subcutaneous tissue is not as richly supplied with blood vessels as muscles; thus drugs are not absorbed as quickly as those given intramuscularly (IM). Anything affecting local blood flow to tissues, such as physical exercise or the local application of hot or cold compresses, influences the rate of drug absorption. Conditions such as circulatory shock or occlusive vascular disease impair clients' blood flow and thus contraindicate Sub-Q injections.

Give only small doses of medications (0.5 to 1 ml) Sub-Q. The tissue is sensitive to irritating solutions and large volumes of medications. Medications collecting within the tissues cause sterile abscesses, which appear as hardened, painful lumps. The best sites for Sub-Q injections include vascular areas around the outer aspect of the upper arms, the abdomen from below the costal margins to the iliac crests, and the anterior aspect of the thighs (Fig. 68-1).

Rotation of injection sites for insulin administration from major site to major site is no longer necessary because the newer human insulins carry a much lower risk for hypertrophy. Therefore clients can choose one anatomical area (e.g., the abdomen) and systematically rotate sites within that region. This helps maintain consistency in insulin absorption from day to day. Once all potential sites within an area are used, the client may choose either to move to another anatomical site (e.g., the thigh) or to start the rotation pattern over in the same anatomical area (ADA, 2004).

Heparin, a drug given Sub-Q, suppresses clot formation. Therefore clients receiving heparin are at risk for bleeding. Be alert for signs of bleeding gums, hematemesis, hematuria, or melena in clients who receive long-term anticoagulation therapy.

Delegation Considerations

Administering Sub-Q injections should not be delegated to assistive personnel (AP).

- Instruct AP about drug reactions (e.g., bleeding) to report or the client's report of pain at the injection site.
- Have AP report any change in the client's condition, including any change in vital signs or level of consciousness.

Fig. 68-1 Common sites for subcutaneous injections.

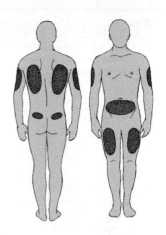

Equipment
- Syringe (1 to 3 ml)
- Needle (25 to 27 gauge, ⅜ to ⅝ inch)
- Alcohol swab
- Small gauze pad (optional)
- Medication ampule or vial
- Disposable gloves
- Medication administration record (MAR) or computer printout

Step	Rationale
1. Complete preprocedure protocol.	
2. Review provider's medication order for client's name, drug name, dose, time, and route of administration against MAR.	Ensures safe and correct administration of medication by verifying order.
3. Check medication's expiration date printed on vial or ampule.	Medications that have expired should not be used because potency of medications changes when medications became outdated.
4. Check name of medication on vial/ampule label against MAR.	First check of label; ensures that client receives correct medication.

Step	Rationale
5. Prepare correct medication dose from ampule or vial (see Skill 49). Check dose carefully.	Ensures that medication is sterile and dose is accurate. Preparation techniques differ for ampule and vial.
6. Compare MAR with prepared drugs and continue.	Reading label second time reduces error.
7. Compare dose in syringe against desired dose on MAR.	Final check ensures correct dosage.
8. Identify client by checking identification bracelet and asking client's name. Compare with MAR.	Ensures that correct client is receiving medication. At least two patient identifiers (neither to be patient's room number) are to be used whenever administering medications (JCAHO, 2004).
9. Keep sheet or gown draped over body parts not requiring exposure.	Respects client's dignity while area to be injected is exposed.
10. Position client and select appropriate injection site. Inspect skin's surface over site for bruises, inflammation, or edema. Palpate site for masses, edema, or tenderness. NOTE:	Injection site should be free of lesions that might interfere with drug absorption.
• When administering heparin Sub-Q, use abdominal injection sites.	Anticoagulant may cause local bleeding and bruising when injected into areas such as arms and legs, which are involved in muscular activity.
• When administering low-molecular-weight (LMW) heparin Sub-Q, choose site on right or left side of abdomen, at least 2 inches away from umbilicus.	Injecting LMW heparin on side of abdomen will help decrease pain and bruising at injection site (Aventis, 2003).
• When administering insulin, rotate injection	Rotating insulin sites within same anatomical area helps maintain

Step	**Rationale**
site within same anatomical area and systematically rotate sites within that area. Once all potential sites within that area are used, move to another anatomical site or start rotation pattern over in same anatomical area.	consistency in insulin absorption from day to day (ADA, 2004).

NURSE ALERT Applying ice to the injection site for 5 minutes before and after the injection may decrease the client's perception of pain (Kuzu and Ucar, 2001).

11. Be sure that needle size is correct by grasping skinfold at site with thumb and forefinger. Measure skinfold from top to bottom; be sure that needle is approximately half this length.	Sub-Q injections can be inadvertently given in muscle, especially in abdomen and thigh sites. Appropriate size of needle ensures that medication will be injected into Sub-Q tissue as ordered.
12. Instruct client to relax arm, leg, or abdomen, depending on site chosen for injection. Talk with client about subject of interest.	Relaxation of area minimizes discomfort during injection. Promoting client's comfort through distraction helps reduce anxiety.
13. Cleanse site with antiseptic swab (Fig. 68-2). Apply swab at center of site, and rotate outward in circular direction for about 5 cm (2 inches).	Mechanical action of swab removes secretions containing microorganisms.
14. Hold swab or square of sterile gauze between third and fourth fingers of nondominant hand.	Swab or gauze remains readily accessible for when needle is withdrawn.
15. Remove safety sheath from needle by pulling it straight off.	Preventing needle from touching sides of sheath prevents contamination.

Step	Rationale

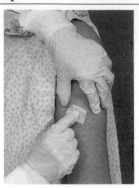

Fig. 68-2 Cleansing site with circular motion.

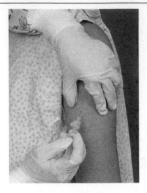

Fig. 68-3 Holding syringe as if grasping a dart

16. Hold syringe between thumb and forefinger of dominant hand as if grasping dart, holding syringe across tops of fingertips (Fig. 68-3).

Quick, smooth injection requires proper manipulation of syringe parts.

17. Administer injection:
    a. For average-size client, spread skin tightly across injection site or pinch skin with nondominant hand.

Needle penetrates tight skin more easily than loose skin. Pinching skin elevates Sub-Q tissue.

    b. Inject needle quickly and firmly at 45- to 90-degree angle (then release skin, if pinched).

Quick, firm insertion minimizes discomfort. (Injecting medication into compressed tissue irritates nerve fibers.)

    c. For obese client, pinch skin at site and inject needle at 90-degree angle below tissue fold.

Obese clients have fatty layer of tissue above Sub-Q layer.

18. After needle enters site, grasp lower end of syringe barrel with nondominant

Properly performed injection requires smooth manipulation of syringe parts. Movement of

Step	Rationale
hand. Move dominant hand to end of plunger, and slowly inject medication. Avoid moving syringe (Fig. 68-4).	syringe may displace needle and cause discomfort.

NURSE ALERT Aspiration before injecting a Sub-Q medication is not necessary. Piercing a blood vessel in a Sub-Q injection is rare. Aspiration before injecting heparin and insulin is not recommended (ADA, 2004; McConnell, 2000).

19. Withdraw needle quickly while placing antiseptic swab or sterile gauze gently above or over site.	Supporting tissues around injection site minimizes discomfort during needle withdrawal. Dry gauze may reduce discomfort associated with alcohol on nonintact skin.
20. Apply gentle pressure to site. *Do not massage site.* (If heparin is given, press alcohol swab or gauze continuously to site for 30 to 60 seconds.)	Aids absorption. Massage can damage underlying tissue.
21. Assist client to comfortable position.	Gives client sense of well-being.
22. Discard uncapped needle or needle enclosed in safety	Prevents injury to client and health care personnel. Recapping

Fig. 68-4   Subcutaneous injection.

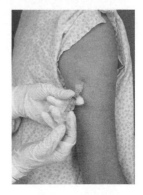

Step	Rationale
shield and attached syringe into sharps receptacle. 23. Complete postprocedure protocol.	needles increases risk of needle-stick injury (OSHA, 2001).

Recording and Reporting

- Immediately after administration, chart medication dose, route, site, time, and date given on MAR. Correctly sign MAR according to institutional policy.
- Record client's response to medication.
- Report any undesirable effects from medication to client's health care provider, and document adverse effects according to institutional policy.

Unexpected Outcomes	Related Interventions
1. Client complains of localized pain or continued burning at injection site.	• Assess injection site for abscess formation. • Monitor client's temperature. • Notify client's health provider, and do not reuse site (Gilsenan, 2000).
2. Client displays signs of adverse reaction, including urticaria, eczema, pruritus, wheezing, and dyspnea.	• Follow institutional policy or guidelines for appropriate response to allergic reactions, and notify client's health care provider immediately.

Suctioning:
Closed (In-line)

Delegation Considerations

The skill of airway suction with a closed (in-line) suction catheter is not routinely delegated to assistive personnel (AP). In special situations, such as suctioning a permanent tracheostomy, this procedure may be delegated to AP. The nurse is responsible for the cardiopulmonary assessment of the client, and before delegation the nurse must:

- Instruct AP regarding any individualized aspects of client care that pertain to suctioning (e.g., position, duration of suction, pressure settings).
- Inform AP about the expected quality, quantity, and color of secretions and to inform the nurse immediately if changes occur (e.g., changes in vital signs, complaints of pain, shortness of breath, confusion, or increased restlessness).

Equipment

- Closed system or in-line suction catheter
- Suction machine
- 6 feet of connecting tubing
- Two clean gloves (optional)
- Face shield

Steps

1. Complete preprocedure protocol and perform assessment as in Skill 70.
2. ✂ Perform hand hygiene, and attach suction.
   a. In many institutions, catheter is attached to mechanical ventilator circuit by respiratory therapist. If catheter is not already in place, open suction catheter package using aseptic technique, attach closed suction catheter to ventilator circuit by removing swivel adapter and placing closed suction catheter apparatus on endotracheal tube (ET) or tracheostomy tube, and connect Y on mechanical ventilator circuit to closed suction catheter with flex tubing (Fig. 69-1).
   b. Connect one end of connecting tubing to suction machine, and connect other to end of closed system or

Steps

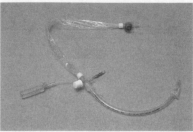

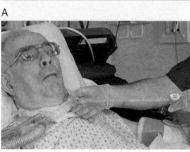

Fig. 69-1 A, Closed system suction catheter attached to endotracheal tube. B, Suctioning tracheostomy with closed system suction catheter.

in-line suction catheter, if not already done. Turn suction device on, and set vacuum regulator to appropriate negative pressure (see manufacturer's directions). Many closed system suction catheters require slightly higher suction pressures; consult manufacturer's guidelines (Connelly and Stone, 1991).

3. Hyperinflate and/or hyperoxygenate client with bag-valve-mask or manual breathing mechanism on mechanical ventilator according to institution protocol and clinical status (usually 100% oxygen).
4. Unlock suction control mechanism if required by manufacturer. Open saline port, and attach saline syringe or vial.
5. Pick up suction catheter enclosed in plastic sleeve with dominant hand.

NURSE ALERT The use of normal saline instillation with closed in-line suction catheters may not be appropriate for all clients and needs further investigation. Normal saline instillation in conjunction with ET suctioning may

Steps

lead to the dispersion of microorganisms into the lower respiratory tract (Fretag and others, 2003; Sole and others, 2003).

6. Insert catheter; use repeating maneuver of pushing catheter and sliding (or pulling) plastic sleeve back between thumb and forefinger until resistance is felt or client coughs.

7. Encourage client to cough, and apply suction by squeezing on suction control mechanism while withdrawing catheter. It is difficult to apply intermittent pulses of suction and nearly impossible to rotate catheter compared with standard catheter. Be sure to withdraw catheter completely into plastic sheath so it does not obstruct airflow.

8. Reassess cardiopulmonary status, including pulse oximetry, to determine need for subsequent suctioning or complications. Repeat Steps 6 and 7 one or two more times to clear secretions. Allow adequate time (at least 1 full minute) between suction passes for ventilation and reoxygenation.

9. When airway is clear, withdraw catheter completely into sheath. Be sure that colored indicator line on catheter is visible in sheath. Squeeze vial or push syringe while applying suction to rinse inner lumen of catheter. Use at least 5 to 10 ml of saline to rinse catheter until it is clear of retained secretions, which can cause bacterial growth and increase risk of infection (Fretag and others, 2003). Lock suction mechanism, if applicable, and turn off suction.

10. If client requires nasal suctioning, perform Skill 70 with separate standard suction catheter.

11. Complete postprocedure protocol.

Suctioning: Nasopharyngeal, Nasotracheal, and Artificial Airway

The major differences between oropharyngeal and tracheal airway suctioning are the depth suctioned and the potential for complications. Tracheal airway suctioning extends into the lower airway and necessitates aseptic technique. Suctioning is necessary to remove respiratory secretions and maintain optimum ventilation and oxygenation in clients who are unable to independently remove these secretions (Moore, 2003). The nurse assesses the client to determine frequency and depth of suctioning. Some clients may require suctioning every hour or two, whereas others need to be suctioned only once or twice a day. How far to insert the suction catheter for tracheal suctioning depends on the size of the client, especially children.

Delegation Considerations

The skills of nasotracheal and artificial airway tube suctioning may be routinely delegated to assistive personnel (AP). When the client is assessed by the nurse to be stable, the skill of performing tracheostomy tube suctioning can be delegated to AP. These situations include clients with permanent tracheostomy tubes and clients receiving mechanical ventilation at home. Before delegating these skills, the nurse must:

- Discuss with AP any unique modifications of the skill, such as the need for supplemental oxygen, the use of a clean versus sterile suction technique, limits for suctioning the tracheostomy tube.
- Instruct AP about signs and symptoms of hypoxemia, such as change in the client's respiratory status, secretions, confusion, and restlessness, and to report these signs immediately to the nurse.

Equipment

- Appropriate size suction catheter (smallest diameter that will remove secretions effectively)
- Nasal or oral airway (if indicated)
- Two sterile gloves or one sterile and one nonsterile glove
- Clean towel or paper drape

- Suction machine
- Mask or face shield
- Connecting tubing (6 feet)
- Small Y-adapter (if catheter does not have a suction control port)
- Water-soluble lubricant
- Sterile basin
- Sterile normal saline solution or water, about 100 ml
- Portable or wall suction apparatus

Step	Rationale
1. Complete preprocedure protocol.	
2. Assess signs and symptoms of upper and lower airway obstruction requiring nasal or oral tracheal suctioning, including wheezes, crackles, or gurgling on inspiration or expiration; restlessness; ineffective coughing; unilateral, segmental, or lobar absent or diminished breath.	Physical signs and symptoms result from decreased oxygen to tissues, as well as pooling of secretions in upper and lower airways. Assessment should be completed before and after suction procedure (Moore, 2003).
3. Determine presence of apprehension, anxiety, decreased level of consciousness, increased fatigue, dizziness, behavioral changes, increased pulse rate, increased rate of breathing, decreased depth of breathing, elevated blood pressure.	Signs and symptoms associated with hypoxia (low oxygen at cellular or tissue level), hypoxemia (low oxygen tension in blood), or hypercapnia (elevated carbon dioxide tension in blood). Clients report sensations of pain and discomfort with suctioning procedure, and as result, anxiety may be present before suctioning. Anxiety and pain consume oxygen and in turn worsen signs of hypoxia (Puntillo and others, 2002).
4. Assess for risk factors for upper or lower airway obstruction.	Presence of these risk factors may impair client's ability to clear secretions from airway and may

Step	Rationale
	necessitate nasopharyngeal or nasotracheal suctioning.
5. Assess the following areas that may influence or affect airway function:	
a. Fluid status.	Fluid overload may increase amount of secretions. Dehydration promotes thicker secretions.
b. Lack of humidity.	Environment influences secretion formation and gas exchange, necessitating airway suctioning when client cannot clear secretions effectively.
c. Infection (e.g., pneumonia).	Clients with respiratory infections are prone to increased secretions that are thicker and sometimes more difficult to expectorate.
6. Identify contraindications to nasotracheal suctioning: a. Facial trauma/surgery. b. Bleeding disorders. c. Nasal bleeding. d. Epiglottitis or croup. e. Laryngospasm. f. Irritable airway.	These conditions are contraindications because passage of catheter through nasal route can cause additional trauma, increase nasal bleeding, or cause severe bleeding in presence of bleeding disorders. In presence of epiglottitis, croup, laryngospasm, or irritable airway, entrance of suction catheter via nasal route can cause intractable coughing, hypoxemia, and severe bronchospasm necessitating emergency intubation or tracheostomy (Moore, 2003).
7. Place towel across client's chest, if needed.	Reduces transmission of microorganisms by protecting gown from secretions.
8. ✈ Perform hand hygiene, and apply face shield if splashing is likely.	Reduces transmission of microorganisms.
9. Connect one end of connecting tubing to	Excessive negative pressure damages nasopharyngeal and

Step	Rationale
suction machine, and place other end in convenient location near client. Turn suction device on, and set vacuum regulator to appropriate negative pressure.	tracheal mucosa and can induce greater hypoxia.
10. If indicated, increase supplemental oxygen therapy to 100% or as ordered by physician. Encourage client deep breathing.	Hyperoxygenation provides some protection from suction-induced decline in oxygenation. Hyperoxygenation is most effective in presence of hyperinflation, such as encouraging client to deep breathe or increasing ventilator tidal volume settings (Moore, 2003).
11. Prepare suction catheter:	
a. One-time-use catheter:	
(1) Open suction kit or catheter with use of aseptic technique. If sterile drape is available, place it across client's chest or on over-bed table.	Maintains asepsis and reduces transmission of microorganisms.
(2) Unwrap or open sterile basin, and place on bedside table. Fill with about 100 ml sterile normal saline solution or water (Fig. 70-1).	Saline or water is used to clean tubing after each suction pass.
(3) Open lubricant. Squeeze small amount onto open sterile catheter package without touching package.	Prepares lubricant while maintaining sterility. Water-soluble lubricant is used to avoid lipoid aspiration pneumonia. Excessive lubricant can occlude catheter.

Step	Rationale

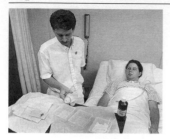

Fig. 70-1 Pouring sterile saline into tray.

NOTE: Lubricant is not necessary for artificial airway suctioning.

b. Closed (in-line) suction catheter: See Skill 69.

12. Turn on suction device, and set regulator to appropriate pressure.

Excessive negative pressure can result in damage to nasopharyngeal and tracheal mucosa and can increase suction-induced hypoxia.

13. Place sterile glove on each hand or place nonsterile glove on nondominant hand and sterile glove on dominant hand.

Reduces transmission of microorganisms and allows nurse to maintain sterility of suction catheter.

14. Pick up suction catheter with dominant hand. Pick up connecting tubing with nondominant hand. Secure catheter to tubing (Fig. 70-2).

Maintains catheter sterility. Connects catheter to suction.

15. Check that equipment is functioning properly by suctioning small amount of normal saline solution from basin.

Ensures equipment function. Lubricates internal catheter and tubing.

16. Suction airway:
   a. Nasopharyngeal and nasotracheal suctioning:

Step	**Rationale**

Fig. 70-2 Attaching catheter to suction.

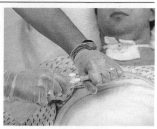

(1) Lightly coat distal 6 to 8 cm (2 to 3 inches) of catheter with water-soluble lubricant.

Lubricates catheter for easier insertion.

(2) Remove oxygen delivery device, Without applying suction and using dominant thumb and forefinger, gently but quickly insert catheter into naris during inhalation, and following natural course of naris, slightly slant catheter downward or through mouth. Do not force through naris (Fig. 70-3).

Application of suction pressure while introducing catheter into trachea increases risk of damage to mucosa and increases risk of hypoxia because of removal of entrained oxygen present in airways.

(a) Nasopharyngeal suctioning (without applying suction): Adults; insert catheter about

Ensures that catheter tip is positioned correctly in pharynx for suctioning.

Step	**Rationale**

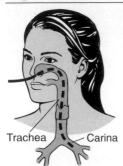

Trachea   Carina

Fig. 70-3 Pathway for nasotracheal catheter progression.

16 cm (6 inches); older children, 8 to 12 cm (3 to 5 inches); infants and young children, 4 to 8 cm (2 to 3 inches).

(b) Nasotracheal suctioning (without applying suction): Adults, insert catheter about 20 cm (8 inches); older children, 14 to 20 cm (5½ to 8 inches); and infants and young children, 8 to 14 cm (3 to 5½ inches).

NURSE ALERT When the catheter is difficult to pass, ask the client to cough or to say "ahh" or try to advance the catheter during inspiration. Coughing or saying "ahh" opens the glottis to permit passage of the catheter into the trachea.

Step	Rationale
(c) Positioning: In some instances, turning client's head to right helps suction left mainstem bronchus; turning head to left helps suction right mainstem bronchus.	Turning client's head to side elevates bronchial passage on opposite side.

NURSE ALERT When performing nasotracheal suctioning, perform tracheal suctioning before pharyngeal suctioning. The mouth and pharynx contain more bacteria than the trachea does. If copious oral secretions are present, suction the oral cavity with a Yankauer catheter first.

(3) Apply intermittent suction for up to 10 seconds (Moore, 2003) by placing and releasing nondominant thumb over vent of catheter and slowly withdrawing catheter while rotating it back and forth between dominant thumb and forefinger.	Intermittent suction and rotation of catheter prevent injury to mucosa. If catheter "grabs" mucosa, remove thumb to release suction. Suctioning longer than 10 seconds can cause cardiopulmonary compromise, usually from hypoxemia or vagal overload.

NURSE ALERT If the client's pulse drops more than 20 beats per minute or increases more than 40 beats per minute or if SpO_2 falls below 90% or 5% from baseline, cease suctioning; perform respiratory assessment, hyperoxygenate, and/or position the client.

(4) Rinse catheter and connecting tubing with normal saline	Secretions that remain in suction catheter or connecting tubing decrease suctioning efficiency.

Step	**Rationale**
or water until cleared.	
(5) Assess for need to repeat suctioning procedure. Observe for alterations in cardiopulmonary status. When possible, allow adequate time (1 to 2 minutes) between suction passes for ventilation and oxygenation. Assist client with deep breathing and coughing.	Suctioning can induce hypoxemia, dysrhythmias, laryngospasm, and bronchospasm. Deep breathing reventilates and reoxygenates alveoli. Repeated passes clear airway of excessive secretions but can also remove oxygen and may induce laryngospasm.
b. Artificial airway suctioning:	
(1) Hyperinflate and/or hyperoxygenate client before suctioning, using manual resuscitation bag connected to oxygen source or sigh mechanism on mechanical ventilator.	Hyperinflation decreases risk for atelectasis caused by negative pressure of suctioning (St. John, 1999). Preoxygenation converts large proportion of resident lung gas to 100% oxygen to offset amount used in metabolic consumption while ventilator or oxygenation is interrupted, as well as to offset volume lost during suction procedure (Day and others, 2002; Wood, 1998).
(2) If client is receiving mechanical ventilation, open swivel adapter or, if necessary, remove oxygen or humidity delivery device with nondominant hand.	Exposes artificial airway.

Step	Rationale
(3) Without applying suction, gently but quickly insert catheter using dominant thumb and forefinger into artificial airway (it is best to try to time catheter insertion into artificial airway with inspiration) until resistance is met or client coughs; then pull back 1 cm ($\frac{1}{2}$ inch).	Application of suction pressure while introducing catheter into trachea increases risk of damage to tracheal mucosa, as well as increased hypoxia related to removal of entrained oxygen present in airways. Pulling back stimulates cough and removes catheter from mucosal wall so that catheter is not resting against tracheal mucosa during suctioning.
(4) Apply intermittent suction by placing and releasing nondominant thumb over vent of catheter; slowly withdraw catheter while rotating it back and forth between dominant thumb and forefinger (Fig. 70-4).	Intermittent suction and rotation of catheter prevent injury to tracheal mucosal lining. If catheter "grabs" mucosa, remove thumb to release suction.
(5) If client is receiving mechanical ventilation, close swivel adapter or replace oxygen delivery device.	Reestablishes artificial airway.
(6) Encourage client to deep breathe, if able. Some clients respond well to	Reoxygenates and reexpands alveoli. Suctioning can cause hypoxemia and atelectasis.

Step	Rationale

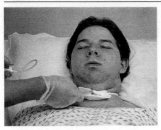

Fig. 70-4 Suctioning tracheostomy.

several manual breaths from mechanical ventilator or bag-valve-mask.

(7) Rinse catheter and connecting tubing with normal saline until clear. Use continuous suction.

Removes catheter secretions. Secretions left in tubing decrease suctioning efficiency and provide environment for microorganism growth.

(8) Assess client's cardiopulmonary status for secretion clearance. Repeat steps once or twice more to clear secretions. Allow adequate time (at least 1 full minute) between suction passes.

Suctioning can induce dysrhythmias, hypoxia, and bronchospasm and impair cerebral circulation or adversely affect hemodynamic stability (Akgul and Akyolcu, 2002; Moore, 2003). Repeated passes with suction catheter clear airway of excessive secretions and promote improved oxygenation (Wood, 1998).

(9) When pharynx and trachea are sufficiently cleared of secretions, perform oropharyngeal suctioning to clear mouth of secretions.

Removes upper airway secretions. More microorganisms are generally present in mouth. Upper airway is considered "clean" and lower airway is considered "sterile." Therefore same catheter can be used to suction from sterile to clean

Step	Rationale
Do not suction nose again after suctioning mouth.	areas (e.g., tracheal suctioning to oropharyngeal suctioning) but not from clean to sterile areas.
17. Complete postprocedure protocol.	
18. If indicated, readjust oxygen to original level because client's blood oxygen level should have returned to baseline.	Prevents absorption atelectasis and oxygen toxicity while allowing client time to reoxygenate blood.
19. Place unopened suction kit on suction machine table or at head of bed.	Provides immediate access to suction catheter for next procedure.
20. Ask client if breathing is easier and if congestion is decreased.	Provides subjective confirmation that airway obstruction is relieved with suctioning procedure.

Recording and Reporting

- Record the amount, consistency, color, and odor of secretions and client's response to suctioning.
- Document client's presuctioning and postsuctioning cardiopulmonary status.

Unexpected Outcomes	Related Interventions
1. Respiratory status worsens.	• Limit length of suctioning. • Determine need for more frequent suctioning, possibly of shorter duration. • Determine need for supplemental oxygen. Supply oxygen between suctioning passes. • Notify physician.
2. Bloody secretions return.	• Determine amount of suction pressure used. May need to be decreased. • Ensure that suctioning uses intermittent suction and catheter rotation. • Evaluate suctioning frequency. • Provide more frequent oral hygiene. • Increase lubrication of catheter.
4. Client has paroxysms of coughing.	• Administer supplemental oxygen. • Allow client to rest between passes of suction catheter. • Consult with physician regarding need for inhaled bronchodilators or topical anesthetics.

Suprapubic Catheter Care

Suprapubic catheters are inserted surgically into the bladder through the lower abdomen above the symphysis pubis. Advantages to the suprapubic catheter are that the client may void naturally when the catheter is clamped and it is more comfortable than the indwelling catheter. The procedure can be performed at the bedside with the client under local anesthesia, or it may be performed in surgery.

The nurse is responsible for maintaining the catheter while the client is in the nursing home or hospital and for teaching the client or caregiver about routine care. Daily care will depend on the institution's policy, but the cleaning and dressing of the catheter site are similar to those for any surgical drain.

Delegation Considerations

The skill of caring for a newly established suprapubic catheter may not be delegated to assistive personnel (AP). However, AP may care for established suprapubic catheters.

■ Instruct AP to report any change in the client's comfort from the tube, appearance of foul-smelling or discolored urine, or fever.

Equipment

■ Gloves, sterile and clean
■ Cleansing agent
■ Sterile gauze for cleaning
■ Sterile drain sponge (split gauze)
■ Tape
■ Dressing bag

Step	Rationale
1. Complete preprocedure protocol.	
2. Assess urine in bag for amount, clarity, color, odor, and sediment.	Abnormal findings may indicate potential complications such as urinary tract infection (UTI), decreased urinary output, and blockage.

Step	Rationale
3. Observe dressing for drainage and intactness.	Drainage indicates potential complication such as infection. Dressing coming off may be caused by tape choice or client picking at dressing.
4. Assess catheter insertion site for signs of inflammation such as redness, swelling, and discharge. Ask client if there is any pain at site.	If insertion is new, slight inflammation may be expected as part of wound healing. May indicate potential infection.
5. Apply sterile gloves.	
6. Use nondominant sterile gloved hand to hold catheter erect while cleaning. Use gauze moistened with cleansing agent to clean site by swabbing in circular motion starting closest to drain and continuing in outward widening circles for approximately 5 cm (2 inches) (Fig. 71-1).	Follows principle of sterile technique to move from area of least contamination to most. Cleanses microorganisms that could migrate to site.
7. Use new piece of moistened gauze to gently clean base of catheter, moving up and away from site of insertion. Do not pull catheter.	Removes microorganisms that reside on any drainage that adheres to tubing.
8. With dominant sterile gloved hand, apply split	Serves to collect secretions.

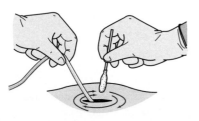

Fig. 71-1 Clean in a circular pattern.

Step	Rationale
gauze around catheter and tape in place.	
9. Secure catheter to abdomen with tape or Velcro multipurpose tube holder to reduce tension on insertion site.	This technique is similar to that used for indwelling urinary catheter. Secures catheter and reduces risk of excessive tension on suture and/or body seal.
10. Check bag and tubing placement.	

NURSE ALERT Be sure there are no obstructions in the tubing. Coil excess tubing on the bed, and fasten it to the bottom sheet with the clip from the kit or with a rubber band and safety pin.

Step	Rationale
11. Ask client whether there is any pain or discomfort from suprapubic catheter.	Determines if bladder is draining and client is free of infection.
12. Observe client's urine for sediment, odor, or discoloration.	Possible signs of infection when present.
13. Inspect dressing at least every shift.	Drainage may indicate infection.
14. Complete postprocedure protocol.	

Recording and Reporting

- Report and record dressing replacement, including assessments of wound and tolerance of client to dressing. Clients may have both indwelling and suprapubic catheters after gynecological or bladder surgery. Urine must be assessed in both drainage systems. (Most urine will be found in suprapubic drainage system.) Record both outputs.

Unexpected Outcomes	Related Interventions
1. Catheter becomes obstructed.	• Catheter is blocked by clots, accumulation of sediment, or position of catheter in bladder. Suprapubic catheter is often small bore and is easily blocked. Encourage client to drink at least 2000 ml of fluids per day if no restrictions. • Notify physician if blockage is persistent.
2. Client develops UTI.	• Encourage fluids, and notify physician. • Observe urine for color, consistency. • Monitor intake and output.
3. Urine leaks at site, and skin breakdown occurs.	• Inspection and dressing changes are important in monitoring for these problems. • Notify physician.

Suture and Staple Removal

Sutures and staples are removed generally within 7 to 10 days after surgery if healing is adequate. Retention sutures usually remain in place 14 to 21 days. Timing the removal of sutures and staples is important. They must remain in place long enough to ensure initial wound closure with enough strength to support internal tissues and organs. Leaving the sutures in too long increases the risk of infection at the puncture sites. Sutures left in longer than 14 days generally leave scar marks (Autio and Olson, 2002). The physician determines and orders removal of all sutures or staples at one time or removal of every other suture or staple as the first phase, with the remainder removed in the second phase.

Delegation Considerations

This skill should not be delegated to assistive personnel (AP). The nurse must:

- Instruct AP to report drainage, bleeding, swelling at the site, or an elevation in the client's temperature to the nurse.
- Instruct AP to report the client's complaints of pain to the nurse.
- Inform AP about any special hygiene practices after suture removal.

Equipment

- Disposable waterproof bag
- Sterile suture removal set (forceps and scissors) or sterile staple extractor
- Sterile applicators or antiseptic swabs
- Steri-Strips or butterfly adhesive strips
- Clean gloves
- Sterile, disposable gloves

Step	Rationale
1. Complete preprocedure protocol.	
2. Identify client with need for suture or staple removal:	

Step	Rationale
a. Review specific directions related to suture or staple removal.	Indicates specifically which sutures are to be removed (e.g., every other suture).
b. Determine history of conditions that may pose risk for impaired wound healing: advanced age, cardiovascular disease, diabetes, immunosuppression, radiation, obesity, smoking, poor cellular nutrition, very deep wounds, and infection.	Preexisting health disorders affect speed of healing and may result in dehiscence.
3. Assess client for history of allergies.	Determines if client is sensitive to antiseptic.
4. Assess client's comfort level or pain on a scale of 0 to 10.	Provides baseline of client's comfort level to determine response to therapy.
5. Assess healing ridge and skin integrity of suture line for uniform closure of wound edges, normal color, and absence of drainage and inflammation.	Indicates adequate wound healing for support of internal structures without continued need for sutures or staples.

NURSE ALERT If wound edges are separated or if signs of infection are present, the wound has not healed properly. Notify the physician because sutures or staples may need to remain in place and/or other wound care initiated.

NURSE ALERT If the client is anxious or has an extensive wound, consider administration of an analgesic 30 minutes before suture/staple removal.

Step	Rationale
6. Expose suture line to ensure that direct lighting is on suture line.	Aids visibility and correct placement of forceps or extractor during removal process, ultimately reducing soft tissue injury.

Step	**Rationale**
7. Place cuffed refuse disposal bag within easy reach.	Provides for easy disposal of contaminated dressings and prevents passing items over sterile work area.
8. Prepare sterile field with dressing change supplies: 　a. Open sterile suture removal tray or staple extractor tray, and slide contents onto prepared field, maintaining sterility of inside surface of wrapper or tray. 　b. Open sterile antiseptic swabs, and place on inside surface of tray. 　c. Open sterile glove package, exposing cuffed ends.	Allows nurse to freely handle sterile supplies.
9. Carefully remove dressing, and discard dressing and clean gloves in prepared refuse disposal bag.	Reduces transmission of infection.
10. Inspect wound.	Determines adequacy of wound healing.
11. Don sterile gloves, if required by policy.	Allows nurse to handle sterile supplies.
12. Cleanse sutures or staples and healed incision with antiseptic swabs.	Removes surface bacteria from incision and sutures or staples.
13. Remove staples: 　a. Place lower tips of staple extractor under first staple. As you close handles, upper tip of extractor depresses center of staple, causing both ends of staple to be bent upward and	Avoids excess pressure to suture line and secures smooth removal of each staple.

Step	**Rationale**

  simultaneously exit
  their insertion sites in
  the dermal layer
  (Fig. 72-1).

  b. Carefully control staple   Avoids suture-line pressure and
  extractor.   pain.

  c. As soon as both ends of   Prevents scratching tender skin
  staple are visible, move   surface with sharp pointed ends
  it away from skin   of staple for comfort and
  surface and continue on   infection control.
  until staple is over
  refuse bag (Fig. 72-2).

  d. Release handles of   Avoids contaminating sterile field
  staple extractor,   with used staples.
  allowing staple to drop
  into refuse bag.

  e. Repeat steps a through
  d until all staples are
  removed.

14. Remove intermittent
  sutures (Fig. 72-3):

  a. Place gauze few inches   Gauze serves as receptacle for
  from suture line. Grasp   removed sutures. Placement of
  scissors in dominant   scissors and forceps allows for
  hand and forceps in   efficient suture removal.
  nondominant hand.

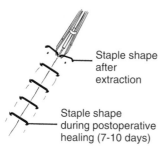

Staple shape
after
extraction

Staple shape
during postoperative
healing (7-10 days)

Fig. 72-1 Staple extractor placed under staple.

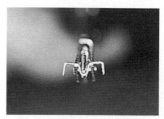

Fig. 72-2 Metal staple removed by extractor.

Step	**Rationale**

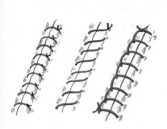

Fig. 72-3 Types of sutures: *Left,*
Intermittent; *middle,* continuous;
right, blanket.

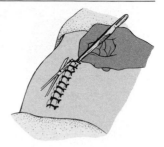

Fig. 72-4 Removal of intermittent
suture. Nurse cuts suture as close
to skin as possible, away from the
knot.

NURSE ALERT Placement of scissor and forceps is very important. Avoid
pinching the skin around the wound when lifting up the suture.

    b. Grasp knot of suture   Releases suture.
       with forceps, and gently
       pull up knot while
       slipping tip of scissors
       under suture near skin
       (Fig. 72-4).
    c. Snip suture as close to
       skin as possible.

NURSE ALERT Never snip both ends of the suture; there will be no way to
remove the part of the suture situated below the surface.

    d. Grasp knotted end   Smoothly removes suture without
       with forceps, and in one   additional tension to suture line.
       continuous smooth
       action pull suture
       through from other side
       (Fig. 72-5). Place
       removed suture on
       gauze.
    e. Repeat steps a through
       d until every other

Step	Rationale

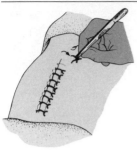

Fig. 72-5 Nurse removes suture and never pulls the contaminated stitch through tissues.

    suture has been
    removed.

  f. Observe healing level.
    Based on observations
    of wound response to
    suture removal and
    physician's original
    order, determine
    whether remaining
    sutures will be removed
    at this time. If so, repeat
    steps a through d until
    all sutures have been
    removed.

Determines status of wound healing and if suture line will remain closed after all sutures are removed.

  g. If any doubt, stop and
    notify physician.

15. Remove continuous
    sutures, including blanket
    stitch sutures:

  a. Place sterile gauze few
    inches from suture line.
    Grasp scissors in
    dominant hand and
    forceps in nondominant
    hand.

Gauze serves as receptacle for removed sutures. Placement of scissors and forceps allows for efficient suture removal.

  b. Snip first suture close to
    skin surface at end
    distal to knot.

Releases suture.

Step	Rationale
c. Snip second suture on same side.	Releases interrupted sutures from knot.
d. Grasp knotted end, and gently pull with continuous smooth action, removing suture from beneath skin. Place suture on gauze compress.	Smoothly removes sutures without additional tension to suture line. Prevents pulling of contaminated portion of suture through skin.
e. Repeat steps a through d in consecutive order until entire line has been removed.	
16. Inspect incision site to make sure that entire suture and all sutures are removed and to identify any trouble areas. Gently wipe suture line with antiseptic swab to remove debris and cleanse wound.	Reduces risk of further incision line separation.
17. To maintain contact between wound edges, apply Steri-Strips if *any* separation greater than two stitches or two staples in width is apparent:	Supports wound by distributing tension across wound and eliminates closure technique scarring (Autio and Olson, 2002).
a. Apply tincture of benzoin or Skin Prep to skin on each side of suture line. Allow to dry.	Promotes increased adherence of Steri-Strips.
b. Cut Steri-Strips to allow strips to extend 4 to 5 cm ($1\frac{1}{2}$ to 2 inches) on each side of the incision.	
c. Inform client to take showers rather than soak in bathtub according to physician's preference.	Steri-Strips are not removed and are allowed to fall off gradually.

Step	Rationale
18. Apply light dressing, or expose to air if no clothing will come in contact with suture line. Instruct client about applying own dressing if it will be needed at home.	Healing by primary intention eliminates need for dressing.
19. Complete postprocedure protocol.	

Recording and Reporting

- Record time sutures or staples were removed; number of sutures or staples removed; cleansing of suture line; appearance of wound; level of healing of wound; type of dressing applied if one is used; and client's response to suture or staple removal.
- Immediately notify physician of suture line separation, dehiscence, evisceration, bleeding, or purulent drainage.

Unexpected Outcomes	Related Interventions
1. Retained suture is present.	• Assess suture line closely to determine if any suture material remains. • Notify physician. • Instruct client to notify physician if signs of suture line infection develop after discharge from agency.
2. Client experiences wound separation or drainage secondary to healing problems.	• Leave remaining sutures or staples in place. • Place supportive butterfly closures across suture line. • Notify physician.

Topical Skin Applications

Locally applied drugs such as lotions, patches, pastes, and ointments can create systemic and local effects if absorbed through the skin. To protect from accidental exposure, apply these drugs using gloves and applicators. If the client's skin is intact, use clean technique when applying lotions, patches, and ointments. If the client has an open wound, use sterile technique.

Skin encrustations and dead tissue harbor microorganisms and block contact of medications with the tissues to be treated. Simply applying new medications over previously applied drugs does little to prevent infection or offer therapeutic benefit. Clean the skin thoroughly before applying medications by washing the area gently with soap and water, soaking an involved site, or locally debriding tissue.

Delegation Considerations

The skill of administering (topical) skin medications should not be delegated to assistive personnel (AP). In some institutions AP may apply ointments or lotions.

- Instruct AP about the expected therapeutic effects and potential side effects of medications and to report their occurrence.
- If AP apply topical agents, ensure that the correct method and site of application are understood, and ensure the "six rights" of medication administration.

Equipment

- Clean gloves (for intact skin) or sterile gloves (for nonintact skin)
- Ordered agent (cream, lotion, ointment, spray, patch)
- Cotton-tipped applicators or tongue blades (optional)
- Basin of warm water
- Washcloth
- Towel
- Nondrying soap
- Sterile dressing, tape (if needed)
- Medication administration record (MAR)
- Soft-tip or felt-tip marker

Step	Rationale
1. Complete preprocedure protocol.	

Step	Rationale
2. Review provider's medication order for client's name, drug name, dose, time, and route of administration against MAR.	Ensures safe and correct administration of medication by verifying order.
3. Remove any old patches or paper measuring guides. Wash site thoroughly with mild, nondrying soap and warm water; rinse; and dry. Be sure any previously applied medication or debris is removed. Also remove any blood, body fluids, secretions, or excretions. Remove and dispose of gloves. Perform hand hygiene.	Cleansing site thoroughly allows nurse to properly assess skin surface. New medication should not be applied over previously applied drug. Overdose can occur with multiple dose papers left in place.
4. Determine amount of topical agent required for application by assessing affected area, reviewing prescriber's order, and reading application directions carefully (thin, even layer is usually adequate).	Excessive amount of topical agent can cause chemical irritation of skin, negate drug's effectiveness, and/or cause adverse systemic effects, such as decreased white cell counts.
5. Check medications' expiration dates on drug packages.	Medications that have expired should not be used because potency of medications changes when mdications become outdated.
6. Check name of medication on drug package label against MAR.	Checking label ensures that client receives correct medication.
7. Check client's identification bracelet, and ask name.	Ensures that correct client receives medication. At least two patient identifiers (neither to be patient's

Step	**Rationale**
	room number) are to be used whenever administering medications (JCAHO, 2004).
8. If skin is broken (e.g., wound), use sterile gloves; otherwise don clean gloves.	Sterile gloves are used when applying agents to open, noninfectious skin lesions. Topical agents are not usually premeasured in medication room. Use of gloves also prevents absorption of medication into nurse's skin.
9. Remove gown or bed linen so as to keep unaffected skin areas draped.	Promotes client's comfort.
10. Compare MAR with drug and continue.	Reduces medication error.
11. Apply topical agent:	
a. Technique for applying creams, ointments, and oil-based lotions:	
(1) Place required amount of medication in palm of gloved hand, and soften by rubbing briskly between hands.	Softening of topical agent makes it easier to spread on skin.
(2) Once medication is softened, spread it evenly over skin surface, using long, even strokes that follow direction of hair growth. Apply to thickness specified by manufacturer's instructions.	Ensures even distribution and sufficient dosage of medication. Technique prevents irritation of hair follicles.
(3) Explain to client that skin may feel	Ointments often contain oils.

Step	Rationale

greasy after
application.

b. Technique for applying
nitroglycerin (an
antianginal) ointment:

(1) Apply desired
number of inches
of ointment over
paper measuring
guide (Fig. 73-1).

Ensures correct dose of
medication. Antianginal
(nitroglycerin) ointments are
usually ordered in inches and
can be measured on small sheets
of paper marked off in 1.25 cm
(½-inch) markings. Unit-dose
packages are available. (*Warning:*
One package equals 2.5 cm
(1 inch); smaller amount should
not be measured from this
package.)

(2) Antianginal
medication may be
applied to chest
area, back, upper
arm, or legs. Do
not apply on hairy
surfaces or over scar
tissue.

If client complains of headaches,
apply ointment farther from
head. Application on hairy
surfaces or scar tissue may
interfere with absorption.

(3) Rotate site when
applying
nitroglycerin pastes.

Prevents skin irritation.

(4) Apply ointment to
skin surface by
holding edge or
back of paper

Minimizes chance of ointment
covering gloves and later
touching nurse's hands.
Medication is designed to absorb

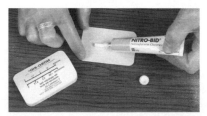

Fig. 73-1 Ointment
spread in inches over
measuring guide.

Step	**Rationale**
measuring guide and placing ointment and wrapper directly on skin. Do not rub or massage ointment into skin.	slowly over several hours; massaging may increase absorption rate.
(5) Date and initial paper, and note time.	Prevents missing doses.
(6) Secure ointment and paper with transparent dressing or strip of tape. Plastic wrap may be used as occlusive dressing.	Prevents staining of clothing or inadvertent removal of medication (McConnell, 2001).
c. Technique for applying a transdermal patch:	
(1) Date and initial outer side of patch before applying it, and note time. Use soft-tip or felt-tip marker pen.	Visual reminder prevents missing or extra doses. It is better to write on patch before it is applied to client's skin. Take care not to damage patch with sharp pen.
(2) Choose clean, dry area of body that is free of hair. Some patches have specific instructions for placement locations (e.g., Testoderm scrotal patches).	Increases absorption. Proper placement ensures correct delivery of drug.

NURSE ALERT Do not try to apply the patch on skin that is oily, burned, broken out, cut, or irritated in any way.

(3) Carefully remove patch from its protective covering.	Touching only edges ensures that patch will adhere and that medication dose has not been

Step	Rationale
Hold patch by edge; do not touch adhesive edges.	changed. Protective covering must be removed to allow medication to be absorbed through skin.
(4) Immediately apply patch, pressing firmly with palm of one hand for 10 seconds. Make sure it sticks well, especially around edges. Apply overlay if provided with patch.	Sufficient pressure is needed to ensure that adhesive will keep patch on skin surface.
(5) When next dose is due, remove old patch and choose different site. Do not apply to previously used sites for at least 1 week.	Rotation of sites reduces skin irritation from medication and adhesive.

NURSE ALERT It is recommended that nitroglycerin transdermal patches be removed after 10 to 12 hours to allow for a nitrate-free interval and reduce the chance of medication tolerance. Check with client's prescriber (Lewis and others, 2004).

Step	Rationale
(6) Dispose of patches by folding in half with sticky sides together. Throw patch in trash away from children and pets. Some agencies require patch to be cut before disposal.	Proper disposal protects others from accidental exposure to medication (Lee and Phillips, 2002).
d. Technique for applying aerosolized medication (spray):	

Step	**Rationale**
(1) Shake container vigorously.	Mixes contents and propellant to ensure distribution of fine, even spray.
(2) Read container's label for distance recommended to hold spray away from area (usually 15 to 30 cm [6 to 12 inches]).	Proper distance ensures that fine spray hits skin surface. Holding container too close results in thin, watery distribution.
(3) If neck or upper chest is to be sprayed, ask client to turn face away from spray or briefly cover face with towel.	Prevents inhalation of spray.
(4) Spray medication evenly over affected site (in some cases spray is timed for select period of seconds).	Entire affected area of skin should be covered with thin spray.
e. Technique for applying suspension-based lotion:	
(1) Shake container vigorously.	Mixes powder throughout liquid to form well-mixed suspension.
(2) Apply small amount of lotion to small gauze dressing or pad, and apply to skin by stroking evenly in direction of hair growth.	Method of application leaves protective film of powder on skin after water base of suspension dries. Technique prevents irritation of hair follicles.
(3) Explain to client that area will feel cool and dry.	Water evaporates to leave thin layer of powder.
12. Complete postprocedure protocol.	

Recording and Reporting

- Describe in nurses' notes condition of skin before topical agent application.
- Immediately after administration, record on MAR actual time each drug was administered, type of agent applied, strength, and site of application. Include initials or signature.
- Report adverse effects/client response and/or withheld drugs to nurse in charge or physician. Depending on medication, immediate prescriber notification may be required.
- Report any abnormalities in condition of skin to nurse in charge or physician.

Unexpected Outcomes	Related Interventions
1. Skin site may appear inflamed and edematous with blistering and oozing of fluid from lesions.	• Notify prescriber; alternative therapies may be needed.
2. Client continues to complain of pruritus and tenderness. Indicates slow or impaired healing.	• Notify prescriber; alternative therapies may be needed.

Tracheostomy Care

Clients who have tracheostomy tubes require specialized nursing care to manage the tube and the stoma. Some clients with a tracheostomy tube are able to cough secretions out of the tracheostomy tube completely, whereas others are able to cough secretions only up into the tracheostomy tube. The latter clients may not require suctioning when an inner cannula is present because it can be safely removed, cleaned, and reinserted. Tracheostomy care includes a comprehensive plan and execution of care that includes properly securing the tube, inflating the cuff to an appropriate pressure, maintaining patency by suctioning, and encouraging communication and oral hygiene (Peers, 2003).

Delegation Considerations

This skill should is not routinely delegated to assistive personnel (AP). In some settings, clients who have well-established tracheostomy tubes may have the care delegated to AP. It is the responsibility of the nurse to assess and ensure that proper artificial airway care is provided. In addition, AP may perform other aspects of the client's care. The nurse should instruct AP about:

- Immediately reporting to the nurse any changes in the client's respiratory status or level of consciousness; any confusion, restlessness, or irritability; any change in level of comfort; or color of tracheal stoma and drainage.

Equipment

- Bedside table
- Towel
- Tracheostomy suction supplies
- Sterile tracheostomy care kit, if available (be sure to collect supplies listed that are not available in kit) or three sterile 4 × 4–inch gauze pads
- Sterile cotton-tipped applicators
- Sterile tracheostomy dressing (precut and sewn surgical dressing)
- Sterile basin
- Small sterile brush (or disposable inner cannula)
- Roll of twill tape, tracheostomy tube ties, or tracheostomy tube holder
- Hydrogen peroxide
- Normal saline solution

- Scissors
- Sterile gloves (two)
- Face shield

Step	Rationale
1. Complete preprocedure protocol.	
2. Observe for signs and symptoms of need to perform tracheostomy care: excess peristomal secretions, excess intratracheal secretions, soiled or damp tracheostomy ties, soiled or damp tracheostomy dressing, diminished airflow through tracheostomy tube, or signs and symptoms of airway obstruction requiring suctioning (see Skill 70).	Signs and symptoms are related to presence of secretions at stoma site or within tracheostomy tube.
3. ![icon] Apply face shield if applicable.	Reduces transmission of microorganisms.
4. Suction tracheostomy (see Skill 70). Before removing gloves, remove soiled tracheostomy dressing and discard in glove with coiled catheter.	Removes secretions to avoid occluding outer cannula while inner cannula is removed. Reduces need for client to cough.
5. While client is replenishing oxygen stores, prepare equipment on bedside table: a. Open sterile tracheostomy kit. Open three packages of 4 × 4–inch gauze using aseptic technique, and pour normal saline on one package and	Prepares equipment and allows for smooth, organized completion of tracheostomy care.

Step	Rationale

hydrogen peroxide on another. Leave third package dry. Open two cotton-tipped swab packages, and pour normal saline on one package and hydrogen peroxide on other. Do not recap hydrogen peroxide and normal saline.

b. Open sterile tracheostomy dressing package.

c. Unwrap sterile basin, and pour about 0.5 to 2 cm ($\frac{1}{2}$ inch) hydrogen peroxide into it.

d. Open package that contains small sterile brush, and place brush aseptically into sterile basin.

e. Prepare length of twill tape long enough to go around client's neck two times, about 60 to 75 cm (24 to 30 inches) for adult. Cut ends on diagonal. Lay aside in dry area.

Cutting ends of tie on diagonal aids in inserting tie through eyelet.

f. If using commercially available tracheostomy tube holder, open package according to manufacturer's directions.

6. Apply sterile gloves. Keep dominant hand sterile throughout procedure.

Reduces transmission of microorganisms.

Step	Rationale
7. Apply oxygen source loosely over tracheostomy if client desaturates during procedure.	Helps reduce amount of desaturation.

NURSE ALERT For a tracheostomy tube with no inner cannula or Kistner button, continue with Step 13.

Step	Rationale
8. Care of tracheostomy with inner cannula:	
a. While touching only outer aspect of tube, remove inner cannula with nondominant hand. Drop inner cannula into hydrogen peroxide basin.	Removes inner cannula for cleaning. Hydrogen peroxide loosens secretions from inner cannula.
b. Place tracheostomy collar, T tube, or ventilator oxygen source over outer cannula. (NOTE: T tube and ventilator oxygen devices cannot be attached to all outer cannulas when inner cannula is removed.)	Maintains supply of oxygen to client.
c. To prevent oxygen desaturation in affected clients, quickly pick up inner cannula and use small brush to remove secretions inside and outside inner cannula.	Tracheostomy brush provides mechanical force to remove thick or dried secretions.
d. Hold inner cannula over basin, and rinse with normal saline, using nondominant hand to pour normal saline.	Removes secretions and hydrogen peroxide from inner cannula.
e. Replace inner cannula, and secure "locking"	Secures inner cannula and reestablishes oxygen supply.

Step	**Rationale**

mechanism (Fig. 74-1). Reapply ventilator or oxygen sources.

9. Tracheostomy with disposable inner cannula:
   a. Remove cannula from manufacturer's packaging.
   b. While touching only outer aspect of tube, withdraw inner cannula and replace with new cannula. Lock into position.
   c. Dispose of contaminated cannula in appropriate receptacle, and apply ventilator or oxygen sources.

10. Using hydrogen peroxide–saturated cotton-tipped swabs and 4 × 4–inch gauze, clean exposed outer cannula surfaces and stoma under faceplate extending 5 to 10 cm (2 to 4 inches) in all directions from stoma. Clean in circular motion from stoma site outward

Aseptically removes secretions from stoma site. Moving in outward circle pulls mucus and other contaminants from stoma to periphery.

Fig. 74-1 Reinserting the inner cannula.

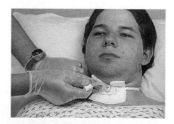

Step	Rationale
using dominant hand to handle sterile supplies.	
11. Using normal saline–saturated cotton-tipped swabs and 4 × 4–inch gauze, rinse hydrogen peroxide from tracheostomy tube and skin surfaces.	Rinses hydrogen peroxide from surfaces. If not removed from skin, hydrogen peroxide can promote tissue injury.
12. Using dry 4 × 4–inch gauze, pat lightly at skin and exposed outer cannula surfaces.	Dry surfaces prohibit formation of moist environment for microorganism growth and skin excoriation.
13. Secure tracheostomy:	Promotes hygiene and reduces transmission of microorganisms. Secures tracheostomy tube. Reduces risk of incidental extubation.

a. Tracheostomy tie
   method:
   (1) Instruct assistant, if
       available, to don
       gloves and securely
       hold tracheostomy
       tube in place. With
       assistant holding
       tracheostomy tube,
       cut old ties.

NURSE ALERT   The assistant must not release hold on the tracheostomy tube until the new ties are firmly tied. If working without an assistant, do not cut the old ties until the new ties are in place and securely tied.

   (2) Insert one end of
       prepared tie
       through faceplate
       eyelet, and pull
       ends even
       (Fig. 74-2).
   (3) Slide both ends of
       tie behind head and
       around neck to

Step	Rationale

Fig. 74-2 Replacing tracheostomy tube ties. Do not remove old tracheostomy tube ties until new ones are secure.

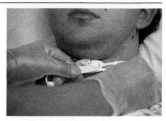

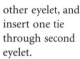

other eyelet, and insert one tie through second eyelet.

(4) Pull snugly.

Ensures that tracheostomy tube will not come out.

(5) Tie ends securely in double square knot, allowing space for only one loose or two snug finger widths in tie.

One finger width of slack prevents ties from being too tight when tracheostomy dressing is in place and prevents movement of tracheostomy tube in lower airway.

(6) Insert fresh tracheostomy dressing under clean ties and faceplate.

Absorbs drainage. Dressing prevents pressure on clavicle heads.

b. Tracheostomy tube holder method:

(1) While wearing gloves, maintain secure hold on tracheostomy tube. This can be done with assistant or, when assistant is not available, leave old tracheostomy tube holder in place until new device is secure.

(2) Align strap under client's neck. Be

Step	Rationale
sure that Velcro attachments are positioned on either side of tracheostomy tube.	
(3) Place narrow end of ties under and through faceplate eyelets. Pull ends even, and secure with Velcro closures.	
(4) Verify that there is space for only one loose or two snug finger widths under neck strap (Fig. 74-3).	
14. Position client comfortably, and assess respiratory status.	Promotes comfort. Some clients may require post–tracheostomy care suctioning.
15. Replace any oxygen delivery sources.	
16. Assess comfort of new tracheostomy ties.	Tracheostomy ties are uncomfortable and place client at risk for injury when they are too loose or too tight.

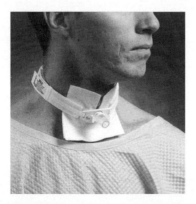

Fig. 74-3 Tracheostomy tube holder in place. (Courtesy Dale Medical Products, Plainesville, Mass.)

Step	Rationale
17. Inspect inner and outer cannulas for secretions.	Presence of secretions on cannulas indicates need for more vigorous tracheostomy care.
18. Assess stoma for signs of infection or skin breakdown.	Broken skin places client at risk for infection. Stomal infection necessitates change in tracheostomy skin care plan.
19. Complete postprocedure protocol.	

Recording and Reporting

- Record respiratory assessments before and after care.
- Record type and size of tracheostomy tube, frequency and extent of care, client tolerance, and special care in event of stomatitis.

Unexpected Outcomes	Related Interventions
1. Stomatitis.	• Increase frequency of tracheostomy care. • Apply topical antibacterial solution, and allow it to dry and provide bacterial barrier. • Apply hydrocolloid or transparent dressing just under stoma to protect skin from breakdown. Consult with skin care specialist.
2. Pressure area around tracheostomy tube.	• Increase frequency of tracheostomy care, and keep dressing under faceplate at all times. • Consider using double dressing or applying hydrocolloid or stoma adhesive dressing around stoma.
3. Accidental decannulation.	• Call for assistance. • Replace old tracheostomy tube with new tube. Some experienced nurses or respiratory therapists may be able to quickly reinsert tracheostomy tube. • Notify physician.

Urinary Catheter: Indwelling, Straight, Care and Removal

Catheterization of the bladder involves introducing a rubber or plastic tube through the urethra and into the bladder. The catheter provides for a continuous flow of urine in clients unable to control micturition or in those with obstruction to urine outflow. Because bladder catheterization carries the risk of the development of urinary tract infection (UTI), it is preferable to rely on less invasive measures to promote bladder emptying.

Delegation Considerations

In some setting, assistive personnel (AP) may insert urinary catheters (see agency policy). Otherwise, AP may assist with positioning the client, focusing lighting for the procedure, and aiding in the client's comfort during the procedure by measures such as holding the client's hand or keeping the client warm.

Equipment
Indwelling or Straight Catheter Insertion

- Catheterization kit containing the following sterile items: gloves (extra pair optional); drapes, one fenestrated; lubricant, antiseptic cleansing solution; cotton balls; forceps; prefilled syringe with sterile water to inflate balloon of indwelling catheter; catheter of correct size and type for procedure (i.e., intermittent or indwelling); sterile drainage tubing with collection bag and multipurpose tube holder or tape, safety pin, and elastic band for securing tubing to bed if client is bedridden (for indwelling catheter); receptacle or basin (usually at the bottom of the catheterization tray); and specimen container
- *Option:* Double- or triple-lumen indwelling catheter if client is to receive catheter irrigation
- Blanket
- Waterproof absorbent pad
- Disposable gloves
- Basin with warm water
- Soap

- Washcloth
- Towel
- Flashlight or other appropriate additional light as needed

Catheter Care

- Soap
- Washcloth
- Basin
- Water (to cleanse perineum before catheter care)
- Graduated cylinder (used if urine collection bag is to be emptied)

Catheter Removal

- Syringe (same size used to inflate balloon); verify balloon size on catheter port
- Waterproof pad
- Appropriate equipment if sterile urine specimen is needed

Step	Rationale
1. Complete preprocedure protocol.	
2. Assess status of client: Time of last urination: ask client and check intake and output (I&O) flowsheet	Determines time of last voiding and indicates likelihood of bladder fullness.
3. Palpate for distended bladder (bladder palpable above symphysis pubis). When bladder is full, palpation causes urge to urinate.	Palpation causes pain. Full bladder with inability to void may indicate need to insert catheter.

NURSE ALERT Assess for allergies to antiseptic, tape, latex, and lubricant. Betadine allergies are common. If the client is unaware of allergy to Betadine, ask if the client is allergic to shellfish.

4. Facing client, stand on left side of bed if right-handed (on right side if left-handed). Clear bedside table, and arrange equipment.	Successful catheter insertion requires nurse to assume comfortable position and all equipment easily accessible.

Step	Rationale
5. If side rails in use, raise side rail on opposite side of bed and lower side rail on working side. Place waterproof pad under client.	Promotes client safety. Prevents soiling of bed linen.
6. Position client:	Provides good visualization of perineal structures.
a. Female client:	
(1) Assist to dorsal recumbent position (supine with knees flexed). Ask client to relax thighs so the hip joints can be externally rotated.	Legs may be supported with pillows to reduce muscle tension and promote comfort.
(2) Position female client in side-lying (Sims') position with upper leg flexed at knee and hip if unable to be supine. If this position is used, nurse must take extra precautions to cover rectal area with drape during procedure to reduce chance of cross contamination.	This alternate position is used if client cannot abduct leg at hip joint (e.g., if client has arthritic joints). Also, this position may be more comfortable for client. Support client with pillows if necessary to maintain position.
b. Male client:	
(1) Assist to supine position with thighs slightly abducted.	Comfortable position for client that aids in visualization of penis.
7. Drape client:	Avoids unnecessary exposure of body parts and maintains client's comfort.

Step	Rationale

   a. Female client:
   - (1) Drape with bath blanket. Place blanket diamond fashion over client, with one corner at client's neck, side corners over each arm and side, and last corner over perineum.

   b. Male client:
   - (1) Drape upper trunk with bath blanket, and cover lower extremities with bed sheet, exposing only genitalia.

8. Wash perineal area with soap and water as needed; dry. Remove gloves.

   Reduces microorganisms near urethral meatus (Haberstich, 2002).

9. Position lamp to illuminate perineal area. (When using flashlight, have assistant hold it.)

   Permits accurate identification and good visualization of urethral meatus.

10. Open package containing drainage system; place drainage bag over edge of bottom bed frame, and bring drainage tube up between side rail and mattress.

   Prepares bag for attachment to catheter.

NURSE ALERT This is necessary only if an indwelling catheter is ordered and a drainage system is not part of the catheterization kit.

11. Open catheterization kit according to directions, keeping bottom of container sterile.

   Prevents transmission of microorganisms from table or work area to sterile supplies. Materials in kit are arranged in sequence of use.

Step	Rationale
12. Place plastic bag that contains kit within reach of work area.	Use as waterproof bag to dispose of used supplies.
13. Don sterile gloves.	Allows nurse to handle sterile supplies without contamination.

NURSE ALERT If an underpad is the first item in the kit, place the pad plastic side down under the client, touching only the edges so as to maintain sterility. Then apply sterile gloves.

Step	Rationale
14. Organize supplies on sterile field. Open inner sterile package containing catheter. Pour sterile antiseptic solution into correct compartment containing sterile cotton balls. Open packet containing lubricant. Remove specimen container (lid should be loosely placed on top) and prefilled syringe from collection compartment of tray, and set them aside on sterile field if needed.	Maintains principles of surgical asepsis and organizes work area.
15. Before inserting indwelling catheter, common practice is to test balloon by injecting fluid from prefilled syringe into balloon port. (Check manufacturer's directions.)	Checks integrity of balloon. Do not use catheter if balloon does not inflate or leaks. This is controversial step. Follow manufacturer's recommendations. Checking balloon in this way may stretch balloon and cause increased trauma on insertion.
16. Lubricate catheter 2.5 to 5 cm (1 to 2 inches) for women and 12.5 to 17.5 cm (5 to 7 inches) for men.	Prevents urethral trauma. Inflamed tissue is more susceptible to infection (Haberstich, 2002).

Step	**Rationale**

NOTE: Some catheter kits will have plastic sheath over catheter that must be removed before lubrication. (*Optional:* Physician may order use of lubricant containing local anesthetic.)

17. Apply sterile drape, keeping gloves sterile:
    a. Female client:

Step	Rationale
(1) Allow top edge of drape to form cuff over both hands. Place drape down on bed between client's thighs. Slip cuffed edge just under buttocks, taking care not to touch contaminated surface with gloves.	Outer surface of drape covering hands remains sterile. Sterile drape against sterile gloves is sterile.
(2) Pick up fenestrated sterile drape, and allow it to unfold without touching unsterile object. Apply drape over perineum, exposing labia and being sure not to touch contaminated surface.	Maintains sterility of work surface.

b. Male client (two methods are used for draping, depending on preference):

	Rationale
	Maintains sterility of work surface.

(1) *First method:* Apply drape over thighs and below penis

Step	Rationale
without completely opening fenestrated drape.	
(2) *Second method:* Apply drape over thighs just below penis. Pick up fenestrated sterile drape, allow it to unfold, and drape it over penis with fenestrated slit resting over penis.	
18. Place sterile tray and contents on sterile drape between legs. Open specimen container. NOTE: Client's size and positioning will dictate exact placement. This method works best with flexible, average-size clients.	Provides easy access to supplies during catheter insertion. Maintains aseptic technique during procedure.
19. Cleanse urethral meatus:	
a. Female client:	
(1) With nondominant hand, carefully retract labia to fully expose urethral meatus. Maintain position of nondominant hand throughout procedure.	Full visualization of urethral meatus is provided. Full retraction prevents contamination of urethral meatus during cleansing.

NURSE ALERT Closure of labia during cleansing requires that the procedure be repeated because the area has become contaminated.

(2) Using forceps in sterile dominant	Cleansing reduces number of microorganisms at urethral

Step	Rationale

hand, pick up cotton ball saturated with antiseptic solution and clean perineal area, wiping front to back from clitoris toward anus. Using a new cotton ball for each area, wipe along the far labial fold, near labial fold, and directly over center of urethral meatus.

meatus. Cleansing moves from area of least contamination to that of most contamination. Dominant hand remains sterile.

b. Male client:

(1) If client is not circumcised, retract foreskin with nondominant hand. Grasp penis at shaft just below glans. Retract urethral meatus between thumb and forefinger. Maintain nondominant hand in this position throughout procedure.

Retraction exposes meatus for catheter insertion. Accidental release of foreskin or dropping of penis during cleansing requires process to be repeated because area has become contaminated.

NURSE ALERT If the foreskin does not remain retracted during insertion, the cleansing procedure must be repeated because the area has become contaminated.

(2) With dominant hand, pick up cotton ball with forceps and clean penis. Move cotton ball in circular

Reduces number of microorganisms at urethral meatus and moves from areas of least to most contamination. Dominant hand remains sterile.

Step	Rationale

motion from
urethral meatus
down to base of
glans. Repeat
cleansing three
more times, using
clean cotton ball
each time.

20. Pick up catheter with
gloved dominant hand 7.5
to 10 cm (3 to 4 inches)
from catheter tip. Hold
end of catheter loosely
coiled in palm of dominant
hand. (*Optional:* May grasp
catheter with forceps.)
Place distal end of catheter
in urine tray receptacle if
straight catheterization is
being done.

21. Insert catheter:
   a. Female client:

   (1) Ask client to bear
   down gently as if to
   void, and slowly
   insert catheter
   through urethral
   meatus (Fig. 75-1).

      Relaxation of external sphincter
   aids in insertion of catheter.

   (2) Advance catheter
   total of 5 to 7.5 cm
   (2 to 3 inches) in
   adult *or until urine
   flows out catheter's
   end.* As soon as
   urine appears,
   advance catheter
   another 2.5 to 5 cm
   (1 to 2 inches). Do
   not force against

      Female urethra is short.
   Appearance of urine indicates
   that catheter tip is in bladder or
   lower urethra. Advancement of
   catheter ensures bladder
   placement.

Step	**Rationale**

Fig. 75-1 Inserting the catheter.

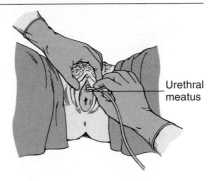

Urethral meatus

resistance. Place end of catheter in urine tray receptacle.	
(3) Release labia, and hold catheter securely with nondominant hand.	Bladder or sphincter contraction may cause accidental expulsion of catheter.
b. Male client:	
(1) Lift penis to position perpendicular to client's body, and apply light traction (Fig. 75-2).	Straightens urethral canal to ease catheter insertion.
(2) Ask client to bear down as if to void, and slowly insert catheter through urethral meatus.	Relaxation of external sphincter aids in insertion of catheter.
(3) Advance catheter 17.5 to 22.5 cm (7 to 9 inches) in adult or *until urine flows out catheter's end.* If resistance is felt,	Adult male urethra is long. It is normal to meet resistance at prostatic sphincter. When resistance is met, nurse should hold catheter firmly against sphincter without forcing

Step	**Rationale**

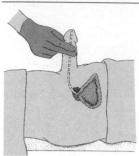

Fig. 75-2 Position penis perpendicular to body for catheter insertion.

withdraw catheter; do not force it through urethra. When urine appears, advance catheter to bifurcation of drainage and balloon inflation port (Fig. 75-3). *Do not use force to insert catheter.*	catheter. After few seconds, sphincter relaxes and catheter is advanced. Appearance of urine indicates catheter tip is in bladder or urethra. Further advancement of catheter to bifurcation of drainage and balloon inflation port ensures proper placement (Daneshgari and others, 2002).
(4) Lower penis, and hold catheter securely in nondominant hand. Place end of catheter in urine tray receptacle.	Catheter may be accidentally expelled by bladder or urethral contraction. Collection of urine prevents soiling and provides output measurement.
(5) Reduce (or reposition) foreskin.	Paraphimosis (retraction and constriction of foreskin behind glans penis) secondary to catheterization may occur if foreskin is not reduced.
22. Collect urine specimen as needed. Fill specimen cup or jar to desired level (20 to	Allows sterile specimen to be obtained for culture analysis.

Step	Rationale

Fig. 75-3 Male anatomy with correct catheter insertion to the bifurcation of the drainage and balloon inflation port.

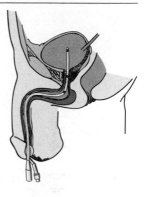

30 ml) by holding end of catheter in dominant hand over cup.

23. Allow bladder to empty fully unless institution policy restricts maximum volume of urine drained with each catheterization (about 800 to 1000 ml).

Retained urine may serve as reservoir for growth of microorganisms.

NURSE ALERT If a straight catheter was used, smoothly and slowly withdraw the catheter.

24. Inflate balloon fully with amount of fluid recommended by manufacturer:

    a. While holding catheter with nondominant hand at urethral meatus, place end of catheter between first two fingers of nondominant hand.

Inflation of balloon anchors catheter tip in place above bladder outlet to prevent removal of catheter (Fig. 75-4). Note size of balloon on catheter. Most commonly, 5-ml balloon is used, but 30-ml balloon may be ordered. A prefilled syringe may be included with kit; use only amount included. Do not

Step	Rationale

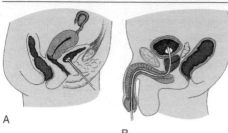

Fig. 75-4
Placement of inflated balloon in bladder.

A

B

overinflate or underinflate balloon.

b. With free dominant hand, attach syringe to injection port at end of catheter.

c. Slowly inject total amount of solution. If client complains of sudden pain, aspirate solution and advance catheter further.

d. After advancing catheter and/or inflating balloon, release catheter and pull gently to feel resistance. Then move catheter slightly back into bladder.

NURSE ALERT If resistance is felt during inflation or if the client complains of pain, the balloon may not be entirely within the bladder. Stop the inflation, aspirate any fluid in the balloon, and advance the catheter before attempting to reinflate.

25. Attach end of catheter to collecting tube of drainage system. Drainage bag must be below level of bladder;

Establishes closed system for urine drainage. Placement on side rails could result in bag being raised above bladder.

Step	**Rationale**
do not place bag on side rails of bed.	
26. Anchor catheter:	
a. Female client:	
(1) Secure catheter tubing to inner thigh with strip of nonallergenic tape (commercial multipurpose tube holders with Velcro strap are also available). Allow for slack so movement of thigh does not create tension on catheter. Clip drainage tubing to edge of mattress.	Anchoring catheter to inner thigh reduces pressure on urethra, thus reducing possibility of tissue injury in this area (Evans, 1999).
b. Male client:	
(1) Secure catheter tubing to top of thigh or lower abdomen (with penis directed toward chest). Allow slack in catheter so movement does not create tension on catheter. Clip drainage tubing to edge of mattress.	Anchoring catheter to lower abdomen reduces pressure on urethra at junction of penis and scrotum, thus reducing possibility of tissue injury in this area.
27. Assist client to comfortable position. Wash and dry perineal area as needed.	Maintains comfort and security.
28. **Catheter care:** Perform catheter care as ordered when indwelling catheter is present:	

Step	Rationale
a. Place waterproof pad under client.	Protects bed from soiling.
b. Provide routine perineal care.	
c. Assess urethral meatus and surrounding tissues for inflammation, swelling, and discharge, and ask client if burning or discomfort is felt.	Determines local infection and status of hygiene.
d. Using clean washcloth, wipe in circular motion along length of catheter for about 10 cm (4 inches).	Reduces presence of secretions or drainage on outside catheter surface.

NURSE ALERT Note the presence of any encrustations, and cleanse thoroughly.

e. Replace, as necessary, adhesive tape or multipurpose tube holder that anchors catheter to client's leg or abdomen. Remove adhesive residue from skin.	Secures catheter, thus reducing risk of catheter being pulled and exposing portion of catheter that was in urethra. Also prevents drag on catheter and avoids creating pressure from balloon on bladder floor.
f. Avoid placing tension on catheter.	Tension causes urethral trauma.
g. Replace tubing and collection bag as necessary and/or according to agency policy, adhering to principles of surgical asepsis.	Urinary tubing and collection bag should be changed if signs of leakage, odor, or sediment buildup are present. Catheterization system, including catheter, may need to be replaced if leaking or blockage occurs.
h. Check drainage tubing and bag to ensure that:	
(1) Tubing is not looped or	Prevents pooling of urine and reflux of urine into bladder.

Step	**Rationale**
positioned above level of bladder.	
(2) Tubing is coiled and secured onto bed linen.	Prevents looping of tubing and subsequent pooling of urine.
(3) Tube is not kinked or clamped.	Prevents stasis of urine in bladder. Also ensures that client is not lying on tubing, causing pressure on skin and increasing risk of pressure ulcer.
(4) Collection bag is positioned appropriately on bed frame.	Ensures appropriate drainage of urine.
i. Collection bag should be emptied as necessary but at least every 8 hours.	Urine in collection bag is excellent medium for growth of microorganisms.
29. Catheter removal:	
a. ✏ Place waterproof pad:	Prevents soiling of bed linen. Provides wrapper to cover contaminated catheter after removal, thus eliminating possibility of urine contaminating nurse's gloved hand.
(1) Between female's thighs (if in supine position).	
(2) Over male's thighs.	
b. Obtain sterile urine specimen if required.	Determines if bacteria are present in urine.
c. Remove adhesive tape or Velcro tube holder used to secure and anchor catheter.	Allows for positioning of catheter for removal.
d. Insert hub of syringe into inflation valve (balloon port). Aspirate	Deflates balloon to allow for removal. If solution is not completely aspirated, partially

Step	Rationale
entire amount of fluid used to inflate balloon.	inflated balloon causes trauma to urethral wall as catheter is removed.
e. Pull catheter out smoothly and slowly.	Prevents trauma to urethral mucosa.

NURSE ALERT If resistance is met, stop pulling the catheter. Aspirate again to ensure that all fluid has been removed. If resistance continues, notify the physician.

f. Wrap contaminated catheter in waterproof pad. Unhook collection bag and drainage tubing from bed.	Prevents contamination of nurse's hands.
30. When catheter care and/or removal is completed:	
a. Reposition client as necessary. Cleanse perineum, and remove any adhesive residue from skin. Lower level of bed, and position side rails accordingly.	Promotes client comfort and safety.
b. Measure and empty contents of collection bag.	Provides accurate recording of urinary output.
31. Palpate bladder.	Determines if distention is relieved, as is case with catheter insertion. Palpation of bladder is needed after catheter removal to ensure bladder emptying.
32. Observe character and amount of urine:	
a. In drainage bag of catheterized client.	Urine in drainage bag determines if urine is flowing into drainage bag adequately.
b. Observe time and amount of first voided specimen after catheter removal.	Indicates return of bladder function.

Step	Rationale
33. Inspect condition of urethra and surrounding tissue, and ask client about discomfort.	Determines if area is irritated or cleansed properly.
34. Complete postprocedure protocol.	

Recording and Reporting

- Report and record type and size of catheter inserted, amount of fluid used to inflate balloon, characteristics of urine, amount of urine, reasons for catheterization, specimen collection, and, if appropriate, client's response to procedure and teaching topics.
- After catheter care, note condition of urethra and surrounding tissues. Indicate any client discomfort associated with the catheter or after catheter removal.
- Record amount of urine in drainage bag every 8 hours; indicate voided amounts after catheter removal. Empty drainage bag and record amounts at least every 8 hours. Initiate I&O records.

Unexpected Outcomes	Related Interventions
1. No urine is present.	• *Female:* Catheter may be in vaginal opening. • *Male:* Catheter may not be advanced far enough through prostatic urethra.
2. Urine is leaking from around catheter.	• Indicates improper catheter placement, possible balloon deflation, or catheter that is too small. Reinflate balloon, or replace catheter.
3. Urethral or perineal irritation is present.	• Observe for urine leaking from catheter; replace if needed. • Ensure that indwelling catheter is secured properly.
4. Fever and/or urine odor is present. Client may void small,	• May indicate UTI. • Obtain sterile specimen.

Unexpected Outcomes	Related Interventions
frequent amounts with sensation of continuing urge to void, burning, or bleeding.	
5. Client is unable to void after catheter removal.	• Provide adequate intake. • Provide for privacy. • Palpate for bladder distention. • Notify physician if client has not been able to void 6 to 8 hours after catheter removal.

Urinary Catheter Irrigation

Catheter irrigations are performed on an intermittent or continuous basis to maintain catheter patency. The two types of irrigation systems are closed bladder irrigation systems and open irrigation systems. A closed bladder irrigation system provides intermittent or continuous irrigation of the system without disrupting the sterile alignment of the catheter and drainage system, thus decreasing the risk of bacteria entering the urinary tract. The closed system is used most frequently in clients who have had genitourinary surgery. These clients are at risk for occlusion of the Foley catheter by small blood clots and mucous fragments; they are also at risk for urinary tract infection (UTI).

The open irrigation system is also used to maintain catheter patency. However, this system is used when bladder irrigations are required less frequently (e.g., every 8 hours) and when no blood clots or large mucous shreds are present in the urinary drainage.

Delegation Considerations

The skill of catheter irrigation should not be delegated to assistive personnel (AP). The nurse provides AP with the following directions:

- Instruct AP to inform the nurse about complaints of pain, discomfort, or fever.
- Instruct AP to inform the nurse about the presence of blood clots in the drainage or a change in color of the drainage.
- Instruct AP to inform the nurse about any decrease in drainage amount.

Equipment
Closed Continuous Method

- Sterile irrigating solution (unless otherwise specified in order) at room temperature
- Irrigation tubing with clamp (with or without Y connector) (clamp regulates irrigation flow rate; Y connector allows intravenous (IV) bags to be connected to tubing)
- IV pole
- Y connector (optional) (used to connect irrigation tubing to double-lumen catheter)

Closed Intermittent Method

- Sterile irrigating solution at room temperature
- Sterile graduated container
- Sterile 30- to 50-ml irrigation or cone syringe (used to instill irrigant into catheter)
- Sterile 19- to 22-gauge 1-inch needle
- Antiseptic swab
- Screw clamp (used to temporarily occlude catheter as irrigant is instilled)

Open Intermittent Method

- Sterile irrigating solution at room temperature (normal saline is most commonly used)
- Disposable sterile irrigation tray and set
- Bulb syringe or 60-ml piston type of syringe
- Sterile collection basin
- Waterproof drape
- Sterile solution container
- Antiseptic swabs
- Gloves
- Tape

Step	Rationale
1. Complete preprocedure protocol.	
2. Check client's record to determine:	
a. Purpose of bladder irrigation.	Allows nurse to anticipate observations to make (e.g., blood or mucus in urine).
b. Type of irrigation: continuous or intermittent.	Allows nurse to select proper equipment. In continuous irrigation, clamp regulates slow, steady flow into bladder. For intermittent irrigation, flow from irrigating solution is clamped for specified time and then opened and designated amount of irrigating solution is allowed to flush into bladder.
c. Type of catheter used (NOTE: Appropriate	Indicates if it is necessary to break system for irrigation.

Step	Rationale

catheter should be inserted at time of original catheterization):

  (1) Single lumen—used primarily with open irrigation.

  (2) Double lumen (one lumen to inflate balloon, one to allow outflow of urine).

  (3) Triple lumen (one lumen to inflate balloon, one to instill irrigant solution, and one to allow outflow of urine) (Fig. 76-1).

3. Assess the following:

  a. Color of urine and presence of mucus, clots, or sediment.

    Indicates if client is bleeding or sloughing tissue and determines necessity for increasing irrigation

Fig. 76-1
Closed continuous irrigation.

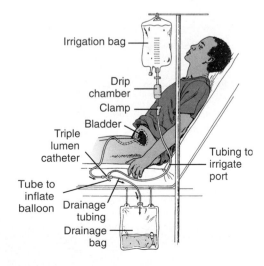

Irrigation bag

Drip chamber

Clamp

Bladder

Triple lumen catheter

Tubing to irrigate port

Tube to inflate balloon

Drainage tubing

Drainage bag

Step	Rationale
	rates with continuous irrigations or increasing irrigation frequency with intermittent irrigations.
b. Palpate bladder.	Determines if urine is draining freely from bladder.
c. Observe existing closed irrigation system:	
(1) Note if fluid entering bladder and fluid draining from bladder are in appropriate proportions.	Determines presence of bladder distention.
(2) Determine that drainage tubing is not kinked, clamped off incorrectly, or looped below bladder level.	Determines if system is obstructed. One would expect more output than fluid instilled because of urine production.
(3) Note amount of fluid remaining in existing irrigating solution container.	Allows nurse to anticipate hanging of new irrigation bag.
4. Review intake and output (I&O) record.	Determines baseline for prior output measures. All clients with continuous bladder irrigations should have I&O measurements.
5. **Closed intermittent irrigation:**	
a. Pour prescribed room-temperature sterile irrigating solution in sterile container. Be sure solution is not cold.	Cold solution may cause bladder spasm.
b. ✄ Clamp indwelling retention catheter below soft injection port or on drainage tubing.	Occlusion of catheter provides resistance against which irrigant can be forcefully instilled into catheter.

Step	Rationale
c. Draw sterile solution into syringe using aseptic technique. Keep tip of syringe sterile.	Ensures sterility of irrigating fluid.
d. Cleanse catheter injection port with antiseptic swab (this same port is used for specimen collections).	Reduces transmission of infection.
e. Insert needle of syringe through port at 30-degree angle. (See manufacturer's instructions for possible variation.)	Ensures that needle tip enters lumen of catheter and that needle does not puncture tubing.
f. Inject fluid into catheter and bladder.	Injection dislodges clots and sediment.

NURSE ALERT If the catheter does not irrigate, the tip may incorrectly be lodged in the urethra and not in the bladder. Use slow, even pressure when injecting fluid. Too much pressure may traumatize the bladder wall.

g. Withdraw syringe, and remove clamp; allow solution to drain into urinary drainage bag. (Tubing is clamped temporarily to allow instilled fluid to remain in bladder, especially if irrigant is medicated.)	Allows drainage to flow via gravity.

6. **Closed continuous irrigation:**
   NOTE: Supplies for closed irrigation system may be kept at bedside. Irrigating solution should be at room temperature. This practice is similar to that used when bag of IV fluid is added to IV infusion. Using principles

Step	Rationale

of medication safety, check that solution, volume, client, route, and time are correct. Discard any sterile solution not used within 24 hours of opening. Check institutional policy. When irrigant is opened, it should be marked with date and time.

a. Insert (spike) tip of sterile irrigation tubing into bag containing irrigation solution.

Reduces transmission of microorganisms.

b. Close clamp on tubing, and hang bag of solution on IV pole.

Prevents loss of irrigating solution.

c. Open clamp, and allow solution to flow through tubing, keeping end of tubing sterile; close clamp, and recap end of tubing.

Removes air from tubing.

d. Use aseptic technique to connect tubing to drainage port of Y connector on double/triple-lumen catheter.

e. For continuous irrigation, calculate drip rate and adjust clamp on irrigation tubing accordingly to begin flow of solution into bladder.

Ensures continuous, even irrigation of catheter system. Prevents accumulation of solution in bladder, which may cause bladder distention and possible injury.

f. For intermittent flow, clamp tubing on drainage system, open clamp on irrigation

Fluid is instilled through catheter in bolus into bladder, flushing system. Fluid drains out after irrigation is complete.

Step	**Rationale**

tubing, and allow prescribed amount of fluid to enter bladder.

NURSE ALERT Do not leave a clamped drainage bag unattended. Check frequently—at least every hour.

7. **Open irrigation:**

a. Open sterile irrigation tray; establish sterile field, and pour required amount of sterile solution into sterile solution container. Replace cap on large container of solution.

   Adheres to principles of surgical asepsis.

b. Position waterproof drape under catheter.

   Prevents soiling of bed linen.

c. Aspirate 30 ml of solution into irrigating syringe. Place syringe in sterile solution container until ready to use.

   Prepares irrigant for instillation into catheter. Maintains sterility of irrigating syringe.

d. Move sterile collection basin close to client's thigh.

   Prevents soiling of bed linen and prohibits reaching over sterile area.

e. Wipe connection point between catheter and tubing with antiseptic wipe before disconnecting.

   Reduces transmission of microorganisms.

f. Disconnect catheter from drainage tubing, allowing urine to flow into sterile collection basin; cover open end of drainage tubing with sterile protective cap, and position tubing so

   Maintains sterility of inner aspect of catheter lumen and drainage tubing; reduces potential of introducing pathogens into bladder.

Step	Rationale
it stays coiled on top of bed.	
g. Maintaining sterility of syringe, insert tip into lumen of catheter, and gently instill solution.	Reduces incidence of bladder spasm but clears catheter of obstruction.
h. Withdraw syringe, lower catheter, and allow solution to drain into basin. Repeat, instilling solution and draining several times until drainage is clear of clots and sediment.	Allows drainage to flow by gravity. Provides for adequate flushing of catheter.
i. If solution does not return, have client turn onto side facing nurse; if changing position does not help, reinsert syringe and gently aspirate solution.	Change in position may move tip of catheter in bladder, increasing likelihood that fluid instilled will flow out.
j. After irrigation is complete, remove protector cap from urinary drainage tubing adapter, cleanse adapter with alcohol swab, and reinsert adapter into lumen of catheter.	Reestablishes closed urinary drainage system.
8. Anchor catheter to client's leg or thigh with tape or Velcro multipurpose tube holder (see Skill 75).	Prevents trauma to urethral tissue.
9. Calculate fluid used to irrigate bladder and catheter, and subtract from volume drained.	Determines accurate urinary output.
10. Observe characteristics of output: viscosity, color, and presence of clots.	Data serve as baseline to judge response to therapy.

Step	Rationale
11. Observe for catheter patency.	Ensures that bladder is emptying freely.
12. Complete postprocedure protocol.	

Recording and Reporting

- Record in nurses' notes and on I&O sheet amount of solution used as irrigant, amount returned as drainage, characteristics of output, and urine output.
- Report catheter occlusion, sudden bleeding, infection, or increased pain to physician.

Unexpected Outcomes	Related Interventions
1. Irrigating solution is not returned or is not flowing at prescribed rate, which indicates possible occlusion of Foley catheter.	• Examine tubing for clots, sediment, and kinks. • Notify physician if irrigant is retained, client complains of pain, or bladder is distended.
2. Signs of fever or cloudy, foul urine is present.	• May indicate infection; physician should be notified. • Monitor vital signs and character of urine.
3. Bladder spasms increase. May indicate occlusion of catheter with foreign object (e.g., blood clot).	• Notify physician if large clots or sediment is returned or if spasms increase or are unrelieved. May need to change from intermittent to continuous irrigation.

Urinary Diversion: Maintaining a Continent Diversion

A continent urinary diversion is a reservoir or pouch that collects urine. Urine is evacuated only when a catheter is inserted into the stoma to empty the urine. This is unlike a conventional urinary diversion such as an ileal conduit, which serves only as a passageway for urine to flow to the outside of the abdomen. The opening (called a *stoma*) into the reservoir generally is placed in the right lower quadrant of the abdomen below where an ileal conduit would be. The stoma is flush with the skin or slightly budded and is reddish pink. The pouch is emptied when the client inserts a catheter or tube into the external stoma to drain the stool. Because the ostomy is continent, the client does not have to wear an external ostomy pouch over the external stoma.

Delegation Considerations

The skill of maintaining a continent diversion may not be delegated to assistive personnel (AP). The nurse should inform AP to:

- Immediately report any leaks of urine or feces seeping around the stoma.
- Report any changes in the client's level of comfort.

Equipment

Varies with recovery phase.

Postoperative Care to 3 Weeks

- Sterile normal saline (NS)
- Sterile catheter tip irrigating syringe
- Sterile gauze pads
- Sterile gloves
- Antiseptic swab (e.g., povidone-iodine or chlorhexidine)
- Sterile specimen cup
- Sterile water
- Towels

Postoperative Care 4 to 6 Weeks

- Sterile NS
- Sterile catheter tip irrigating syringe

- Sterile gauze pads
- Sterile gloves
- Antiseptic swab (e.g., povidone-iodine or chlorhexidine)
- Sterile basin
- Sterile 14 to 16 Fr red rubber catheter
- Water-soluble lubricant
- Stoma cover (commercial or adhesive strip or nonstick dressing)
- Liquid antimicrobial soap
- Towels

Step	Rationale
1. Complete preprocedure protocol.	
2. Observe all tubes for intactness and patency, nature of drainage, and connection to appropriate collection system.	Clients return immediately after surgery with catheter in stoma. Avoids errors in input and output record. Minimum acceptable urine output is 30 ml/hr from all sites.
3. Observe stoma for color, peristomal skin for maceration, and condition of all external suture lines.	Determines potential circulatory problems and reflects healing progress. Stoma should be red or pink, glistening with mucous coating. Dusky or bluish stoma has compromised circulation (Lewis and others, 2004).
4. Auscultate bowel sounds and lung sounds. Obtain serum values of chloride and creatinine.	Manipulation of large portions of bowel may lead to ileus. Under-ventilation by client after surgery may lead to respiratory complications. Immediately after surgery, intestinal segment used for reservoir may absorb chloride and hydrogen ions. Creatinine measures effectiveness of kidney function (Pagana and Pagana, 2004).
5. Palpate lightly around stoma, noting any localized tenderness or guarding.	May be sign of infection along internal suture lines.
6. Initiate care of continent diversion:	

Step	Rationale
a. **Postoperative care to 3 weeks:**	
(1) Position client supine or sitting, and drape with towels.	Facilitates instilling NS into reservoir; sitting is better position for drainage. Maintains client's dignity.
(2) Perform hand hygiene, and open sterile equipment. Remove lid from sterile specimen cup, and place lid with open side up. Pour 20 to 30 ml sterile NS into sterile specimen cup. Open sterile syringe and antiseptic swabs, and position them for use.	Reduces transmission of microorganisms.
(3) Don sterile gloves, and draw 20 to 30 ml sterile NS into syringe. Cleanse connection point of indwelling stomal catheter and drainage tubing with antiseptic swabs using circular motion; use each swab once; wait 30 seconds.	Reduces risk of nosocomial infection.
(4) Disconnect catheter and tubing, and gently irrigate stomal catheter by infusing NS; do not contaminate tip of	Large numbers of internal surgical sites require strict asepsis during postoperative phase. Reflux into ureters may cause infection (Lewis and others, 2004).

Step	Rationale
drainage tubing. If new urinary diversion, gently irrigate to avoid forcing solution and retained urine into implanted ureters.	
(5) Reconnect drainage system. Record volume used for irrigation. For urinary diversions, subtract this from total urine output at end of each shift. Follow agency protocol for changing bedside urinary drainage bags.	Keeps accurate urinary output record. Reduces risk of colonization of microorganisms.
(6) Using remaining antiseptic swabs, cleanse "face" of stoma around catheter. Use another swab, and cleanse skin around base of stoma; allow to dry 30 seconds, and gently remove antiseptic with gauze pad moistened with sterile water.	Mucus accumulates on face of stoma and seeps onto skin. Maintains skin integrity and reduces risk of infection. Some clients are allergic to iodine, so assess for allergy to iodine or shellfish before this step (Lewis and others, 2004).
(7) Discard soiled equipment; remove gloves. Maintain sterile specimen cup and sterile NS and water containers for next irrigation.	Reduces transmission of microorganisms. Maintains sterility of cup so it can be used for 8 hours. Some supplies can stay at bedside for 8 hours if strict aseptic technique is followed; this helps contain costs.

Step	Rationale
Label these with date, time, and nurse's initials.	
NOTE: Hospital protocols vary; generally, immediately after surgery, continent diversions are gently irrigated every 2 to 4 hours to maintain patency of stomal catheter, allowing urine to drain freely.	
b. **Postoperative care 4 to 6 weeks:**	
(1) Follow steps 1 and 2 in preceding section. Omit setting up sterile specimen cup.	Generally, stoma catheter is removed third postoperative week.
(2) Open sterile basin, and maintain inside of wrapper as sterile field. Pour 30 to 60 ml of sterile NS into basin. Open gauze pads onto sterile wrapper; squeeze small amount of water-soluble lubricant onto gauze pad. Open wrapper of sterile red catheter for use, or place catheter onto sterile basin wrapper.	Maintains strict aseptic technique to reduce risk of nosocomial infection during recovery phase.
(3) Don sterile gloves, and draw 30 to 60 ml of sterile NS into syringe. Cleanse "face" of	Reduces risk of nosocomial infection; removes any accumulation of mucus.

Step	**Rationale**
stoma with antiseptic swab starting from center and using circular movements to outer edge; wait 30 seconds.	
(4) Lubricate tip of catheter well. Insert into stoma by gently rotating during insertion; insert until urine starts to drain.	Reduces trauma to continence mechanism (valve) during insertion; some resistance to insertion is normal as catheter passes through layer of abdominal fascia. Client may need to change position to facilitate insertion. Taking slow, deep breaths also helps by relaxing abdominal muscles.
(5) If no effluent starts to drain, problem solving is needed. For example, try moving catheter in and out slightly, have client move side to side, or ask client to cough. If these actions do not cause drainage, then gently irrigate catheter with 30 to 60 ml of sterile NS.	Mucus may plug catheter. Catheter may need to be irrigated to establish flow.
(6) Before withdrawing catheter, have client cough three or four times; then slowly remove.	Positive pressure inside abdomen clears residual urine or stool from pouch and continence valve; clears mucus from catheter.
(7) Gently cleanse peristomal skin with gauze pads and liquid	Reduces bacterial colonization and removes any dried mucus to maintain skin integrity.

Step	Rationale
antimicrobial soap; rinse; pat dry.	
(8) Cover stoma with stomal covering.	Some leakage of effluent occurs until full recovery from surgery; mucus will always be produced.
(9) Discard soiled equipment; remove gloves. Maintain sterile NS; label with date, time, and nurse's initials.	Reduces transmission of microorganisms. Some equipment can stay at bedside for 8 hours if strict aseptic technique is followed; this helps contain costs.
7. Record output and amount used for irrigation.	Keeps accurate output record.
8. Note appearance of stoma, peristomal skin, and abdominal suture lines.	Determines condition of stoma and peristomal skin and progress of wound healing.
9. Complete postprocedure protocol.	

Recording and Reporting

- Record time of irrigation and/or intubation, size of catheter used, ease of intubation, amount of NS used, amount and character of output, and client's tolerance. Include client's and family's responses and their level of participation in care.
- Report abnormalities of stoma and peristomal skin.

Unexpected Outcomes	Related Interventions
1. Continence valve leaks excessively and continuously after stomal catheter is removed.	• Replace valve. • Empty reservoir more often to avoid overdistention.
2. Catheter cannot be inserted.	• Remove catheter, and start again. • Pouch may be overdistended; empty pouch more frequently.
3. Stool is especially thick.	• Encourage client not to take laxative but rather to increase daily fluid intake, including intake of prune juice.

Urinary Diversion: Pouching an Incontinent Urinary Diversion

Because urine flows continuously from an incontinent urinary diversion, a urinary pouch is usually placed over the opening immediately after surgery. Placement of the pouch may be more challenging than the enterostomy because urine flow keeps the skin moist and in the immediate postoperative period, urinary stents may be in place in the stoma.

The stoma of a urinary diversion is normally reddish. It is made from a portion of the gastrointestinal (GI) tract, either the ileum or the colon, and has the same mucosal surface. Ideally, the stoma should protrude 1.25 to 2 cm ($\frac{1}{2}$ to $\frac{3}{4}$ inch) above the skin. An ileal conduit is usually located in the right lower quadrant; a colon conduit is usually located in the left lower quadrant. Ureterostomies are usually performed in infants, and a conduit is performed when the child approaches school age.

Delegation Considerations

The skill of pouching a new incontinent urinary diversion may not be delegated to assistive personnel (AP). Care of an established incontinent urinary diversion can be delegated. When delegating this skill, the nurse must inform AP about:

- The baseline assessment findings of the client's ostomy and when to report changes.
- Expected amount and character of the output, and when to report changes.
- Special equipment needed to complete procedure.

Equipment

- Pouch, urinary (with antireflux flap) and skin barrier
  NOTE: Use two-piece system (pouch and flange) if stents are present; use measuring guide to measure the stoma to determine the correct size of pouch and skin barrier
- Bedside urinary drainage bag
- Clean, disposable gloves (sterile gloves optional)
- Hand-held hair dryer
- Sterile gauze pads

- Towel or disposable waterproof barrier
- Basin with warm tap water
- Scissors
- Skin-sealant wipes
- Sterile forceps (if stents present)
- Vinegar

Step	Rationale
1. Complete preprocedure protocol.	
2. ▰ Check pouch for leakage, length of time in place; ask client about skin tenderness or discomfort. Check stoma for color, healing. Check abdominal incision (if present) for relationship to stoma for proper placement of pouch. To prevent skin irritation, one-piece pouch or skin barrier from two-piece system should be changed, if not leaking, every 3 to 7 days or when checking for skin irritation.	Pouches should be emptied when one-third to one-half full because weight of urine in pouch may weaken or dislodge skin seal (Thompson, 2000). Stoma should be moist and reddish pink; immediately after surgery, it is edematous and usually has urinary stents in place (Fig. 78-1).
3. Observe output from stoma. Immediately after surgery, ureteral stents are	Urinary output must be monitored on all postoperative clients with urinary diversions to

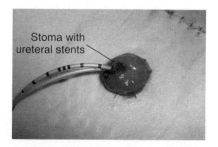

Stoma with
ureteral stents

Fig. 78-1 Viable ileal conduit stoma with stents present and normal peristomal skin and pouch. (Courtesy Hollister, Inc, Libertyville, Ill.)

Step	**Rationale**
in place and remain for up to 10 to 14 days.	monitor renal status and patency of stents and whether volume of output is within acceptable limits (minimum of 30 ml/hr). Stents (internal support device) are used to maintain patency of ureters at surgical anastomoses.
4. Assess abdomen for best type of pouch to use. After pouch is off, assess skin around stoma, observing scars, folds, skin breakdown; also check peristomal suture line if present. Discard gloves.	Maximizes secure fit and minimizes chance of leakage. Pouch and skin barrier are changed with any leakage. Determines need for barrier paste and additional intervention.
5. Position client standing or supine, and drape. Some clients may prefer to do pouch change while sitting because this may make it easier for them to see stoma. However, when skin barrier and pouch are applied in sitting position, skin may have folds and wrinkles. Because of this, skin barriers and pouches applied with client in sitting position may leak.	When client is supine, fewer wrinkles occur, allowing for ease of pouch application; maintains client's dignity.
6. Prepare pouch by removing backing from barrier and adhesive; if using cut-to-fit, cut opening $\frac{1}{16}$ to $\frac{1}{8}$ inch larger than stoma before removing backing.	Barrier facilitates seal and protects skin; size of opening keeps urine off skin and lessens risk of maceration with skin irritation; avoids risk of damage to stoma. Stoma shrinks and does not reach optimal size for 6 to 8 weeks (Thompson, 2000).
7. Place towel or disposable waterproof barrier under client.	Protects bed linen. Rolled gauze pads used to absorb urine during pouch change.

Step	Rationale
Tightly roll several gauze pads separately (should resemble tampon). (*Optional:* If gauze pads [called "wicks"] are to come in contact with stents, roll with sterile gloves on. Place wicks on sterile barrier [can use the inside of gauze wrapper].)	
8. Remove used pouch carefully and gently by pushing skin away from barrier. If stents are present, *do not pull on them*. Immediately place wick or sterile gauze pad over stomal opening. If stents are present, place sterile gauze pad underneath tips.	Reduces risk of trauma to skin and risk of injury to ureters if stents are present; jerking irritates skin and can cause skin tears. Keeps urine from leaking onto skin. Immediately after surgery, copious mucus exists over stoma because bowel has not adjusted to presence of urine.
9. Cleanse peristomal skin gently with warm tap water using gauze pads; do not scrub skin. Dry skin.	Avoid soap. It leaves residue on skin, which interferes with pouch adhesion (Thompson, 2000). Pouch does not adhere to wet skin. Stents are sutured in place to decrease risk of damage. Do not be alarmed if small amount of blood appears on stoma because stomal surface may ooze blood if rubbed. Bleeding into pouch is abnormal.

NURSE ALERT   If uric crystals are present on the skin, apply washcloth with a vinegar soak ($1/3$ vinegar with $2/3$ warm water) to peristomal skin. Rinse with warm tap water, and dry completely.

10. Wick stoma continuously during pouch measurement and change. Place tip of gauze at stomal opening. Measure stoma.	Using wick at stoma tip prevents peristomal skin from becoming wet with urine during pouching-change procedure.

Step	Rationale
a. If creases form next to stoma, use barrier paste or seal to fill in; let dry 1 to 2 minutes.	Flattening of creases with paste or seal creates smooth surface for pouch placement (Thompson, 2000).
b. Apply skin sealant in circular area around base of stoma to any skin not protected by barrier; let dry. Hold pouch by barrier, center over stoma and stents, and press down gently on barrier. Bottom of pouch should be angled slightly to attach to bedside urinary drainage bag. Use another skin sealant on skin coming in contact with adhesive; allow to dry. Press adhesive backing smoothly against skin, starting from bottom and working up and around sides. Never use karaya skin barrier with urinary diversion.	Urine renders karaya in skin barrier ineffective and results in leakage.
c. Maintain gentle finger pressure around barrier for 1 to 2 minutes.	Helps ensure molding and adherence of skin barrier.
d. If using two-piece pouch, apply flange (barrier with adhesive) as above; then snap on pouch. If client is out of bed and ambulatory most of the time, apply pouch vertically.	Urine drains almost continuously. Flange waterproofs any skin that may contact urine. Creates wrinkle-free, secure seal. Angling pouch avoids uneven twisting, which can disrupt seal. Prevents trauma to skin.
11. During night, open drain spout, attach specific	Constant flow of urine results in frequent emptying; overfilling of

Step	Rationale
manufacturer adapter piece to end of pouch, and then attach this to bedside urinary bag. Place bag at point close to foot of bed.	pouch may break skin seal. Placing night bag at foot of bed maximizes straight drainage that avoids urine accumulation in pouch.
12. Observe appearance of stoma, peristomal skin, and suture line during pouch change.	Determines condition of stoma and peristomal skin and progress of wound healing.
13. Evaluate character and volume of urinary drainage.	Determines if stoma and/or stents are patent. Character of urine can reveal degree of concentration and alterations in renal function.
14. Complete postprocedure protocol.	

Recording and Reporting

- Record type of pouch, time of change, condition and appearance of stoma and peristomal skin, character of urine, volume of urinary output; include client's, family's, or significant other's reaction to stoma and level of participation.
- Report abnormalities in stoma or peristomal structures and absence of urinary output to nurse in charge or physician.

Unexpected Outcomes	Related Interventions
1. Peristomal skin is irritated, reddened, or tender or has overgrowth.	• Keep peristomal skin dry. • Determine if client has allergy to barrier and adhesive or infection. • Remeasure stoma before each change to ensure best fit of pouch.
2. No urinary output for several hours or output is less than 30 ml/hr. Urine has foul odor.	• Determine patency of stents or stoma. • Obtain urine specimen for culture and sensitivity to test for possible infection. • Notify physician.

Unexpected Outcomes	Related Interventions
3. Client reports burning sensation around base of stoma.	• Assess for presence of yeast infection around stoma, which causes itching, burning; appears as reddened area with maculopapular rash (Erwin-Toth, 2000).

Vaginal Instillations

Vaginal medications are available in foam, jelly, cream, and suppository form and by douche. Caution clients about excessive use of douches, because the therapy can lead to vaginal irritation. Vaginal suppositories are oval shaped and come individually packaged in foil wrappers. They are larger and more oval than rectal suppositories. Storage in a refrigerator prevents the solid suppositories from melting.

Delegation Considerations

The skill of vaginal instillations should not be delegated to assistive personnel (AP).

- Instruct AP about potential side effects of medications and to report their occurrence.
- Instruct AP to report any change in comfort level and any new or increased vaginal discharge or bleeding to the nurse.

Equipment

- Vaginal cream, foam, jelly, tablet, or suppository or irrigating solution
- Applicators (if needed)
- Disposable gloves
- Tissues
- Towels and/or washcloths
- Perineal pad
- Drape or sheet
- Water-soluble lubricants
- Bedpan, absorbent pad
- Irrigation or douche container (if needed)
- Medication administration record (MAR)

Step	Rationale
1. Complete preprocedure protocol.	
2. Review prescriber's medication order, including client's name, drug name, form (foam, jelly, cream, tablet, suppository, or irrigating solution), route,	Ensures safe and correct administration of medication.

Step	**Rationale**
dosage, and time of administration against MAR.	
3. Have client void.	Empties bladder and promotes comfort during insertion.
4. Assess client's ability to manipulate applicator, suppository, or irrigation equipment and to properly position self to insert medication (may be done just before insertion).	Mobility restriction indicates level of assistance required from nurse.
5. Check medication's expiration date on drug package.	Medications that have expired should not be used because potency of medication changes when medication becomes outdated.
6. Check name of medication on drug package label against MAR.	Checking label ensures that client receives correct medication.
7. Check client's identification bracelet, and ask name.	Ensures that correct client receives medication. At least two patient identifiers (neither to be patient's room number) are to be used whenever administering medications (JCAHO, 2004).
8. Explain procedure to client. Be specific if client plans on self-administering medication.	Promotes client's understanding. Enables client to self-administer drug if physically able.
9. Compare MAR with drug and continue.	Reduces medication error.
10. Assist client with lying in dorsal recumbent position. Clients with restricted mobility in knees or hips may lie supine with legs abducted.	Position provides easy access to and good exposure of vaginal canal. Dependent position also allows suppository to dissolve in vagina without escaping.
11. Keep abdomen and lower extremities draped.	Minimizes client's embarrassment by limiting exposure.

Step	Rationale

12. Be sure vaginal orifice is well illuminated by room light. Otherwise, position portable gooseneck lamp.

Proper insertion requires visualization of external genitalia if not self-administered.

13. Inspect condition of external genitalia and vaginal canal.

Provides baseline to monitor effect of medication.

14. For suppository insertion:

   a. Remove suppository from wrapper, and apply liberal amount of water-soluble lubricant to smooth or rounded end. Be sure that suppository is at room temperature. Lubricate gloved index finger of dominant hand.

Lubrication reduces friction against mucosal surfaces during insertion. Use of petroleum jelly may leave residue that harbors bacteria and yeast fungi.

   b. With nondominant gloved hand, gently separate labial folds in front-to-back direction.

Exposes vaginal orifice.

   c. Insert rounded end of suppository along posterior wall of vaginal canal entire length of finger (7.5 to 10 cm or 3 to 4 inches) (Fig. 79-1).

Proper placement of suppository ensures equal distribution of medication along walls of vaginal cavity.

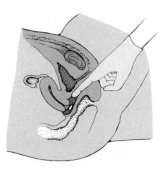

Fig. 79-1   Angle of vaginal suppository insertion.

Step	Rationale
d. Withdraw finger, and wipe away remaining lubricant from around orifice and labia with tissue or cloth.	Maintains comfort.
15. For application of cream or foam:	
a. Fill cream or foam applicator following package directions.	Dose is instilled based on volume in applicator.
b. With nondominant gloved hand, gently separate labial folds.	Exposes vaginal orifice.
c. With dominant gloved hand, insert applicator approximately 5 to 7.5 cm (2 to 3 inches). Push applicator plunger to deposit medication into vagina (Fig. 79-2).	Allows equal distribution of medication along vaginal walls.
d. Withdraw applicator, and place on paper towel. Wipe off residual cream from labia or vaginal orifice with tissue or cloth.	Maintains client comfort. Residual cream on applicator may contain microorganisms.

Fig. 79-2 Applicator inserted into vaginal canal. Plunger pushed to instill medication.

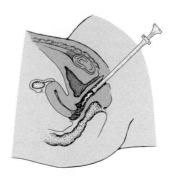

Step	Rationale
16. For irrigation and douche:	
a. Place client on bedpan with absorbent pad underneath.	Allows hips to be higher than shoulders and solution reaches posterior wall of vagina. Bedpan collects solution.
b. Be sure fluid is at body temperature. Run fluid through container nozzle (priming tubing).	Body temperature promotes client comfort. Priming tubing removes air and moistens nozzle tip.
c. Gently separate labial folds, and direct nozzle toward sacrum, following floor of vagina.	Correct angle allows nozzle access into vagina.
d. Raise container approximately 30 to 50 cm (12 to 20 inches) above level of vagina. Insert nozzle 7 to 10 cm (3 to 4 inches). Allow solution to flow while rotating nozzle. Administer all irrigating solution.	Rotating nozzle allows irrigation of all areas in vagina.
e. Withdraw nozzle, and assist client to comfortable sitting position.	Remaining solution drains by gravity.
f. Allow client to remain on bedpan for few minutes. Cleanse perineum with soap and water.	Ensures that all solution drains from vagina. Provides comfort for client.
g. Assist client off bedpan. Dry perineal area.	
17. Instruct client who received suppository, cream, or tablet to remain on her back for at least 10 minutes. If applicator is used, wash with soap and warm water,	Allows melting and spreading of medication throughout vaginal cavity and prevents loss through orifice. Vaginal cavity is not sterile. Soap and water assist in removal of

Step	Rationale
rinse, and store for future use.	bacteria and residual cream from applicator.
18. Offer perineal pad when client resumes ambulation.	Provides client comfort.
19. Complete postprocedure protocol.	
20. Have client demonstrate administration of next dose.	Reflects learning of technique.

Recording and Reporting

- Record in nurses' notes appearance of vaginal canal and genitalia, and report any unusual findings.
- Immediately after administration, record on MAR actual time each drug solution was administered, form of medication, and route. Include initials or signature.
- If symptoms do not disappear or if they get worse, report to prescriber.
- Report adverse effects/client response and/or withheld drugs to nurse in charge or physician.

Unexpected Outcomes	Related Interventions
1. Thick, white, patchy, curdlike discharge is clinging to vaginal walls. Vaginal walls appear bright pink or inflamed.	• Continue medication administration, and report if symptoms continue or appear to get worse.
2. Client reports localized pruritus and burning.	• Monitor symptoms; report to physician if they worsen.
3. Client is unable to self-administer medications.	• Reinstruct as necessary.

Venipuncture: Collecting Blood Specimens and Cultures by Syringe and Vacutainer Method

Nurses are often responsible for collecting blood specimens; however, many institutions have specially trained phlebotomists. As a nurse, be familiar with your institution's policies and procedures and your state's Nurse Practice Act regarding guidelines for drawing blood samples.

The three primary methods of obtaining blood specimens are venipuncture, skin puncture, and arterial stick. Venipuncture, the most common method, involves inserting a hollow-bore needle into the lumen of a large vein to obtain a specimen. Use a needle and syringe or a special Vacutainer tube connected to a needle housing that allows the drawing of multiple blood samples. Because veins are major sources of blood for laboratory testing and routes for intravenous (IV) fluid or blood replacement, maintaining their integrity is essential. Always try to avoid unnecessary injury to veins.

When drawing blood cultures, it is important that at least two culture specimens be drawn from two different sites. Because bacteremia may be accompanied by fever and chills, draw blood cultures when the client is experiencing these clinical signs (Pagana and Pagana, 2002). If only one culture produces bacteria, the assumption is that the bacteria are skin contaminants rather than the infectious agent. Bacteremia (infection of the blood) exists when both cultures grow the infectious agent you are testing for.

Because culture specimens obtained through an IV catheter are frequently contaminated, tests using them should not be performed unless you are testing for catheter sepsis. Cultures should be drawn before antibiotic therapy is started, because the antibiotic may interrupt the organism's growth in the laboratory. If the client is receiving antibiotics, notify the laboratory and report what specific antibiotics the client is receiving (Pagana and Pagana, 2005).

Delegation Considerations

The skill of collecting blood specimens by venipuncture is often delegated to specially trained assistive personnel (AP). In some institutions, phlebotomists are responsible for obtaining venipuncture samples. Agency policies differ regarding personnel who may draw blood specimens.

Equipment

- Alcohol or antiseptic swab (e.g., chlorhexidine)
- Disposable gloves
- Small pillow or folded towel
- Sterile gauze pads (2 × 2 inch)
- Rubber tourniquet
- Adhesive bandage or adhesive tape
- Appropriate blood tubes or culture bottles
- Completed identification labels according to agency policy
- Completed laboratory requisition (date, time, type of test)
- Plastic bag for delivery of specimen to laboratory (or container as specified by agency)

Syringe Method

- Sterile needles: 20- to 21-gauge for adults; 23- to 25-gauge for children
- Sterile syringe of appropriate size

Vacutainer Method

- Vacutainer tube with needle holder
- Sterile double-ended safety needles: 20- to 21-gauge for adults; 23- to 25-gauge for children

Blood Cultures

- Antiseptic swabs (check agency policy for specific antiseptic solution)
- 70% alcohol (check agency policy)
- Sterile needles: 20- to 21-gauge for adults; 23- to 25-gauge for children
- Sterile syringe of appropriate size

Step	Rationale
1. Complete preprocedure protocol.	
2. Determine if special conditions need to be met before specimen collection.	Some tests require meeting specific conditions to obtain accurate measurement of blood

Step	Rationale
	elements (e.g., fasting blood sugar, drug peak and trough level). Test results are more accurate with desired amount of blood.

NURSE ALERT Special collection requirements must be met for certain specimens before or after specimen collection; for example:
- Cryoglobulin levels: Use prewarmed test tubes.
- Ammonia levels: Tube must be placed in ice for delivery to laboratory.
- Lactic acid levels: Do not use tourniquet.
- Vitamin levels: Avoid exposure of test tube to light.

Step	Rationale
3. Assess client for possible risks associated with venipuncture: anticoagulant therapy, low platelet count, bleeding disorders (history of hemophilia). Review medication history.	Client history may include abnormal clotting abilities caused by low platelet count, hemophilia, or medications that increase risk for bleeding and hematoma formation.
4. Assess client for contraindicated sites for venipuncture: presence of IV fluids, hematoma at potential site, arm on side of mastectomy, or hemodialysis shunt.	Drawing specimens from such sites can result in false test results or may injure client. Samples taken from vein near IV infusion may be diluted or may contain concentrations of IV fluids. Postmastectomy client may have reduced lymphatic drainage in arm on operative side, increasing risk of infection from needle sticks. Arteriovenous shunt should never be used to obtain specimens because of risks of clotting and bleeding. Hematoma indicates existing injury to vessel's wall.
5. Don disposable gloves. If glove(s) become contaminated with blood,	Reduces risk of exposure to blood-borne bacteria.

Step	Rationale

replace with clean pair after proper disposal of contaminated gloves.

6. Apply tourniquet 5 to 10 cm (2 to 4 inches) above venipuncture site selected (antecubital fossa site is used most often).

Tourniquet blocks venous return to heart from extremity, causing veins to dilate for easier visibility.

NURSE ALERT Palpate distal pulse (e.g., brachial) below tourniquet. If pulse is not palpable, reapply tourniquet more loosely. If tourniquet is too tight, pressure will impede arterial blood flow.

7. Keep tourniquet on client no longer than 1 minute.

Prolonged tourniquet application may cause stasis, localized acidemia, and hemoconcentration (Malarkey and McMorrow, 2000).

8. Ask client to open and close fist several times, finally leaving fist clenched.

Facilitates distention of veins by forcing blood up from distal veins.

9. Quickly inspect extremity for best venipuncture site, looking for straight, prominent vein without swelling or hematoma.

Straight and intact veins are easiest to puncture.

10. Palpate selected vein with fingers. Note if vein is firm and rebounds when palpated or if vein feels rigid and cordlike and rolls when palpated (Fig. 80-1).

Patent, healthy vein is elastic and rebounds on palpation. Thrombosed vein is rigid, rolls easily, and is difficult to puncture.

11. Select venipuncture site. In case of blood cultures, two different sites are selected. If tourniquet has been in place longer than 1 minute, remove and assess other extremity or wait 60 seconds before

Prevents discomfort to client and inaccurate test results (Malarkey and McMorrow, 2000). Heat causes local dilation.

Step	Rationale

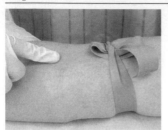

Fig. 80-1 Palpation of vein.

reapplying. (If vein cannot be palpated or viewed easily, remove tourniquet and apply warm, wet compress over extremity for 10 minutes.)

12. Obtain blood sample:
    a. Syringe method:
        (1) Have appropriate-size syringe with appropriate needle securely attached.

        (2) Cleanse venipuncture site with antiseptic swabs, moving in circular motion from site for approximately 5 cm (2 inches). Allow to dry.
           (a) If drawing sample for blood alcohol level or blood cultures, use only antiseptic swab rather than alcohol swab.

Needle must not dislodge from syringe during venipuncture.

Antimicrobial agent cleans skin surface of resident bacteria so organisms do not enter puncture site. Allowing antiseptic to dry completes its antimicrobial task and reduces "sting" of venipuncture. Alcohol left on skin can cause hemolysis of sample.

Ensures accurate test results.

Step	Rationale
(3) Remove needle cover, and inform client that "stick" lasting only few seconds will be felt.	Client has better control over anxiety when prepared about what to expect.

NURSE ALERT Observe the needle for defects, such as burrs, which cause increased discomfort and damage to the client's vein.

Step	Rationale
(4) Place thumb or forefinger of nondominant hand 2.5 cm (1 inch) below site, and gently pull skin taut. Stretch skin down until vein is stabilized.	Stabilizes vein and prevents rolling during needle insertion.
(5) Hold syringe and needle at 15- to 30-degree angle from client's arm with bevel up.	Reduces chance of penetrating both sides of vein during insertion. Keeping bevel up reduces vein trauma.
(6) Slowly insert needle into vein (Fig. 80-2). With experience, nurse will feel "pop" as needle enters vein.	Prevents puncture through vein to opposite side.

Fig. 80-2 Inserting needle into vein.

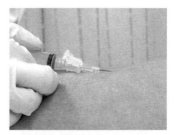

Step	**Rationale**
	If plunger is pulled back too quickly, pressure may cause vein to collapse.
(7) Hold syringe securely, and pull back gently on plunger.	Syringe held securely prevents needle from advancing. Pulling on plunger creates vacuum needed to draw blood into syringe.
(8) Look for blood return.	If blood flow fails to appear, needle is not in vein.
(9) Obtain desired amount of blood, keeping needle stabilized.	Some tests cannot be performed without minimum blood requirement. Movement of needle increases discomfort.
(10) After specimen is obtained, release tourniquet.	Reduces bleeding at site when needle is withdrawn.
(11) Apply 2 × 2–inch gauze pad or alcohol swab over puncture site without applying pressure. Quickly but carefully withdraw needle from vein, and apply pressure after removal of needle.	Pressure over needle can cause discomfort. Careful removal of needle minimizes discomfort and vein trauma.
(12) Activate needle safety cover, and discard needle in sharps container.	Reduces risk of needle-stick injury.
b. Vacutainer method (vacuum tube system method):	
(1) Attach double-ended needle to Vacutainer tube.	Long end of needle is used to puncture vein. Short end fits into blood tubes.

Step	**Rationale**
(2) Have proper blood specimen tube resting inside Vacutainer, but do not puncture rubber stopper.	Puncturing causes loss of tube's vacuum.
(3) Cleanse venipuncture site with antiseptic swab, moving in circular motion out from site for approximately 5 cm (2 inches). Allow to dry.	Cleans skin surface of resident bacteria so that organisms do not enter puncture site. Drying ensures maximal antimicrobial activity.
(4) Remove needle cover, and inform client that "stick" lasting only few seconds will be felt.	Client has better control over anxiety when prepared about what to expect.
(5) Place thumb or forefinger of nondominant hand 2.5 cm (1 inch) below site, and pull skin taut. Stretch skin down until vein is stabilized.	Helps stabilize vein and prevent rolling during needle insertion.
(6) Hold Vacutainer needle at 15- to 30-degree angle from arm with bevel up.	Reduces chance of penetrating both sides of vein during insertion. Keeping bevel up causes less trauma to vein.
(7) Slowly insert needle into vein.	Prevents puncture on opposite side.
(8) Grasp Vacutainer securely, and advance specimen tube into needle of holder (do not	Pushing needle through stopper breaks vacuum and causes flow of blood into tube. If needle in vein advances, vein may become punctured on other side.

Step	Rationale

advance needle in vein).

(9) Note flow of blood into tube (should be fairly rapid) (Fig. 80-3).

Failure of blood to appear indicates that vacuum in tube is lost or needle is not in vein.

(10) After specimen tube is filled, grasp Vacutainer firmly and remove tube. Insert additional specimen tubes as needed.

Prevents needle from advancing or dislodging. Tube should fill completely because additives in certain tubes are measured in proportion to filled tube. Tubes with additives should be inverted as soon as possible.

(11) After last tube is filled and removed from Vacutainer, release tourniquet.

Reduces bleeding at site when needle is withdrawn.

(12) Apply 2 × 2–inch gauze pad over puncture site without applying pressure, and quickly but carefully withdraw needle from vein.

Pressure over needle can cause discomfort. Careful removal of needle minimizes discomfort and vein trauma.

c. Immediately apply pressure over venipuncture site with gauze or antiseptic pad for 2 to 3 minutes or

Direct pressure minimizes bleeding and prevents hematoma formation. Pressure dressing controls bleeding.

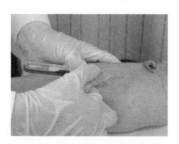

Fig. 80-3 Blood flowing into tube.

Step	**Rationale**

until bleeding stops.
Apply pressure over site,
and tape gauze dressing
securely.

d. For blood obtained by
   syringe, transfer
   specimen to tubes:

   (1) Using one-handed
      technique, insert
      needle through
      stopper of blood
      tube and allow
      vacuum to fill tube.
      Do not force
      blood into tube.

Prevents needle-stick injury.

   (2) Alternative
      method is to
      remove needle
      from syringe and
      stopper to each
      test tube. Gently
      inject required
      amount of blood
      into each tube.
      Reapply stopper.

Forcing blood into tube may cause
hemolysis of red blood cells. Risk
of blood splashing exists.

e. Rotate blood tubes
   containing additives
   gently back and forth
   8 to 10 times.

Additives should be mixed with
blood to prevent clotting.
Shaking can cause hemolysis of
red blood cells, producing
inaccurate test results.

f. Inspect puncture site
   for bleeding, and apply
   adhesive tape with
   gauze.

Keeps puncture site clean and
controls any final oozing.

g. Check tubes for any
   sign of external
   contamination with
   blood. Decontaminate
   with 70% alcohol if
   necessary.

Prevents cross contamination.
Reduces risk of exposure to
pathogens present in blood.

Step	Rationale
h. Securely attach properly completed identification label to each tube, and affix proper requisition.	Incorrect identification of specimen could result in diagnostic or therapeutic errors.
i. Place specimens in bag to be sent to laboratory.	
j. Perform postprocedure protocol.	
13. Obtain blood cultures:	
a. Carefully prepare proposed sites with antiseptic swab (check agency policy). Allow antiseptic to dry.	Antimicrobial agent cleans skin surface so organisms do not enter puncture site or contaminate culture. Drying ensures complete antimicrobial action.
b. Clean bottle tops of vacuum tubes or culture bottles. Check agency policy regarding cleaning with 70% alcohol after cleaning with antiseptic solution and air-drying.	Ensures that specimen is sterile.
c. Collect 10 to 15 ml of venous blood by venipuncture in 20-ml syringe from each venipuncture site.	Ensures that a positive blood culture indicates infection and not false confirmation.
d. Discard needle on syringe; replace with new sterile needle before injecting blood sample into culture bottle.	Maintains sterile technique and prevents contamination of specimen.
e. If both aerobic and anaerobic cultures are needed, inoculate anaerobic first.	Anaerobic organisms may take longer to grow (Pagana and Pagana, 2002).
f. Mix gently after inoculation.	Mixes medium and blood.

Step	Rationale
g. Immediately apply pressure over venipuncture site with gauze or antiseptic pad for 2 to 3 minutes or until bleeding stops. Apply pressure over site, and tape gauze dressing securely.	Direct pressure minimizes bleeding and prevents hematoma.
h. Label specimen with client's name, date, time, and tentative diagnosis. Indicate on laboratory slip any medications (e.g., antibiotics) taken. Place in appropriate bag for transfer.	Ensures correct processing and accurate reporting of results. Antibiotics may affect results.
i. Transport culture bottles immediately to laboratory (or at least within 30 minutes) (Pagana and Pagana, 2002).	Cultures should be prepared quickly for accurate results.
j. Perform postprocedure protocol.	

Recording and Reporting

- Record date and time of venipuncture, samples obtained, and disposition of specimen.
- Describe venipuncture site in nurse's notes.
- Report any "stat" test results to physician.
- Report any abnormal test results to physician.

Unexpected Outcomes	Related Interventions
1. Hematoma forms at venipuncture site.	• Apply pressure. • Continue to monitor client for pain and discomfort.
2. Bleeding at site continues.	• Apply pressure to site. • Instruct client to apply pressure. • Monitor client. • Notify physician.
3. Client becomes dizzy or faints during or after venipuncture.	• Lower client's head between knees. • Remain with client.

Wound Drainage Devices: Jackson-Pratt, Hemovac

Wound healing is delayed when drainage accumulates in a wound bed. A wound drainage device is inserted directly through the suture line into the wound or through a small stab wound near the suture line into the wound.

An open drain system (e.g., a Penrose drain [Fig. 81-1]) removes drainage from the wound and deposits it onto the skin surface. A sterile safety pin inserted through the drain, outside the skin, prevents the tubing from moving into the wound. To remove the Penrose drain, the physician advances the tubing in stages as the wound heals from the bottom up.

A closed drain system (e.g., the Jackson-Pratt drain [Fig. 81-2]), Hemovac drain (Fig. 81-3), VacuDrain, or Constavac) relies on the presence of a vacuum to withdraw accumulated drainage from a wound bed. The drain system connects to a clear plastic drain with multiple perforations. Drainage collects in a closed reservoir, suction bladder, or bag.

Delegation Considerations

Assessment of wound drainage and maintenance of drains and the drainage system should not be delegated to assistive personnel (AP). However, emptying a closed drainage container or pouch, measuring the amount of drainage, and reporting the amount on the client's intake and output (I&O) record may be delegated to AP.

- Discuss with AP any modification of the skill such as increased frequency of emptying the drain other than once a shift.
- Instruct AP to report any change in amount, color, or odor of drainage.

Equipment

- Graduated measuring container
- Alcohol sponge
- Gauze sponges
- Goggles if risk of splashing
- Sterile specimen container, if culture is needed

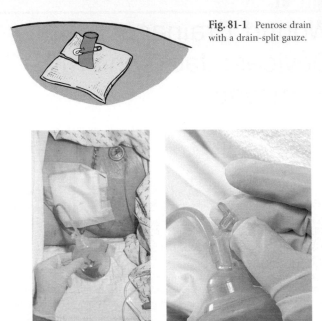

Fig. 81-1 Penrose drain with a drain-split gauze.

A

B

Fig. 81-2 A, Jackson-Pratt wound drainage system. B, Emptying Jackson-Pratt device.

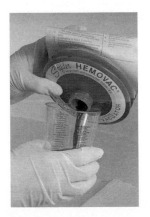

Fig. 81-3 Hemovac contents drained into sterile measuring container.

- Sterile dressings or pouch, if drain is needed
- Clean disposable gloves
- Safety pin(s)

Step	Rationale
1. Complete preprocedure protocol.	
2. Identify presence, location, and purpose of closed wound drain and drainage system. Note whether suction is in place and type of tubing.	Ensures proper management and prevents accidental drain dislocation.
3. Identify *number* of wound drain tubes and what drainage each one ought to be draining. Label each drain tube with number or label.	Assigning labeling system to each drain helps with consistent documentation when client has multiple drainage tubes.
4. Be sure Penrose drain has sterile safety pin in place. Penrose drains may be covered with gauze dressing or wound pouch. Use caution and do not accidentally pull on drain while positioning gauze.	Pin prevents drain from being pulled below skin's surface.

NURSE ALERT Attach the drainage tubing with tape or tube fixation device to the client's gown so that it does not pull on insertion site.

Step	Rationale
5. ⬛ Place open specimen container or graduated measuring container on bed between you and client.	Permits measuring and discarding of wound drainage.
6. When emptying evacuator, maintain asepsis while opening port:	Avoids entry of pathogens.
a. Hemovac (see Fig. 81-3):	
(1) Open plug on port indicated for emptying drainage reservoir.	Vacuum will be broken, and reservoir will pull air in until chamber is fully expanded.

Step	Rationale
(2) Tilt evacuator in direction of plug.	Drains fluid toward plug.
(3) Slowly squeeze two flat surfaces together while draining into sterile laboratory specimen container if culture is ordered; then drain remainder into graduated cylinder. Cover specimen container.	Prevents splashing of contaminated drainage.
(4) Hold an opened alcohol sponge in dominant hand; place evacuator on flat surface with open outlet facing upward; continue pressing downward until bottom and top are in contact; hold surfaces together with one hand, and quickly cleanse opening and plug with other hand; immediately replace plug; secure evacuator on client's bed.	Compression of surface of Hemovac reestablishes vacuum. Cleansing of plug reduces transmission of microorganisms into drainage evacuator.
(5) Check evacuator for reestablishment of vacuum, patency of drainage tubing, and absence of stress on tubing.	Facilitates wound drainage and prevents tension on drainage tubing.

b. Jackson-Pratt evacuator (see Fig. 81-2, *A*):

Step	Rationale
(1) Open emptying cap on side of bulb-shaped reservoir (see Fig. 81-2, *B*).	Breaks vacuum for drain.
(2) Tilt drain toward direction of plug, and drain toward opening. Empty drainage from evacuator into measuring container.	
(3) Compress bulb over drainage container. Cleanse ends of emptying port with alcohol sponge while continuing to compress container. Replace cap immediately. Secure evacuator below wound site with safety pin through client's gown.	Reestablishes vacuum. Reduces transmission of microorganisms into drainage evacuator and prevents tension on drainage tubing.
7. Place and secure drainage reservoirs to prevent any pull on tubing insertion sites.	Pinning drainage tubing to client's gown will prevent tension or pulling on tubing and insertion site.

NURSE ALERT Be sure there is slack in tubing from reservoir to wound.

8. Send labeled specimen to laboratory if ordered by physician or if purulence is noted. All other drainage is measured as fluid output.	Allows for culture testing to reveal infection.
9. Complete postprocedure protocol.	

Recording and Reporting

- Chart in the nurses' notes emptying of drainage evacuator; reestablishment of vacuum in evacuator; amount, color, odor of drainage; dressing change to drain site; and appearance of drain insertion site.
- Record amount of drainage on I&O record.
- Immediately report to physician sudden change in amount or character of drainage.

Unexpected Outcomes	Related Interventions
1. Wound develops purulent, foul smelling drainage; white blood cell count increases.	• Notify physician about signs of infection. • Use aseptic technique when changing dressings.
2. Bleeding appears.	• Determine amount of bleeding, and notify physician if excessive. • Assess for tension on client's drainage tubing. • Secure tubing to prevent pulling and pain.
3. Drainage evacuator system is not accumulating drainage.	• Assess drainage tubing for clots. • Assess drainage system for air leaks or kinks. • Notify physician.

Wound Irrigation

Wound cleansing and irrigation (Table 82-1) require sterile technique for surgical wounds or clean technique for some chronic wounds. Introduce the cleansing solution directly into the wound with a syringe, syringe and catheter, shower, or whirlpool. Principles of basic wound irrigation include cleansing in a direction from the least contaminated area to the most contaminated. When using a syringe, the tip should remain 2.5 cm (1 inch) above the wound. If the client has a deep wound with a narrow opening, attach a soft 19-gauge catheter to the syringe to permit the fluid to enter the wound. Irrigation should not cause tissue injury or discomfort. Avoid fluid retention within the wound by positioning the client on the side to encourage the flow of the irrigant away from the wound.

Delegation Considerations

The skill of wound irrigation should not be delegated to assistive personnel (AP). However, cleansing of chronic wounds using clean technique can be delegated.

- Discuss with AP modifications of the skill such as increased frequency of wound cleansing other than once a shift.
- Instruct AP what to report when a wound is cleansed (e.g., wound color, presence of bleeding, drainage).
- Instruct AP to report the status of client's pain.

Equipment

- Irrigant/cleansing solution (volume 1.2 to 2 times the estimated wound volume)
- Irrigation delivery system, depending on amount of pressure desired: sterile irrigation 35-ml syringe with sterile soft angiocatheter or 19-gauge needle (AHCPR, 1994) or hand-held shower or whirlpool
- Clean or sterile gloves
- Waterproof underpad, if needed
- Dressing supplies (see Skills 17 and 18)
- Disposable waterproof biohazard bag
- Gown
- Goggles
- Extra towels and padding (to protect bed)

TABLE 82-1 Wound Cleansing Protocol

	Mechanical Force	
	High Pressure (for Inflammatory Phase of Healing)	Low Pressure (for Proliferative Phase of Healing)
Wound base characteristics	Presence of necrotic tissue (eschar, fibrin slough), debris, or other particulate matter Significant bacterial burden Moderate/large amount of exudate Residue from wound care products	Presence of granulation tissue or new epithelial cells No/minimum serous or serosanguineous exudate Residue from wound care products
Clinical outcomes	Loosen, soften, and remove devitalized tissue from wound Separate eschar from fibrotic tissue/fibrotic tissue from granulating base Remove wound care product residue	Prevent trauma to viable wound tissue Remove wound care product residue
Solutions: Wound cleansers	Normal saline Volume of solution depends on size of wound	Normal saline Volume of solution depends on size of wound
Delivery systems*	35-ml syringe/19-gauge angiocatheter Irrijet® DS Pleurovac	Pouring saline directly from a bottle Bulb syringe Piston syringe

Used with permission of HMP Communications. Modified from Barr JE: Principles of wound cleansing, *Ostomy Wound Manage* 7A(suppl 41):15S, 1995.

*This is not an all-inclusive list of delivery systems available. Inclusion does not imply endorsement.

Step	Rationale
1. Complete preprocedure protocol.	
2. Administer prescribed analgesic 30 to 45 minutes before starting wound irrigation procedure.	Promotes pain control and permits client to move more easily and be positioned to facilitate wound irrigation (Dochterman and Bulechek, 2004).
3. Position client:	
a. Position comfortably to permit gravitational flow of irrigating solution through wound and into collection receptacle (Fig. 82-1).	Directing solution from top to bottom of wound and from clean to contaminated area prevents further infection. Position client during planning stage, keeping in mind bed surfaces needed for later preparation of equipment.
b. Position client so that wound is vertical to collection basin. Place container of irrigant/ cleansing solution in basin of hot water to warm solution to body temperature.	Warmed solution increases comfort and reduces vascular constriction response in tissues.
c. Place padding or extra towel in bed.	Protects bedding.
d. Expose wound only.	Prevents chilling of client.
4. Form cuff on waterproof biohazard bag, and place it near bed.	Cuffing helps maintain large opening, thereby permitting placement of contaminated dressing without touching refuse bag itself.

Fig. 82-1 Client position for wound irrigation.

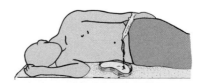

Step	Rationale
5. Don gown and goggles.	Protects nurse from splashes or sprays of blood and body fluids (CDC, 1997).
6. Remove soiled dressing and discard in waterproof bag. Discard gloves.	Reduces transmission of microorganisms.
7. Prepare equipment; open sterile supplies.	
8. Don sterile gloves.	Prevents transfer of microorganisms to wound surface.
9. To irrigate wound with wide opening:	
a. Fill 35-ml syringe with irrigation solution.	Flushing wound helps remove debris and facilitates healing by secondary intention.
b. Attach 19-gauge angiocatheter.	Catheter lumen delivers ideal pressure for cleansing and removal of debris (Ramundo and Wells, 2000).
c. Hold syringe tip 2.5 cm (1 inch) above upper end of wound and over area being cleansed.	Prevents syringe contamination. Careful placement of syringe prevents unsafe pressure of flowing solution.
d. Using continuous pressure, flush wound; repeat steps a, b, and c until solution draining into basin is clear.	Clear solution indicates that all debris has been removed.
10. To irrigate deep wound with very small opening:	
a. Attach soft 19-gauge angiocatheter to filled irrigating syringe.	Catheter permits direct flow of irrigant into wound. Expect wound to take longer to empty when opening is small.
b. Lubricate tip of catheter with irrigating solution; then gently insert tip of catheter and pull out about 1 cm (½ inch).	Removes tip from fragile inner wall of wound.

Step	**Rationale**

NURSE ALERT Do not force the catheter into the wound because this could damage tissue.

c. Using slow, continuous pressure, flush wound.	Use of slow mechanical force of stream of solution loosens particulate matter on wound surface and promotes healing (Ramundo and Wells, 2000).

NURSE ALERT *CAUTION:* Splashing may occur during this step.

d. Pinch off catheter just below syringe while keeping catheter in place.	Prevents aspiration of solution into syringe and contamination of sterile solution (Dochterman and Bulechek, 2004).
e. Remove and refill syringe. Reconnect to catheter, and repeat until solution draining into basin is clear.	

NURSE ALERT Pulsatile high-pressure lavage may be the irrigation of choice for necrotic wounds. The amount of irrigant is wound-size dependent. Pressure settings on the device should remain between 4 and 15 psi. Do not use pulsatile high-pressure lavage on exposed blood vessels, muscle, tendon, and bone. This type of irrigation should not be used with graft sites and should be used with caution in clients receiving anticoagulant therapy (Ramundo and Wells, 2000).

11. To cleanse wound with hand-held shower:

a. With client seated comfortably in shower chair, adjust spray to gentle flow; water temperature should be warm.	Useful for clients able to shower with assistance or independently. May be accomplished at home. Shower table is helpful for bed-bound or acutely ill clients.
b. Cover showerhead with clean washcloth if needed.	Reduces pressure released at showerhead.

Step	**Rationale**
c. Shower for 5 to 10 minutes with showerhead 30 cm (12 inches) from wound.	Ensures that wound is thoroughly cleansed.
12. To cleanse wound with whirlpool:	
a. Adjust water level and temperature; add prescribed cleansing agent.	Wound is hypersensitive to hot temperature.
b. Assist client into whirlpool, or place extremity into whirlpool. Position client so that water jets are not directly over clean, granulating wound tissue.	
c. Allow client to remain in whirlpool for prescribed interval.	Ensures thorough wound cleansing.

NURSE ALERT   Clients who are confused, have poor activity tolerance, or have impaired mobility should never be left alone in the whirlpool.

13. When indicated, obtain cultures after cleansing with nonbacteriostatic saline. Consider culture if client is febrile; wound has foul, purulent odor; inflammation surrounds wound; or nondraining wound begins to drain.	Routine culturing of open wounds is not recommended by AHCPR (1994). AHCPR (1994) recommends using quantitative bacterial cultures (tissue biopsy or wound fluid by needle aspiration) rather than swab cultures, which often detect only surface bacterial contaminants.
14. Dry wound edges with gauze; dry client if shower or whirlpool is used.	Prevents maceration of surrounding tissue from excess moisture.
15. Apply appropriate dressing (see Skills 17 and 18).	Maintains protective barrier and healing environment for wound.
16. Complete postprocedure protocol.	

Recording and Reporting

- Chart in nurses' notes wound assessment before and after irrigation; amount, color, and odor of drainage on dressing removed; amount and type of solution used; irrigation device used; client's tolerance of procedure; type of dressing applied after irrigation.
- Immediately report to attending physician any evidence of fresh bleeding, sharp increase in pain, retention of irrigant, or signs of shock.

Unexpected Outcomes	Related Interventions
1. Bleeding or serosanguineous drainage appears.	• Flush wound during next irrigation using less pressure. • Notify physician of bleeding.
2. Retained fluid and debris appear.	• Increase amount of fluid used during irrigation. • Increase amount of pressure when flushing wound. • Make sure wound is clear of retained fluid and debris before applying dressing.
3. Suture line opening extends.	• Notify physician. • Reevaluate amount of pressure to use for next wound irrigation.

Wound Vacuum Assisted Closure

Wound Vacuum Assisted Closure (V.A.C.®) speeds wound healing by applying localized negative pressure to draw the edges of a wound together (Figs. 83-1 and 83-2). V.A.C.® accelerates wound healing by promoting the formation of granulation tissue, collagen, fibroblasts, and inflammatory cells to completely close or improve the health of a wound. Often the treatment prepares a wound for a skin graft. The use of negative pressure removes fluid from the area surrounding the wound, thus reducing local peripheral edema and improving circulation to the area (Chua and others, 2000). In addition, V.A.C.® reduces bacterial counts in wounds, which improves healing because the body can focus on healing rather than fighting infection (Mendez-Eastman, 2001).

The cycle and amount of negative pressure to the wound are ordered by the physician or wound care specialist (Mendez-Eastman, 2001). The target negative pressures for wound healing range from 50 mm Hg to 125 mm Hg. The negative pressure can be continuous or intermittent, depending on the stage of wound healing. To optimize wound healing, negative pressure should be maintained 22 of 24 hours per day (KCI, 2003). As the wound heals, the settings may change.

Delegation Considerations

The skill of Wound V.A.C.® should not be delegated to assistive personnel (AP).

- Instruct AP to use caution in positioning or turning the client to avoid tubing displacement.

Equipment

- V.A.C.® ATS System
- V.A.C.® foam dressing
- Tubing for connection between V.A.C.® ATS System and V.A.C.® dressing
- Gloves, clean and sterile
- Scissors, sterile
- Waterproof bag for disposal
- Skin preparation/skin barrier
- Moist washcloth

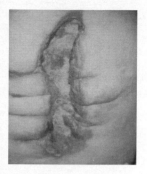

Fig. 83-1 Dehisced wound before V.A.C.® therapy. (Courtesy KCI USA, Inc., San Antonio, Tex.)

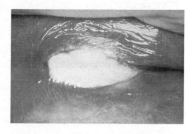

Fig. 83-2 Dehisced wound after V.A.C.® therapy. (Courtesy KCI USA, Inc., San Antonio, Tex.)

- Linen bag
- Protection gown, mask, goggles (used when spray from wound is a risk)

Step	Rationale
1. Complete preprocedure protocol.	
2. Review physician's orders for frequency of dressing change, type of foam to use, and amount of negative pressure to use.	Physician orders frequency of dressing changes and special instructions.
3. Position client, expose wound site, and cover client.	Draping provides access to wound while minimizing exposure. Positioning ensures client's comfort during procedure.
4. Cuff top of disposable waterproof bag, and place within reach of work area.	Cuff prevents accidental contamination of top of outer bag.
5. ✦ If risk of spray exists, don protective gown, goggles, and mask.	Reduces transmission of infectious organisms.
6. Push therapy on/off button on V.A.C.® ATS System.	Deactivates therapy.

Step	Rationale
7. Raise tubing connectors above level of V.A.C.® ATS System and disconnect tubes from each other to drain fluids into canister. Before lowering, tighten clamp on canister tube.	Allows for proper drainage of fluid in drainage tubing (KCI, 2003). V.A.C.® ATS canister unit should be changed when full or at least once a week to control odor (KCI, 2003).
8. With dressing tube unclamped, introduce 10 to 30 ml of normal saline, if ordered, into tubing to soak underneath foam. Let set for 15 to 30 minutes.	Facilitates loosening of foam when tissue adheres to foam (KCI, 2003; Krasner, 2002).
9. Gently stretch transparent film horizontally, and slowly pull up from skin.	Reduces stress on suture line or wound edges and reduces irritation and discomfort.
10. Remove old V.A.C.® dressing, observing appearance and drainage on dressing. Use caution to remove dressing around drains. Dispose of soiled dressings in waterproof bag. Remove gloves by pulling them inside out, and dispose of them in waterproof bag. Avoid having client see old dressing because sight of wound drainage may upset client. Perform hand hygiene.	Determines dressings needed for replacement. Avoids accidental removal of drains. Reduces transmission of microorganisms.
11. 🖐 Don sterile or clean gloves. Irrigate wound with normal saline or other solution ordered by physician. Gently blot to dry (see Skill 82).	Irrigation removes wound debris and cleanses wound bed.
12. Measure wound as ordered: at baseline, first dressing	Provides objective measure of progress of wound healing in

Step	Rationale
change, weekly, and discharge from therapy. Remove and discard gloves. Perform hand hygiene.	response to negative pressure therapy (KCI, 2003).

NURSE ALERT Wound cultures may be ordered at this time. Obtain a wound culture during the dressing change when the drainage looks purulent, when the amount or color changes, or when the drainage has a foul odor (Chua and others, 2000).

Step	Rationale
13. Depending on type of wound, don sterile or new clean gloves.	Fresh sterile wounds require sterile gloves. Chronic wounds may require clean technique. Do not use same gloves worn to clean wound, because cross-contamination may occur.
14. Select appropriate foam dressing depending on wound type and stage of healing. Use sterile scissors to cut foam to exact wound size, making sure to fit size and shape of wound, including tunnels and undermined areas.	Black polyurethane (PU) foam has larger pores and is most effective in stimulating granulation tissue and wound contraction. White polyvinyl alcohol (PVA) soft foam is denser with smaller pores and is used when growth of granulation tissue needs to be restricted (KCI, 2003; Mendez-Eastman, 2001).

NURSE ALERT Use of black foam causes clients to experience more pain because of excessive wound contraction. You may need to switch to the PVA soft foam for the client.

Step	Rationale
15. Gently place foam in wound, being sure that foam is in contact with entire wound base, margins, and tunneled and undermined areas.	Maintains negative pressure to entire wound. Edges of foam dressing must be in direct contact with client's skin (Mendez-Eastman, 2001).
16. Apply tubing to foam in wound.	Connects negative pressure from V.A.C.® ATS System to wound foam.

Step	Rationale

NURSE ALERT For deep wounds, regularly reposition tubing to minimize pressure on wound edges. Clients with restricted mobility or sensation must be repositioned frequently so that they do not lie on the tubing, which could damage the skin (KCI, 2003).

17. Apply skin protectant, such as skin prep or Stomahesive wafer, to skin around wound.	Protects periwound skin from injury that may result from occlusive dressing and will help decrease pain associated with wound margins (Krasner, 2002).
18. Apply V.A.C.® transparent dressing, covering V.A.C.® foam and 3 to 5 cm ($1^1/_4$ to 2 inches) of surrounding healthy tissue. Make sure transparent dressing is wrinkle-free. Secure tubing to transparent film, aligning drainage hole to ensure an occlusive seal (Fig. 83-3). Do not apply tension to drape and tubing.	Ensure that wound is properly covered and negative pressure seal can be achieved (Box 83-1). Excessive tension may compress foam dressing, impede wound healing, and produce shear force on periwound area (KCI, 2003).
19. Secure tubing several centimeters away from dressing.	Prevents pull on primary dressing, which can cause leaks in negative pressure system (Chua and others, 2000; KCI, 2003).
20. After wound is completely covered, connect tubing from dressing to tubing from canister and V.A.C.® ATS system.	Intermittent or continuous negative pressure can be administered at 50 mm Hg to 175 mm Hg, according to physician's orders and client's comfort. Average is 125 mm Hg (Chua and others, 2000; KCI, 2003).
21. Remove canister from sterile packaging, and push into V.A.C.® ATS System until click is heard. *Alarm will sound if canister is not properly engaged.*	

Step	**Rationale**

Fig. 83-3 Foam dressing, transparent dressing, and V.A.C.® tubing secured over existing wound. (Courtesy KCI USA, Inc., San Antonio, Tex.)

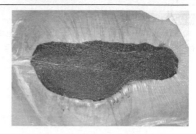

22. Connect dressing tubing to canister tubing. Make sure both clamps are open.

23. Place V.A.C.® ATS System on level surface or hang from foot of bed. V.A.C.® ATS System will alarm and deactivate therapy if unit is tilted beyond 45 degrees.

24. Press in green-lit power button, and set pressure as ordered. — Activates negative pressure.

25. Complete postprocedure protocol.

26. Inspect V.A.C.® ATS System to verify that negative pressure is achieved. — Negative pressure is achieved when airtight seal is achieved (see Box 83-1).

   a. Verify that display screen reads "THERAPY ON."

   b. Be sure clamps are open and tubing is patent.

   c. Identify air leaks by listening with stethoscope or by moving hand around edges of wound while applying light pressure.

   d. If leak is present, use strips of transparent film to patch areas around edges of wound.

BOX 83-1   Maintaining an Airtight Seal

Once the V.A.C.® ATS System is initiated, the wound must stay sealed to avoid wound desiccation. Wounds around joints and near the sacrum are problem areas to seal. The following points may assist in maintaining an airtight seal:

- Shave hair around wound.
- Cut transparent film to extend 3 to 5 cm ($1^{1}/_{4}$ to 2 inches) beyond wound perimeter.
- Avoid wrinkles in transparent film.
- Patch leaks with transparent film.
- Use multiple small strips of transparent film to hold dressing in place before covering dressing with large piece of transparent film.
- Avoid adhesive remover because it leaves a residue that hinders film adherence.

Modified from Chua PC and others: Vacuum-assisted wound closure, *Am J Nurs* 100(12):46, 2000.

Recording and Reporting

- Chart in nurses' notes appearance of wound, color, characteristics of any drainage, presence of wound healing augmentation such as V.A.C®, dressing change, and client's response to dressing change.
- Record date and time of dressing change on new dressing.
- Report brisk, bright red bleeding; evidence of poor wound healing; evisceration or dehiscence; and possible wound infection to physician.

Unexpected Outcomes	Related Interventions
1. Wound appears inflamed and tender, drainage has increased, and odor is present.	• Notify physician. • Obtain wound culture. • Increase frequency of dressing changes.
2. Negative pressure seal has broken.	• Take preventive measures (see Box 83-1). • Shave surrounding skin.

Appendix

Overview of CDC Hand Hygiene Guidelines

In 2002 the Centers for Disease Control and Prevention (CDC) released recommendations for hand hygiene in health care settings. *Hand hygiene* is a general term that applies to hand washing, antiseptic hand wash, antiseptic hand rub, or surgical hand antisepsis. *Hand washing* refers to washing hands thoroughly with plain soap and water. *Antiseptic hand wash* is defined as washing hands with water and soap containing an antiseptic agent. Antimicrobials effectively reduce bacterial counts on the hands and often have residual antimicrobial effects for several hours. An antiseptic hand rub is an application of an antiseptic alcohol-based waterless product to all surfaces of the hands to reduce the number of microorganisms present. Surgical hand antisepsis is an antiseptic hand wash or antiseptic hand rub performed preoperatively by surgical personnel.

Evidence suggests that hand antisepsis, the cleansing of hands with an antiseptic hand rub, is more effective in reducing nosocomial infections than plain hand washing.

Guidelines in the Care of All Patients

Wash hands when hands are visibly dirty or contaminated with proteinaceous material or are visibly soiled with blood or other body fluids. Wash hands preferably with an antimicrobial soap and water or with a nonantimicrobial soap and water. The recommended duration for lathering hands is *at least 15 seconds* and preferably 30 seconds.

- Wash hands with soap and water before eating.
- Wash hands with soap and water after using the restroom.
- Wash hands if exposed to spore-forming organisms such as *Clostridium difficile* or *Bacillus anthracis.* The physical action of washing and rinsing hands is recommended because alcohols, chlorhexidine, iodophors, and other antiseptic agents have poor activity against spores.

If hands are not visibly soiled, use an alcohol-based hand rub for routinely decontaminating the hands in all of the following clinical situations:

- Before having direct contact with clients
- Before donning sterile gloves
- Before inserting indwelling urinary catheters, peripheral vascular catheters, or other invasive devices that do not require a surgical procedure
- After contact with a client's intact skin (e.g., after taking a pulse or blood pressure, after lifting a client)
- After contact with body fluids or excretions, mucous membranes, nonintact skin, and wound dressings *if hands are not visibly soiled*
- When moving from a contaminated body site to a clean body site during client care
- After contact with inanimate objects (e.g., medical equipment) in the immediate vicinity of the client
- After removing gloves

Note that an antiseptic hand wash may be performed in all situations in which an alcohol-based hand rub is indicated. Antimicrobial-impregnated wipes (i.e., towelettes) are not a substitute for using an alcohol-based hand rub or antimicrobial soap.

Method for Decontaminating Hands

When using an alcohol-based hand rub, apply product to palm of one hands and rub hands together, covering all surfaces of hands and fingers, until hands are dry. Follow the manufacturer's recommendations regarding the volume of product to use.

Guidelines for Surgical Hand Antisepsis

Surgical hand antisepsis reduces the resident microbial count on the hands to a minimum.

- The CDC recommends using an antimicrobial soap and to scrub hands and forearms for the length of time recommended by the manufacturer, usually 2 to 6 minutes. Refer to agency policy for time required.
- When using an alcohol-based surgical hand-scrub product with persistent activity, follow the manufacturer's instructions. Before applying the alcohol solution, prewash hands and forearms with a nonantimicrobial soap and dry hands and forearms completely. After application of the alcohol-based product as recommended, allow hands and forearms to dry thoroughly before donning sterile gloves.

General Recommendations for Hand Hygiene

- Use hand lotions or creams to minimize the occurrence of irritant contact dermatitis associated with hand antisepsis or hand washing.
- Do not wear artificial fingernails or extenders when having direct contact with clients at high risk (e.g., those in intensive care units or operating rooms).
- Keep natural nail tips less than 1/4 inch long.
- Wear gloves when contact with blood or other potentially infectious materials, mucous membranes, and nonintact skin could occur.
- Remove gloves after caring for a client. Do not wear the same pair of gloves for the care of more than one client.
- Change gloves during client care if moving from a contaminated body site to a clean body site. This includes when working under isolation precautions.

(Data from Centers for Disease Control and Prevention: *Morbidity and Mortality Weekly Report [MMWR],* October 25, 51[RR16]:1–44, 2000. Available at www.cdc.gov/handhygiene; and Centers for Disease Control and Prevention, Hospital Infection Control Practice Advisory Committee, and the HICPAC/SHEA/APIC/IDSA Hand Hygiene Task Force: Guideline for hand hygiene in health-care settings, *MMWR Morb Mortal Wkly Rep: Recommendations and Reports* 51(RR16), 2002.)

Bibliography

Acute Pain Management Guideline Panel: *Acute pain management: operative or medical procedures and trauma.* Clinical practice guideline, AHCPR Pub. No. 92-0032, Rockville, Md, 1992, Agency for Health Care Policy and Research, Public Health Service, U.S. Department of Health and Human Services.

Agency for Health Care Policy and Research (AHCPR), Panel for the Treatment of Pressure Ulcers: *Treatment of pressure ulcers,* Clinical practice guideline No. 15, AHCPR Pub. No. 95-0652, Rockville, Md, 1994, U.S. Department of Health and Human Services.

Agency for Health Care Policy and Research (AHCPR): *Treatment of pressure ulcers*, Clinical practice guideline No. 15, Rockville, Md, 1994, U.S. Department of Health and Human Services, Public Health Service.

AHCPR Panel for the Prediction and Prevention of Pressure Ulcers in Adults: *Pressure ulcers in adults: prediction and prevention,* Clinical practice guideline No. 3, Pub. No. 92-0047, Rockville, Md, 1992, Public Health Service, U.S. Department of Health and Human Services.

AHCPR Panel for the Treatment of Pressure Ulcers in Adults: *Treatment of pressure ulcers,* Clinical practice guideline No. 15, Pub. No. 95-0653, Rockville, Md, 1994, Public Health Service, U.S. Department of Health and Human Services.

Airaksinen O and others: Efficacy of cold gel for soft tissue injuries, *Am J Sports Med* 31(5):680, 2003.

Akgul S, Akyolcu N: Effects of normal saline on endotracheal suctioning, *J Clin Nurs* 11(6):826, 2002.

Allibone L: Nursing management of chest drains, *Nurs Stand* 17(22):45, 2003.

American Association of Blood Banks (AABB): *Technical manual,* ed 14, Bethesda, Md, 2002, The Association.

American Diabetes Association (ADA): Insulin administration: position statement, *Diabetes Care* 27(suppl 1):S106, 2004.

American Diabetes Association: *Diabetes forecast: the foot care top ten tips,* http://www.diabetes.org/diabetes-forecast/may2003/ feet.jsp. Retrieved Oct. 2005.

American Diabetes Association: Position statement on preventive foot care in people with diabetes: clinical practice recommendations 1999, *Diabetes Care* 22(Suppl 1):1, 1999.

American Heart Association (AHA): *Guidelines 2000 for cardiopulmonary resuscitation and emergency cardiovascular care: international consensus on science,* Dallas, 2000, The Association.

American Nurses Association (ANA): *Position statement on elimination of manual patient handling to prevent work-related musculoskeletal disorders,* www.nursingworld.org.readroom/position/workplac/pathand.htm, June 2003.

American Pain Society: *Analgesic use in the treatment of acute pain and cancer pain,* ed 6, Glenview, Ill, 2003, American Pain Society.

American Society for Parenteral and Enteral Nutrition (ASPEN): Guidelines for the use of parenteral and enteral nutrition in adult and pediatric patients, *JPEN J Parenter Enteral Nutr* 26:1SA, 2002.

American Society for Parenteral and Enteral Nutrition (ASPEN): *The science and practice of nutrition support: a case-based core curriculum,* Dubuque, Iowa, 2001, Kendall Hunt.

Armstrong DG, Lavery LA: Diabetic foot ulcers: prevention, diagnosis and classification, *Am Fam Physician* 57(6):1425, 1998.

Autio L, Olson KK: The four S's of wound management: staples, sutures, Steri-Strips, and sticky stuff, *Holist Nurs Pract* 16(2):80, 2002.

Aventis: *Lovenox: enoxaparin sodium injection,* 2003, http://www.lovenox.com/. Retrieved July 6, 2004.

Ayello EA and others: Pressure ulcers. In Baranoski S, Ayello EA, editors: *Wound care essentials: practice principles,* Philadelphia, 2004, Lippincott Williams and Wilkins.

Ayello EA, Braden B: How and why to do pressure ulcer risk assessment, *Adv Wound Care* 15(3):125, 2002.

Babis GC and others: Poor outcomes of isolated tibial insert exchange and arthrolysis for the management of stiffness following total knee arthroplasty, *J Bone Joint Surg Am* 83-A(10):1534, 2001.

Bach PB and others: Management of acute exacerbations of chronic obstructive pulmonary disease: a summary and appraisal of published evidence, *Ann Intern Med* 134(7):600, 2001.

Barabas G, Molstad S: No association between elevated post-void residual volume and bacteriuria in residents of nursing homes, *Scand J Prim Health Care* 23:53, 2005.

Baranoski S, Ayello EA: Wound treatment options. In Baranoski S, Ayello EA, editors: *Wound care essentials: practice principles,* Philadelphia, 2004, Lippincott Williams and Wilkins.

Barr JE: Principles of wound cleansing, *Ostomy Wound Manage* 7A(Suppl 41):15S, 1995.

Bates-Jensen B: New pressure ulcer status tool, *Decubitus* 3(3):14, 1990.

Beevers G and others: ABC's of hypertension. I. Blood pressure measurement, *Br Med J* 322(7292):981, 2001a.

Beevers G and others: ABC's of hypertension. II. Blood pressure measurement, *Br Med J* 322(7293):1043, 2001b.

Beitz JM, Bates-Jensen B: Algorithms, critical pathways, and computer software for wound care: contemporary status and future potential, *Ostomy Wound Manage* 47(4):33, 2001.

Bennett MA: Report of the task force on the implications for darkly pigmented intact skin in the prediction and prevention of pressure ulcers, *Adv Wound Care* 8(6):34, 1995.

Benya R and others: Diarrhea associated with tube feeding: the importance of using objective criteria, *J Clin Gastroenterol* 13:167, 1991.

Bergstrom N and others: Multisite study of incidence of pressure ulcers and the relationship between risk level, demographic characteristics, diagnoses, and prescription of preventive interventions, *J Am Geriatr Soc* 44:22, 1996.

Bergstrom N and others: Predicting pressure ulcer risk: a multisite study of the predictive validity of the Braden scale, *Nur Res* 47(5):261, 1998.

Bergstrom N, Demuth PJ, Braden BJ: A clinical trial of the Braden scale for predicting pressure sore risk, *Nurs Clin North Am* 22(2):417, 1987.

Bernard L and others: Bacterial contamination of hospital physicians' stethoscopes, *Infect Control Hosp Epidemiol* 20(9):626, 1999.

Bernier M and others: Preoperative teaching received and valued in a day surgery setting, *AORN J* 77(3):563, 2003.

Boccalon H and others: Clinical outcomes and cost of hospital vs. home treatment of proximal deep vein thrombosis with low-molecular-weight heparin, *Arch Intern Med* 160(12):1769, 2000.

Borrie MJ and others: Urinary retention in patients in a geriatric rehabilitation unit: prevalence, risk factors, and validity of bladder scan evaluation. *Rehabil Nurs* 26(5):187, 2001.

Braden BJ, Bergstrom N: Clinical utility of the Braden scale for predicting pressure sore risk, *Decubitus* 2(3):44, 1989.

Braden BJ, Bergstrom N: Predictive utility of the Braden scale for predicting pressure sore risk, *Res Nurs Health* 17:459, 1994.

Breen P: DVT. What every nurse should know, *RN* 63(4):58, 2000.

Brians LK and others: The development of the RISK tool for fall prevention, *Rehabil Nurs* 16(2):67, 1991.

Brody R and others: *Newark Beth Israel Medical Center nutrition screening, and reassessment policy and procedure,* Newark, NJ, 2000a, Newark Beth Israel Medical Center.

Brody R and others: Role of registered dietitians in dysphagia screening, *J Am Diet Assoc* 100(9):1029, 2000b.

Bryant RA: *Acute and chronic wounds: nursing management,* ed 2, St Louis, 2000, Mosby.

Burt S: What you need to know about latex allergy, *Nursing* 28(10):33, 1998.

Campany E and others: Nurses' knowledge of wound irrigation and pressures generated during simulated wound irrigation, *J Wound Ostomy Continence Nurs* 27:296, 2000.

Capasso V, Munro VH: The cost and efficacy of two wound treatments, *AORN J* 77(5):984, 2003.

Carroll P: A guide to mobile chest drains, *RN* 65(5):56, 2002.

Carroll PF: What's new in chest-tube management, *RN* 54(5):34, 1991.

Catney MR and others: Relationship between peripheral intravenous catheter dwell time and the development of phlebitis and infiltration, *J Infus Nurs* 24(5):332, 2001.

Centers for Disease Control and Prevention (CDC), Hospital Infection Control Practice Advisory Committee: Guidelines for isolation precautions in hospitals, *Am J Infect Control* 24:24, 1996.

Centers for Disease Control and Prevention (CDC): Guidelines for the prevention of intravascular catheter-related infections, *MMWR Morb Mortal Wkly Rep* 51(No. RR-10):1-26, 2002.

Centers for Disease Control and Prevention (CDC): *Mantoux tuberculin skin test facilitator guide,* 2004, www.cdc.gov/nchstp/tb/pubs/Mantoux/images/Mantoux.pdf. Retrieved March 21, 2004.

Centers for Disease Control and Prevention (CDC): Part II: *Recommendations for isolation precautions in hospitals,* 1997, http://wonder.cdc.gov/wonder/prevguid/p000049/p0000419.asp.

Centers for Disease Control and Prevention (CDC): Web-based Injury Statistics Query and Reporting System (WISQARS) [online], National Center for Injury Prevention and Control, Centers for Disease Control and Prevention (producer), http://www.cdc.gov/ncipc/wisqars. Cited Nov. 24, 2003.

Centers for Medicare and Medicaid Services (CMS): *Conditions of participation: interpretive guidelines,* Bethesda, Md, 2004, U.S. Department of Health and Human Services.

Chan H: Effects of injection duration on site-pain intensity and bruising associated with subcutaneous heparin, *J Adv Nurs* 35(6):882, 2001.

Chua PC and others: Vacuum-assisted wound closure, *Am J Nurs* 100(12):45, 2000.

Chukhraev AM, Grekov IG: Local complications of nursing interventions on peripheral veins, *J Infus Nurs* 23(3):167, 2000.

Collier M: Brevet tx: anti-embolism stockings for prevention and treatment of DVT, *Br J Nurs* 8(1):44, 1999.

Connelly M, Stone K: Descriptive determination of negative airway pressure with closed system suctioning, *Heart Lung* 20(3):298, 1991.

Cooper DM: Assessment, measurement, and evaluation: their pivotal roles in wound healing. In Bryant RA, editor: *Acute and chronic wounds: nursing management,* ed 2, St Louis, 2000, Mosby.

Cosentino B: Epidural pain management, *Nurs Spectr* 12A(4):NJ1, 2000.

Cox F: Clinical care of patients with epidural infusions, *Prof Nurse* 16(10):1429, 2001.

Crosby CT, Mares AK: Skin antisepsis past, present, and future, *JVAD* 6(2):26-27, 2001.

Crosby CT, Mares AK: Skin antisepsis past, present, and future, *JVAD* 6(2), 2001.

Cullum N and others: Beds, mattresses and cushions for pressure sore prevention and treatment, *Cochrane Review,* The Cochrane Library, Issue 3, 2000.

Cullum N and others: Beds, mattresses and cushions for pressure sore prevention and treatment, *Cochrane Database Syst Rev* 1(1), most recent update April 2003.

Cummins RO, editor: *ACLS provider manual,* Dallas, 2001, American Heart Association.

Cuzzell J: Wound assessment and evaluation wound dressings—confusion or choice? *Dermatol Nurs* 14(3):187, 2002.

Dallan LE and others: Pain management and wounds. In Baranoski S, Ayello EA, editors: *Wound care essentials: practice principles,* Philadelphia, 2004, Lippincott Williams and Wilkins.

Daneshgari F and others: Evidence based multidisciplinary practice: improving the safety and standards of male bladder catheterization, *Medsurg Nurs* 11(5):236, 2002.

Dangerfield L, Sullivan R: Screening for and managing dysphagia after stroke, *Nurs Times* 95(19):44, 1999.

Daniels S and others: Clinical predictors of dysphagia and aspiration risk: outcome measures in acute stroke patients, *Arch Phys Med Rehabil* 81:1030, 2000.

Dawkins L and others: A randomized trial of winged Vialon cannulae and metal butterfly needles, *Int J Palliat Nurs* 6(3):110, 2000.

Day T and others: Tracheal suctioning: an exploration of nurses' knowledge and competence in acute and high dependency ward areas, *J Adv Nurs* 39(1):35, 2002.

DeCastro M: Aseptic technique. In *APIC text of infection control epidemiology,* Chicago, revised 2002, Association for Professionals in Infection Control and Epidemiology, Inc.

Dochterman JC, Bulechek GM: *Nursing interventions classification (NIC),* ed 4, St Louis, 2004, Mosby.

Dosh SA: Evaluation and treatment of constipation, *J Fam Pract* 51(6):555, 2002.

Edwards SJ, Metheny NA: Measurement of gastric residual volume: state of the science, *Medsurg Nurs* 9:25, 2000.

Eisenberg P: An overview of diarrhea in the patient receiving enteral nutrition, *Gastroenterol Nurs* 25:95, 2002.

Elmstahl S and others: Treatment of dysphagia improves nutritional conditions in stroke patients, *Dysphagia* 14:61, 1999.

Engstrom JL and others: Procedures used to prepare and administer intramuscular injections: a study of infertility nurses, *J Obstet Gynecol Neonatal Nurs* 29(2):159, 2000.

Erwin-Toth P: Caring for a stoma is more than skin deep, *Nursing* 31(5):36, 2001.

Erwin-Toth P: Ostomies and fistulas: prevention and management of peristomal skin complications, *Adv Skin Wound Care* 13(4):175, 2000.

Erwin-Toth P: Ostomy pearls, *Adv Skin Wound Care* 16(3):146, 2003.

Evans E: Indwelling catheter care: dispelling the misconceptions, *Geriatr Nurs* 20(5):85, 1999.

Fabian B: Intravenous complication: infiltration, *J Intraven Nurs* 23(4):229, 2000.

Feldt K: The checklist of nonverbal pain indicators (CNPI), *Pain Manag Nurs* 1(1):35, 2000.

Fink JB, Mahlmeister MJ: High frequency oscillation of the airway and chest wall, *Resp Care* 47(7):797, 2002.

Fitch JA and others: Oral care in the adult intensive care unit, *Am J Crit Care* 8(2):314, 1999.

Fretag CC and others: Prolonged application of closed in-line suction catheters increases microbial colonization of lower respiratory tract bacterial growth on catheter surface, *Infection* 31(1):31, 2003.

Gilsenan I: A practical guide to giving injections, *Nurs Times* 96(33):43, 2000.

Godden J: Managing the patient with a chest drain: a review, *Nurs Stand* 12(32):35, 1998.

Gordon PA and others: Positioning of chest tubes: effects on pressure and drainage, *Am J Crit Care* 6:33, 1997.

Gottschlich MM and others: The 2002 Clinical Research Award: an evaluation of the safety of early vs. delayed enteral support and effects on clinical, nutritional, and endocrine outcomes after severe burns, *J Burn Care Rehabil* 23:401, 2002.

Grap MJ and others: Oral care interventions in critical care: frequency and documentation, *Am J Crit Care* 12(2):114, 2003.

Grap MJ: Pulse oximetry, *Crit Care Nurse* 22(3):69, 2002.

Gray M, Doughty DB: Clean versus sterile technique when changing wound dressings, *J Wound Ostomy Continence Nurs* 28(3):125, 2001.

Groher M: *Dysphagia: diagnosis and management,* Boston, 1997, Butterworth-Heinemann.

Guenter PA and others: Tube feeding–related diarrhea in acutely ill patients, *JPEN J Parenter Enteral Nutr* 15:277, 1991.

Guiliano KK and others: Temperature measurement in critically ill adults: a comparison of tympanic and oral methods, *Am J Crit Care* 9(4):254, 2000.

Haberstich N: Protecting catheterized patients from infection, *Nurs Residential Care* 4(10):482, 2002.

Hammesfahr R, Serafino M: Early motion gets the worm: continuous passive motion following total hip arthroplasty can aid in alleviating pain, edema, stiffness, deep vein thrombosis, and dislocation, and in controlling cost, *Rehab Manag* 15(2):20, 2002.

Hammond C and others: Assessment of aspiration risk in stroke patients with quantification of voluntary cough, *Neurology* 56:502, 2001.

Hankins J and others: *Infusion therapy in clinical practice,* Philadelphia, 2001, Saunders.

Heitz UE, Horne MM: *Pocket guide to fluid, electrolyte, and acid-base balance,* ed 4, St Louis, 2001, Mosby.

Henderson CT and others: Draft definition of stage I pressure ulcers: inclusion of persons with darkly pigmented skin, *Adv Wound Care* 10(5):16, 1997.

Hess CT: How to use gauze dressings, *Nursing* 30(9):88, 2000.

Heyland D and others: Enteral nutrition in the critically ill patient: a prospective survey, *Crit Care Med* 23:1055, 1995.

Heyland D, Mandell LA: Gastric colonization by gram-negative bacilli and nosocomial pneumonia in the intensive care unit patient: evidence for causation, *Chest* 101:187, 1992.

Hignett S: Systematic review of patient handling activities starting in lying, sitting and standing positions, *J Adv Nurs* 41(6):545, 2003.

Hockenberry MJ and others: *Wong's essentials of pediatric nursing,* ed 7, St Louis, 2003, Mosby.

Hockenberry MJ and others: *Wong's nursing care of infants and children,* ed 7, St Louis, 2003, Mosby.

Hoeman S: *Rehabilitation nursing process, application, and outcomes,* ed 3, St Louis, 2002, Mosby.

Holland AE and others: Non-invasive ventilation assists chest physiotherapy in adults with acute exacerbations of cystic fibrosis, *Thorax* 58:880, 2003.

Ignatavicius DD, Workman ML: *Medical-surgical nursing: critical thinking for collaborative care,* Philadelphia, 2002, Saunders.

Institute for Safe Medicine Practices (ISMP): Hazard alert! Asphyxiation possible with syringe tip caps. *ISMP medication safety alert,* Aug. 2001, http://www.ismp.org/MSAarticles/Hypodermic.html. Retrieved July 11, 2004.

Intravenous Nurses Society (INS): Infusion nursing standards of practice, *J Intraven Nurs* 23(6S):556, 2000.

Jeffries C, MacKay AT: Improving stoma management in the low-vision patient, *J Wound Ostomy Continence Nurs* 24(6):302, 1997.

Jevon P, Ewens B: Assessment of a breathless patient, *Nurs Stand* 15(16):48, 2001.

Jiricka MK and others: Pressure ulcer risk factors in an ICU population, *Am J Crit Care* 4(5):361, 1995.

Joint Commission on Accreditation of Healthcare Organizations (JCAHO): 2005 National Patient Safety Goals. *2006 Critical access hospitals' national patient safety goals,* www.jcipatientsafety.org. Retrieved Sept. 21, 2006.

Joint Commission on Accreditation of Healthcare Organizations (JCAHO): *Comprehensive accreditation manual for hospitals,* Chicago, 2004, The Commission.

Joint National Committee: The seventh report of the Joint National Committee on Prevention, Detection, Evaluation and Treatment of High Blood Pressure, *JAMA* 289:2560, 2003.

Jones V and others: Acute and chronic wound healing: pressure ulcers. In Baranoski S, Ayello EA, editors: *Wound care essentials: practice principles,* Philadelphia, 2004, Lippincott Williams and Wilkins.

Katsma DL, Katsma R: The myth of the 90°-angle intramuscular injection, *Nurse Educ* 25(1):34, 2000.

KCI USA: *The V.A.C.: Vacuum Assisted Closure: V.A.C. therapy clinical guidelines,* product information, San Antonio, Tex, 2003.

Keele-Smith R, Price-Daniels C: Effects of crossing legs on blood pressure measurement, *Clin Nurs Res* 10(2):202, 2001.

Kenny R: Advances in the treatment of orthostatic hypotension, *Clin Geriatr* 8(7, Suppl):S1, 2000.

Kittinger JW and others: Efficacy of metoclopramide as an adjunct to duodenal placement of small-bore feeding tubes: a randomized, placebo-controlled, double-blind study, *JPEN J Parenter Enteral Nutr* 11:33, 1987.

Knoerl D and others: Preoperative PCA teaching program to manage postoperative pain, *Medsurg Nurs* 8(1):26, 1999.

Konradi D, Anglin D: Moderate-intensity exercise: for our patients, for ourselves, *Orthop Nurs* 20(1):47, 2001.

Krasner DL: Managing wound pain in patients with vacuum-assisted closure devices, *Ostomy Wound Manage* 48(5):38, 2002.

Krouskop T, van Rijswijk L: Standardizing performance-based criteria for support surfaces, *Ostomy Wound Manage* 41(1):34, 1995.

Kuckelkorn R and others: Emergency treatment of chemical and thermal eye burns, *Acta Ophthalmol Scand* 80:4, 2002.

Kudsk KA and others: Enteral versus parenteral feeding: effects on septic morbidity after blunt and penetrating abdominal trauma, *Ann Surg* 215:503, 1992.

Kuzu N, Ucar H: The effect of cold on the occurrence of bruising, haematoma and pain at the injection site in subcutaneous low molecular weight heparin, *Int J Nurs Stud* 38(1):51, 2001.

Lambert V: Patient restraints, *FDA Consum* 26(8):9, 1992.

Lancaster L: *ANNA: curriculum for nephrology nursing,* ed 4, Pitman, NJ, 2001, Anthony J. Janetti.

Lance R and others: Comparison of different methods of obtaining orthostatic vital signs, *Clin Nurse Res* 9(4):479, 2000.

Langenderfer B: Alternatives to percussion and postural drainage: a review of mucus clearance therapies—percussion and postural drainage, autogenic, positive expiratory pressure, flutter valve, intrapulmonary percussive ventilation, and high-frequency chest compression with the ThAIRapy Vest, *J Cardiopulm Rehabil* 18(4):282, 1998.

Lavender S and others: Postural analysis of paramedics simulating frequently performed strenuous work tasks, *Appl Ergon* 3(1):45, 2000.

Leavitt S: Using patient-controlled analgesia (PCA) for acute pain management, http://www.baxter.com/services/professional-education/. Retrieved Dec. 3, 2003.

Lee M, Phillips J: Transdermal patches: high risk for error? *FDA safety page—drug topics,* April 1, 2002, http://www.fda.gov/cder/drug/MedErrors/transdermal.pdf. Retrieved July 11, 2004.

Lehr V, BeVier P: Patient-controlled analgesia for the pediatric patient, *Orthop Nurs* 22(4):298, 2003.

Lembo A, Camilleri M: Current concepts: chronic constipation, *N Engl J Med* 349(14):1360, 2003.

Lewis M and others: *Medical-surgical nursing: assessment and management of clinical problems,* ed 6, St Louis, 2004, Mosby.

Lewis SL and others: *Medical-surgical nursing: assessment and management of clinical problems,* ed 5, St Louis, 2000, Mosby.

Lilley LL and others: *Pharmacology and the nursing process,* ed 4, St Louis, 2005, Mosby.

Lombardo M, Hartwig M: Central nervous system injury. In Price S, Wilson L: *Patho-physiology: clinical concepts of disease,* ed 6, St Louis, 2003, Mosby.

Lueckenotte AG: *Gerontologic nursing,* St Louis, 2000, Mosby.

Lyder CH and others: Validating the Braden scale for the prediction of pressure ulcer risk in Black and Latino/Hispanic elders: a pilot study, *Ostomy Wound Manage* 44(Suppl A):42s, 1998.

Mahan LK, Escott-Stump S: *Krause's food, nutrition, and diet therapy*, ed 11, Philadelphia, 2004, Saunders.

Malarkey LM, McMorrow ME: *Nurse's manual of laboratory tests and diagnostic procedures,* ed 2, Philadelphia, 2000, Saunders.

Maloney J, Metheny N: Controversy in using blue dye in enteral tube feeding as a method of detecting pulmonary aspiration, *Crit Care Nurse* 22:84, 2002.

Marion B: A turn for the better: prone positioning of patients with ARDS, *Am J Nurs* 101(5):26, 2001.

Marsh P, Martin M: *Oral microbiology,* ed 3, London, 1992, Chapman Hall.

McCaffery M, Pasero C: *Pain: clinical manual,* ed 2, St Louis, 1999, Mosby.

McClave SA and others: North American Summit on Aspiration in the Critically Ill Patient: consensus statement, *JPEN J Parenter Enteral Nutr* 26:S80, 2002.

McClave SA and others: Use of residual volume as a marker for enteral feeding intolerance: prospective blinded comparison with physical examination and radiographic findings, *JPEN J Parenter Enteral Nutr* 16:99, 1992.

McConnell EA: Administering subcutaneous heparin, *Nursing* 36(6):17, 2000.

McConnell EA: Clinical do's and don'ts: applying nitroglycerin ointment, *Nursing* 31(6):17, 2001.

McKenry LM, Salerno E: *Pharmacology in nursing,* revised ed 21, St Louis, 2003, Mosby.

MedTronic MiniMed: *Pump infusion set overview,* 2004, http://www.minimed.com. Retrieved Sept. 21, 2006.

Mendez-Eastman S: Guideline for using negative pressure wound therapy, *Adv Skin Wound Care* 14(6):314, 2001.

Merli G: Low-molecular-weight heparin versus unfractionated heparin in the treatment of deep vein thrombosis and pulmonary embolism, *Am J Phys Med Rehabil* 79(Suppl):S9, 2000.

Metheny N: *Fluid and electrolyte balance: nursing considerations*, ed 4, Philadelphia, 2000, Lippincott.

Metheny N and others: Effect of feeding tube properties and three irrigants on clogging rates, *Nurs Res* 37:165, 1988.

Metheny N and others: Effectiveness of pH measurements in predicting feeding tube placement: an update, *Nurs Res* 42:324, 1993.

Metheny N and others: Visual characteristics of aspirates from feeding tubes as a method for predicting tube location, *Nurs Res* 43:282, 1994.

Metheny N and others: pH, color, and feeding tubes, *RN* 61(1):277, 1998.

Metheny NA and others: pH and concentration of bilirubin in feeding tube aspirates as predictors of tube placement, *Nurs Res* 48:189, 1994.

Metheny NA and others: Efficacy of dye-stained enteral formula in detecting pulmonary aspiration, *Chest* 122:276, 2002.

Metheny N, Titler M: Assessing placement of feeding tubes, *Am J Nurs* 101(5):36, 2001.

Miller D, Miller H: To crush or not to crush. *Nursing* 30(2):51, 2000.

Moody LE, Lowry L, Yarandi H, Voss A: Psychophysiologic predictors of weaning from mechanical ventilation in chronic bronchitis and emphysema, *Clin Nurs Res* 6(4):311, 1997.

Moore FA and others: TEN versus TPN following major abdominal trauma—reduced septic morbidity, *J Trauma* 29:916, 1989.

Moore T: Suctioning techniques for the removal of respiratory secretions, *Nurs Stand* 18(9):47, 2003.

Moppett S: Administration of an enema, *Nurs Times* 95:insert 2p, 1999.

Murphy LM, Bickford V: Gastric residuals in tube feeding: how much is too much? *Nutr Clin Pract* 14:304, 1999.

Myer AH: The effects of aging on wound healing, *Top Geriatr Rehabil* 19(2):1, 2000.

National Dysphagia Diet Task Force: *National dysphagia diet: standardization for optimal care*, Chicago, 2002, American Dietetic Association.

National Heart, Lung, and Blood Institute: *Nurses: partners in asthma care*, NIH Pub. No. 95-3308, Oct. 1994, http://www.nhlbi.nih.gov/health/prof/lung/asthma/nurs_gde.htm. Retrieved July 11, 2004.

National Institute of Neurological Disorders and Stroke: *Seizures and epilepsy: hope through research*, Bethesda, Md, 2001, National Institutes of Health.

National Pressure Ulcer Advisory Panel (NPUAP): Pressure Ulcer Stages. Revised by NPUAP, February 2007.

Nelson DB, Dilloway MA: Principles, products and practical aspects of wound care, *Crit Care Nurs Q* 25(1):33, 2002.

Netea RT and others: Both body and arm position significantly influence blood pressure measurement, *J Hum Hypertens* 17(7):459, 2003.

Nicoll L: Heat in motion: evaluating and managing temperature, *Nursing* 32(5):s1, 2002.

Nicoll LH, Hesby A: Intramuscular injection: an integrative research review and guideline for evidence-based practice, *Appl Nurs Res* 16(2):149, 2002.

O'Shea HS: Teaching the adult ostomy patient, *J Wound Ostomy Continence Nurs* 28(1):47, 2001.

Occupational Safety and Health Administration (OSHA): Occupational exposure to blood borne pathogens, needlestick, and other sharps injuries: final rule, *Federal Register*, CFR 29, part 1910 (*Federal Register* 66:5317, Jan 18, 2001), http://www.osha.gov/pls/oshaweb/owadisp.show_document?p_table=STANDARDS&p _id=10051.

Odderson I and others: Swallow management in patients on an acute stroke pathway: quality is cost effective, *Arch Phys Med Rehabil* 76:1130, 1995.

Ovington LG: Hanging wet-to-dry dressing out to dry, *Home Healthc Nurse* 19(8):477, 2001.

Owen S, Gould D: Underwater seal chest drains: the patient's experience, *J Clin Nurs* 6(3):215, 1997.

Owens B: Preventing injuries using an ergonomic approach, *AORN J* 72(6):1031, 2000.

Owens B and others: What are we teaching about lifting and transferring patients? *Res Nurs Health* 22:3, 1999.

Padula CA and others: Enteral feedings: what the evidence says, *Am J Nurs* 104:62, 2004.

Pagana K, Pagana T: *Mosby's manual of diagnostic and laboratory tests*, St Louis, 2002, Mosby.

Pagana KD, Pagana TJ: *Mosby's diagnostic and laboratory test reference,* ed 6, St Louis, 2004, Mosby.

Pan C, Freivalos A: Ergonomic evaluation of a new patient handling device, Proceedings of the IEA2000/HFES 2000 Congress: the human factors and ergonomics society 4:274, 2000.

Pancorbo-Hidalgo PL, Garcia-Fernandez FP, Ramirez-Perez C: Complications associated with enteral nutrition by nasogastric tube in an internal medicine unit, *J Clin Nurs* 10:482, 2001.

Parkin C: A retrospective audit of chest drain practice in a specialist cardiothoracic center and current review of chest drain literature, *Nurs Crit Care* 7(1):30, 2002.

Pasero C: Continuous local anesthetics, *Am J Nurs* 100(8):22, 2000.

Pasero C: Subcutaneous opioid infusion, *Am J Nurs* 102(7):61, 2002.

Pasero C: Epidural analgesia for postoperative pain, *Am J Nurs* 103(10):62, 2003.

Pasero C: *Intravenous patient-controlled analgesia for acute pain management*, Self-directed learning module, Pensacola, Fla, 2003, American Society for Pain Management Nursing.

Pasero C, Portenoy R, McCaffery M: Using continuous infusion with PCA, *Am J Nurs* 99(2):22, 1999.

Pearce CB, Duncan HD: Enteral feeding: nasogastric, nasojejunal, percutaneous endoscopic gastrostomy, or jejunostomy—its indications and limitations, *Postgrad Med J* 78:198, 2002.

Peers K: Cuff pressures, *Nurs Stand* 17(36):20, 2003.

Perkins L, Shortall SP: Ventilation without intubation, *RN* 63(1):34, 2000.

Perry L: Screening swallowing function of patients with acute stroke. I. Identification, implementation, and initial evaluation of a screening tool for use by nurses, *J Clin Nurs* 10:463, 2001a.

Perry L: Screening swallowing function of patients with acute stroke. II. Detailed evaluation of the tool used by nurses, *J Clin Nurs* 10:474, 2001b.

Perry L, Love C: Screening for dysphagia and aspiration in acute stroke: a systematic review, *Dysphagia* 16:7, 2001.

Perry L, McLaren S: Eating difficulties after stroke, *J Adv Nurs* 43(4):360, 2003.

Phillips D: *Manual of IV therapeutics,* ed 3, Philadelphia, 2001, FA Davis.

Phipps W and others: *Medical-surgical nursing: health and illness perspectives,* ed 7, St Louis, 2003, Mosby.

Phipps WJ and others, editors: *Medical-surgical nursing: concepts and clinical practice,* ed 6, St Louis, 1999, Mosby.

Pickering TG: Self-monitoring of blood pressure. In White WB, editor: *Blood pressure monitoring in cardiovascular medicine and therapeutics,* Totowa, NJ, 2001, Humana Press.

Pieper B: Mechanical forces: pressure, shear, and friction. In Bryant RA: *Acute and chronic wounds: nursing management,* ed 2, St Louis, 2000, Mosby.

Poddar S: Heat or ice for acute ankle sprain, *J Fam Pract* 52(8):642, 2003.

Powell KS and others: Aspirating gastric residuals causes occlusion of small-bore feeding tubes, *JPEN J Parenter Enteral Nutr* 17:243, 1993.

Prather CM, Ortiz-Camacho CP: Evaluation and treatment of constipation and fecal impaction in adults, *Mayo Clin Proc* 73(9):881, 1998.

Preston R: Introducing non-invasive positive pressure ventilation, *Nurs Stand* 15(26):42, 2001.

Puntillo K: Pain assessment and management in the critically ill: wizardry or science? *Am J Crit Care* 12(4):10, 2003.

Puntillo KA and others: Practices and predictors of analgesic interventions for adults undergoing painful procedures, *Am J Crit Care* 11(5):415, 2002.

Ramundo J, Wells J: Wound debridement. In Bryant RA: *Acute and chronic wounds: nursing management,* St Louis, 2000, Mosby.

Regional anesthesia in the anticoagulated patient: defining the risk, http://www. asra.com/Consensus_Conferences/Consensus_Statements.shtml, 2003. Retrieved Dec. 20, 2003,

Rodger MA, King L: Drawing up and administering intramuscular injections: a review of the literature, *J Adv Nurs* 31(3):574, 2000.

Rolstad B and others: Wound care product formulary. In Bryant RA: *Acute and chronic wounds: nursing management,* St Louis, 2000, Mosby.

Rudolph DM: Why won't this wound heal? Understand the causes of and interventions for chronic wounds, *Am J Nurs* 102(2):24, 2002.

Ruffolo D: Hypothermia in trauma, *RN* 65(2): 46, 2002.

Sager P: Nutritional care to prevent and heal pressure ulcers, *Isr Med Assoc J* 4(9):713, 2002.

Saltzstein R and others: Anorectal injuries incident to enema administration: a recurring avoidable problem, *Am J Phys Med Rehabil* 67:186, 1988.

Schmelz JO and others: Effects of position of chest drainage tube on volume drained and pressure, *Am J Crit Care* 8(5):319, 1999.

Schott-Baer FD, Reaume L: Accuracy of ultrasound estimates of urine volume, *Urol Nurs* 21(3):193, 2001.

Scott M: Caring for the orthopaedic patient receiving continuous ambulatory peritoneal dialysis, *Orthop Nurs* 18(4):59, 1999.

Seay SJ and others: Tracheostomy emergencies: correcting accidental decannulation or displaced tracheostomy tube, *Am J Nurs* 102(3):59, 2002.

Secord C and others: Adjusting to life with an ostomy. *Canadian Nurse* 97(1):29, 2001.

Seidel HM and others: *Mosby's guide to physical examination,* ed 5, St Louis, 2003, Mosby.

Seifert CF and others: Drug administration through enteral feeding catheters, *Am J Health Syst Pharm* 59:378, 2002.

Shuldham C: A review of the impact of pre-operative education on recovery from surgery, *Int J Nurs Stud* 36:171, 1999.

Shuster PM: Chest tubes: to clamp or not to clamp, *Nurse Educ* 23(3):9, 1998.

Slovenkai NP: Getting and keeping a leg up on diabetes-related foot problems, *J Musculoskel Med* 15(12):46, 1998.

Smithard D and others: Complications and outcome after acute stroke: does dysphagia matter? *Stroke* 27(7):1200, 1996.

Snow V and others: The evidence base for management of acute exacerbations of COPD: clinical practice guideline, part I, *Chest* 119(4):1185, 2001.

Sole ML and others: A multisite survey of suction techniques and airway management practices, *Am J Crit Care* 12(3):220, 2003.

Soroksky A, Stav D, Shipirer I: A pilot prospective, randomized, placebo-controlled trial of bilevel positive airway pressure in acute asthmatic attack, *Chest* 123(4):1018, 2003.

Sorrentino SA: *Assisting with patient care,* St Louis, 1999, Mosby.

Sorrentino SA: *Mosby's textbook for nursing assistants,* ed 5, St Louis, 2000, Mosby.

Sparks L: Taking the "ouch" out of injections for children, *MCN Am J Matern Child Nurs* 26(2):72, 2001.

Sprigle S and others: Clinical skin temperature measurement to predict incipient pressure ulcers, *Adv Skin Wound Care* 14(3):133, 2001.

St. John RE: Airway management, *Crit Care Nurse* 19(4):79, 1999.

Sterling DA and others: Geriatric falls: injury severity is high and disproportionate to mechanism, *J Trauma* 50(1):116, 2001.

Stiefel KA and others: Improving oral hygiene for the seriously ill patient: implementing research-based practice, *Medsurg Nurs* 9(1):40, 2000.

Stitik T, Nadler S: I. When—and how—to use cold most effectively, *Consultant* 38(12):2881, 1998.

Stitik TP, Nadler SF: Sports injuries: when and how to apply heat, *Consultant* 39(1):144, 1999.

Strauss MB: Diabetic foot problems: keys to effective, aggressive prevention. *Consultant* 41(14):1693, 2001.

Strauss MB, Hart JD, Winant DM: Preventive foot care: a user friendly system for patients and physicians, *Postgrad Med* 103(5):233, 1998.

Suchinski G and others: Treating urinary infections in the elderly. *Dimens Crit Care Nurs* 18(2): 21, 1999.

Sund-Levander M, Forsberg C, Wahren LK: Normal oral, rectal, tympanic and axillary body temperature in adult men and women: a systematic literature review, *Scand J Caring Sci* 16(2):122-128, 2002.

Szor JK, Bourguignon C: Description of pressure ulcer pain at rest and dressing change, *J Wound Ostomy Continence Nurs* 26(3):115, 1999.

Thomas C: Specialty beds: decision-making made easy, *Ostomy Wound Manage* 23:51, 1989.

Thomas DR and others: Pressure ulcer scale for healing: derivation and validation of the PUSH tool, *Adv Wound Care* 10(5):96, 1997.

Thomas SA and others: A review of nursing research on blood pressure, *J Nurs Scholarsh* 34(4):313, 2002.

Thomason SS: Promoting outcomes for patients with spinal cord impairments and ostomies, *Medsurg Nurs* 9(2):77, 2000.

Thompson A and others: Oxygen therapy in acute medical care: the potential dangers of hyperoxia need to be recognised, *Br Med J* 324(7351):1406, 2002.

Thompson J: A practical ostomy guide, part I, *RN* 63(11):61, 2000.

Tinetti ME: Preventing falls in elderly persons, *N Engl J Med* 348(1):42, 2003.

Togger DA, Brenner PS: Metered dose inhalers, *Am J Nurs* 101(10):26, 2001.

Tomaselli N, Goldberg E, Wind S: Pressure-reducing devices: lateral rotation therapy. In Lynn-McHale DJ, Carlson KK, editors: *AACN procedural manual for critical care,* ed 4, Philadelphia, 2001, Saunders.

Torre MC: Subcutaneous infusion: non-metal cannulae vs. metal butterfly needles, *Br J Community Nurs* 7(7):365, 2002.

Trelease CC: Developing standards for wound care, *Ostomy Wound Manage* 26:50, 1988.

U.S. National Library of Medicine: Medline Plus: *Eye emergencies,* 2003, http://www.nlm.nih.gov/medlineplus/ency/article/ 000054.htm. Retrieved Jan. 10, 2004.

United States Department of Labor, Occupational Safety and Health Administration: *Guidelines for nursing homes: ergonomics for the prevention of musculoskeletal disorders,* Washington, DC, 2003.

Vanderberg JT and others: Large-diameter suction system reduces oropharyngeal evacuation time, *J Emerg Med* 17(6):941, 1999.

Volsko TA, DiFiore JM, Chatburn RL: Performance comparison of two oscillating positive expiratory pressure devices: acapella versus flutter, *Resp Care* 48(2):124, 2003.

Waldrop J, Doughty DB: Wound healing physiology. In Bryant RA, editor: *Acute and chronic wounds: nursing management,* ed 2, St Louis, 2000, Mosby.

Weissberg-Benchell J and others: Insulin pump therapy: a meta-analysis, *Diabetes Care* 26(4):1079, 2003.

West JM, Gimbel M: Acute surgical and traumatic wound healing. In Bryant RA: *Acute and chronic wounds: nursing management,* St Louis, 2000, Mosby.

Wood CJ: Endotracheal suctioning: a literature review, *Intensive Crit Care Nurs* 14(9):124, 1998.

Wood P, Emick-Herring B: Dysphagia: a screening tool for stroke patients, *J Neurosci Nurs* 29(5):325, 1997.

Woodrow P: Using non-invasive ventilation in acute wards, part I, *Nurs Stand* 18(1):39, 2003a.

Woodrow P: Using non-invasive ventilation in acute wards, part II, *Nurs Stand* 18(2):41, 2003b.

Woodruff DW: Pneumothorax, *RN* 62(9):62, 1999.

Wound, Ostomy, and Continence Nurses (WOCN) Society: *Guideline for prevention and management of pressure ulcers,* WOCN clinical practice guidelines series, Glenview, Ill, 2003, The Association.

Wound, Ostomy, and Continence Nurses (WOCN) Society: *Stoma complications, best practices for clinicians,* Glenview, Illinois, 2005, The Association.

Wysocki AB: Evaluating and managing open skin wounds: colonization versus infection, *AACN Clin Issues* 13(3):382, 2002.

Young-McCaughan A, Miaskowski C: Measurement of opioid-induced sedation, *Pain Manage Nurs* 2(4):132, 2001.

Yucha CB: Ambulatory blood pressure monitoring: measurement implications for research, *J Nurs Meas* 9(1):49, 2001.

Zhuang Z and others: Psychophysical assessment of assistive devices for transferring patients/residents, *Appl Ergon* 31(1):35, 2000.

Zurlinden J: Double check IV push, *Nurs Spectr* 15(25IL):16, 2002.

Index

Page numbers followed by *b* indicate box, by *f*
indicate figure, and by *t* indicate table.

This logo identifies when the use of clean gloves is recommended. Clean gloves can protect both caregivers and clients. However, gloves are not 100% effective. Personnel should wear clean, disposable gloves when touching blood, body fluids, mucous membranes, nonintact skin, secretions, excretions, and contaminated items. Gloves should be changed between skills on a client involving contact with material that might contain a high concentration of microorganisms.

Preprocedure Protocol

1. Verify physician orders and if consent form is needed.
2. Introduce yourself to client by both name and title or role, and explain what you plan to do.
3. Check client's identification bracelet and ask name. At least two client identifiers must be used (neither identifier may be client's room number).
4. Explain procedure and reason it is to be done in terms that client can understand.
5. Assess client to determine that the intervention is still appropriate and whether adaptations to skill are needed.
6. Gather equipment.
7. Perform hand hygiene before each new client contact.
8. Adjust bed or chair to appropriate working height as needed.
9. Make sure that client is comfortable and that you have sufficient room to perform procedure.
10. Make sure that you have sufficient lighting to perform procedure.
11. If client is in bed and a side rail is raised, lower rail on side nearest you to access client.
12. Provide privacy. Close door, use privacy curtain, and position and drape client as needed.

During Skill Protocol

1. Promote client involvement and comfort.
2. Communicate during skill to allay client's anxiety, and explain sources of any discomfort.
3. Assess client's tolerance throughout procedure.